PHYSIOLOGY REVIEW 2

DR.RABIA SIDDIQUI

To my mother for all her support

TABLE OF CONTENTS:

CENTRAL NERVOUS SYSTEM:

1.	Anterolateral System and Dorsal Column Medial Leminiscal System	1
2.	Autonomic Nervous System	4
3.	Basal Ganglia	15
4.	Blood Supply of Brain	21
5.	Brain Stem	25
6.	Cerebellum	27
7.	Cerebral areas and their functions	38
8.	Corticospinal tract	41
9.	CSF	43
10.	Headache	46
11.	Learning and Memory	48
12.	Limbic System	56
13.	Meninges of the Brain	59
14.	Nerve Fiber	60
15.	Neurons	65
16.	Pain Physiology	66
17.	Receptors	78
18.	Reticular Activating System	84
19.	Sleep and EEG	87
20.	Speech and Language	98
21.	Spinal Cord	104
22.	Stretch reflex	110
23.	Upper Motor Neuron and Lower Motor Neuron	120

GASTROINTESTINAL SYSTEM AND TEMERATURE REGULATION

1.	Functional and Structural Organization of GIT	124
2.	Functions of GIT	127
3.	Enteric Nervous System	128
4.	Physiology of Mastication	130

5.	Physiology of Swallowing	132
6.	Saliva	135
7.	Gastric Acid Secretion	139
8.	Phases of Gastric Acid Secretion	142
9.	Regulation of Gastric Emptying	145
10.	Small Intestine	147
11.	Large Intestine	153
12.	Bile and Gallbladder	159
13.	Liver and Pancreas	163
14.	Malabsorption	173
15.	GI Hormones	183
16.	GI Motility	188
17.	GI Reflexes	194
18.	Temperature Regulation	198

KIDNEY:

1.	Body fluids	207
2.	Functions of different segments of Nephron	216
3.	Principles of Renal Tubular Reabsorption	218
4.	Tubular reabsorption of Sodium	221
5.	Tubular Handling of Potassium	223
6.	Renal regulation of Urea, Phosphate, Calcium and Magnesium	228
7.	Renal Mechanism for Handling Acid Base Disorders	238
8.	GFR and its regulation	244
9.	Renal Clearance	248
10.	Autoregulation of renal blood flow	254
11.	Countercurrent Mechanism	257
12.	Hormonal control of Kidney Function	261
13.	Micturition reflex	264
14.	Acid base disorders	269
15.	Anion gap of Plasma	271
16.	Dialysis and Transplantation	272

ENDOCRINOLOGY:

1.	Introduction of Endocrinology	276
2.	Classification and Mechanism of Action	276
3.	Regulation of Hormone Synthesis	283
4.	Regulation of Hormone Receptors	289
5.	Endocrine role of Hypothalamus	291
6.	Anterior Pituitary Hormones	293
7.	Growth Hormone	293
8.	Posterior pituitary hormones	297
9.	Prolactin	303
10.	Insulin	305
11.	Glucagon	311
12.	Parathyroid hormone, Vitamin D and Calcitonin	314
13.	Thyroid hormones	318
14.	Adrenocortical Hormones	337
15.	Adrenal Medulla	348

REPRODUCTION:

1.	Male Reproductive System	349
2.	Female reproductive System	366
3.	Pregnancy and Lactation	393

SPECIAL SENSES:

1.	Introduction to vision	408
2.	Layers of Retina	410
3.	Phototransduction	412
4.	Physiology of Vision	417
5.	Visual Pathway	418
6.	Physiology of Gustation	422
7.	Physiology of Olfaction	429
8.	Physiology of Hearing	434

PREFACE:

There are several textbooks of physiology to consult for the medical and non-medical students but the most books are too big and have scattered knowledge. Guyton and Hall have difficult to follow concepts with many concepts imbibed in irrelevant detail and unnecessary repetition along with too much emphasis on experimental physiology. There are textbooks of physiology available in the market which are again big books which is difficult to finish by medical students in 2 years. Sherwood physiology goes into molecular details of concepts, again making many things irrelevant and many chapters are very concise like CNS. BRS physiology is a short review book which cannot be easily followed by a beginner in physiology therefore cannot be relied entirely to cover the course syllabus and again the chapter on Blood is omitted from this book. Kaplan lecture notes is not introduced to the students as it is of interest to medical students who are appearing for USMLE step 1 only. All topics are not given equally well explained in all textbooks as some topics are covered nicely in some books and some topics are left unexplained only touching the main features.

After outlining the course content of second year MBBS to which I am the course coordinator in BUMDC, for each topic I consulted the different textbooks (Indukhurana, Costanzo, Sherwood, BRS, Kaplan Lecture notes)on physiology and made notes from the book which had easier explanations and easier way of conveying concepts which is required by a teacher. Therefore the notes were only meant to facilitate me but seemingly enough, it came about to help the students also. This short review book is actually my interactive notes. These are also my teaching notes which I consult regularly to facilitate myself for my teaching sessions. These notes were meant to facilitate me for my sessions actually helped students of 2nd year MBBS in understanding difficult concepts and passing theory and BCQ exams. Our way of assessment of students in medical universities may not prepare the students for the post graduate exams but certainly pass students on demonstrating the basic knowledge of key concepts of the subject being tested.

I have personally followed the student agony of consulting a big book and not being able to understand and learn key concepts even with the objectives laid in front of them. I know this because they come to me saying that their time is going out of their hands and still they cannot manage to cover the syllabus with a big book. These interactive notes have been running among students for past six years now in BUMDC.

We assess students on the basis of theory and via exams. Theory consists of Short answer questions and BCQ's. Second year MBBS result comes out to be around 90-95% each year making only few students failing the final exams. I am bringing out these interactive notes in the form of book to facilitate students with your help as publishers.

ALS AND DCML SYSTEM:

RECEPTOR	FREE NERVE ENDINGS	MEISSNER'S CORPUSCLE PACINIAN CORPUSCLE MUSLCE SPINDLE GOLGI TENDON ORGANS
SENSATIONS	PAIN, TEMPERATURE, TOUCH AND PRESSURE	DISCRIMINATIVE TOUCH, VIBRATION, PROPRIOCEPTION
NERVE FIBERS	A delta C	A beta
FIRST ORDER NEURON	POSTERIOR ROOT GANGLION	POSTERIOR ROOT GANGLION
SECOND ORDER NEURON	SUBSTANTIA GELATINOSA	NUCLEUS GRACILUS AND CUNEATUS
THIRD ORDER NEURON	VPL OF THALAMUS	VPL OF THALAMUS
DESTINATION	POST CENTRAL GYRUS	POST CENTRAL GYRUS
DECUSSATION	SPINAL CORD	MEDULLA OBLONGATA
PATHWAY	SPINAL LEMINISCUS	MEDIAL LEMINISCUS

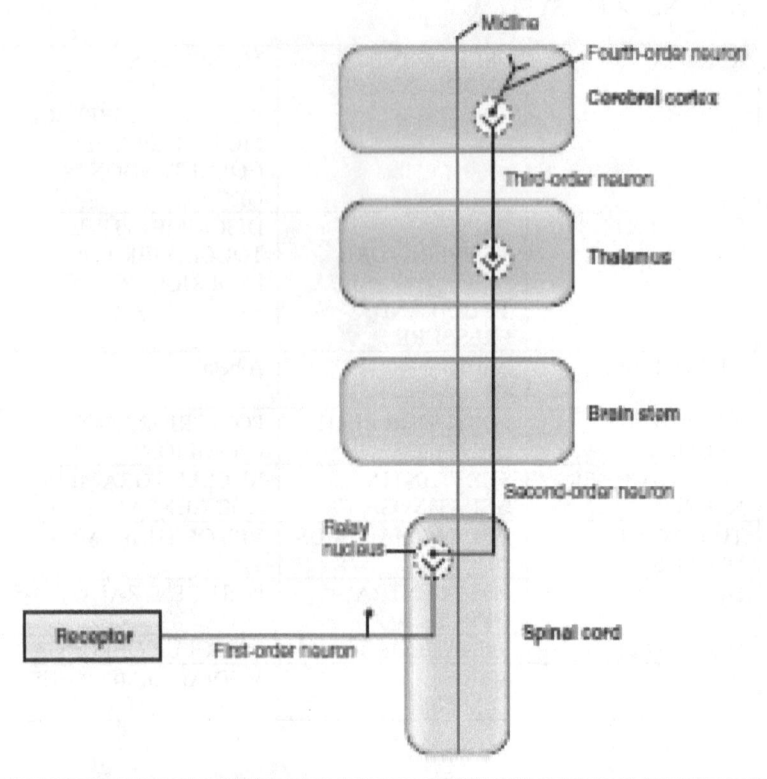

SCHEMATIC DIAGRAM OF SENSORY PATHWAYS

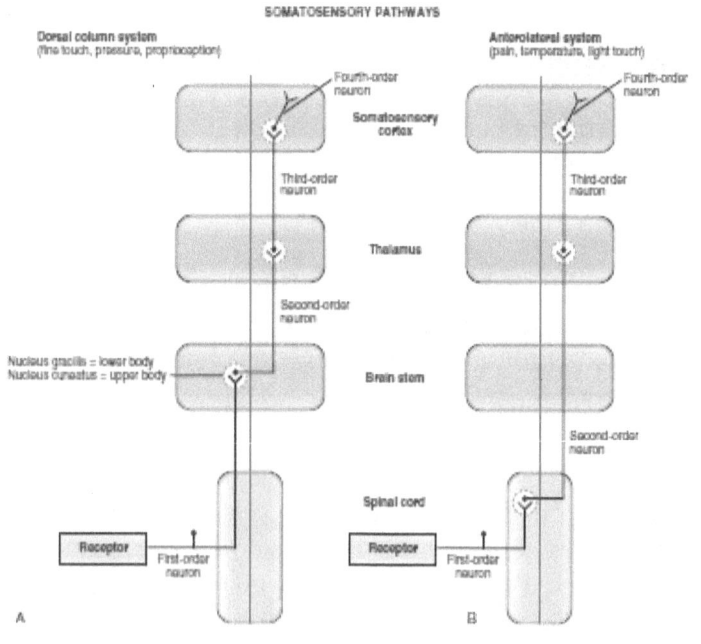

COMPARISON OF SOMATOSENSORY PATHWAYS (ALS AND DCML)

AUTONOMIC NERVOUS SYSTEM

The motor efferent nervous system has two components:

A. Somatic
B. Autonomic

SOMATIC NERVOUS SYSTEM: This is a voluntary nervous system under conscious control consisting of a single motor neuron innervating effector organ, the skeletal muscle fibers.

AUTONOMIC NERVOUS SYSTEM:

It controls the functions of smooth muscle, glands and heart. The efferent pathway in the autonomic nervous system consists of two neurons: a preganglionic neuron and a post ganglionic neuron. The cell bodies of the preganglionic neuron lie in the CNS. The axons of these preganglionic neurons synapse on the cell bodies of the post ganglionic neurons in one of the many autonomic ganglia located outside the CNS. The axons of the postganglionic neurons travel to the periphery, where they synapse on visceral effector organs such as heart, bronchioles, vascular smooth muscle, gastrointestinal tract, bladder, and genitalia. All preganglionic neurons of the autonomic nervous system release acetylcholine. Post ganglionic neurons release either acetylcholine or norepinephrine.

ORGANIZATION OF GENERAL FEATURES OF THE AUTONOMIC NERVOUS SYSTEM:

The autonomic nervous system has two major divisions: the sympathetic and the parasympathetic, which often complement each other in the regulation of organ system function. The sympathetic division is thoracolumbar referring to its origin in the spinal cord. The parasympathetic division is craniosacral, referring to its origin in the brain stem and sacral spinal cord.

Efferent pathways in the autonomic nervous system consist of a preganglionic and a postganglionic neuron, which synapse in autonomic ganglia. The axons of postganglionic neurons travel to the periphery to innervate the effector organs. The adrenal medulla is a specialized of the sympathetic division: when stimulated, it secretes catecholamines into the circulation.

Often the sympathetic and the parasympathetic innervations of organ system have reciprocal effects. These effects are coordinated by autonomic centers in the brain stem.

Receptors for neurotransmitters in the autonomic nervous system is either adrenergic (adrenoceptors) or cholinergic (cholinoceptors). Adrenoceptors are activated by the catechoalmines, norepinephrine and epinephrine. Cholinoceptors are activated by acetylcholine.

SYMPATHETIC NERVOUS SYSTEM:

Operates continuously to modulate the functions of many organ systems e.g.; heart, blood vessels, GIT, bronchi and sweat glands .Stressful stimulation activates SNS leads to a response known as "fight or flight": increased arterial pressure, blood flow, blood glucose, metabolic rate and mental activity
Sympathetic preganglionic neurons originate from thoracolumbar spinal cord (T1-L3).SNS ganglia are located near the spinal cord either in the paravertebral ganglia (sympathetic chain) or in the prevertebral ganglia. Preganglionic neurons are short and the post ganglionic neurons are long.

NEUROTRANSMITTERS AND TYPES OF RECEPTORS:

Preganglionic neurons are always cholinergic in nature. They release Ach, interacts with nicotinic receptors on the cell body of postganglionic neurons. Postganglionic neurons are adrenergic except in thermoregulatory sweat glands (muscarinic, cholinergic). The Adrenergic neurons affect adrenorecepters: alpha1, alpha2, beta1, beta2

PARASYMPATHETIC NERVOUS SYSTEM:

Preganglionic fibers originate from cranial nuclei in brain stem (mid brain, pons, and medulla) and in sacral segments (S2-S4) (craniosacral).Parasympathetic ganglia are located on or in the effecter organs. Preganglionic neuron has long axon and postganglionic neuron has short axon.

NEUROTRANSMITTERS AND TYPES OF RECEPTORS:

All preganglionic neurons are cholinergic, release Ach which interacts with nicotinic receptors. Postganglionic neurons are cholinergic, release Ach which interacts with muscarinic receptors

SYMAPTHETIC AND PARASYMPATHETIC NERVOUS SYSTEM:

Smooth muscle, cardiac muscle and glands are innervated by the ANS. The sympathetic and parasympathetic divisions have efferent (output) that evoke or modulate contraction, secretory and metabolic responses throughout the body. The ANS has central components in hypothalamus and brainstem autonomic nuclei that receive input from visceral and somatic afferents as well as more rostral brain regions. In the sympathetic and parasympathetic systems, the final efferent pathways consists of central preganglionic neurons which synapse onto peripheral post ganglionic neurons, which synapse onto effector cells in target organs. In the sympathetic system, the preganglionic cell bodies are in the lateral grey column of the spinal cord between T1 and L3 (thoracolumbar). The post ganglionic cell bodies are in either the nearby paraverteberal ganglia or the most distant preverteberal ganglia. Each preganglionic sympathetic fiber synapses with many post-ganglionic neurons across several ganglia. The sympathetic postganglionic neurons usually send very long axons to effector organs.

In the parasympathetic system, the preganglionic cell bodies reside in the nuclei of the medulla, pons and midbrain and spinal segments S2 through S4 (craniosacral) and send long axons to synapse with relatively few postganglionic neurons in the terminal ganglia, which are close to or are embedded in the walls of their target organs. The sympathetic and parasympathetic system has opposite effects on the visceral targets. Massive activation of sympathetic system enhances the capacity for immediate physical activity (e.g. exercise and flight or fight response). The parasympathetic activity enhances the functions of organs active during quiescent states (rest and digest functions).

All preganglionic fibers (sym and para) release acetylcholine at synapses in autonomic ganglia. The acetylcholine binds to nicotinic receptors and excites post-ganglionic neurons. Nearly all sympathetic postganglionic neurons release norepinephrine on target organs. The major exceptions are the sympathetic fibers innervating the sweat glands which release acetylcholine (binding to muscarinic receptors) and the cells in the adrenal medulla which are homologous with sympathetic postganglionic neurons but release epinephrine and some norepinephrine into the blood stream.

The major classes of receptors for norepinephrine and epinephrine are:
Alpha 1-bloodvessels,
Alpha 2- preganglionic terminals of sympathetic postganglionic axons.
Beta 1-heart
Beta 2- bronchial smooth muscle.

All parasympathetic post ganglionic neurons release acetylcholine which binds to muscarinic receptors on effector cells.

Both muscarinic and adrenergic receptors are linked positively or negatively by G proteins to adenyl cyclase or phospholipase C, which alters cAMP or Ca levels in target cells.

AUTONOMIC RECEPTORS:

1. ADRENOCEPTORS:

   a. **α1 receptor**: found in vascular smooth muscle, G.I sphincters and bladder, radial muscle of iris

Activation of α1: contraction or excitation. They are equally sensitive to norepinephrine and epinephrine. However only norepinephrine released from adrenergic neurons is present in high enough concentrations to activate α1 receptor

Mechanism of action: Gq protein, stimulation of phospholipase C, and increase in inositol 1,4,5-triphosphate (IP3) and intracellular [Ca2+].

b. **α2 Receptors:**
They are located on sympathetic postganglionic nerve terminals (autoreceptors), platelets,
fat cells, and the walls of the GI tract (heteroreceptors). They often produce inhibition (e.g., relaxation or dilation).

Mechanism of action: Gi protein inhibition of adenylate cyclase and decrease in cyclic adenosine monophosphate (cAMP).

c. **β1 Receptors**
They are located in the sinoatrial (SA) node, atrioventricular (AV) node, and ventricular muscle of the heart. They produce excitation (e.g., increased heart rate, increased conduction velocity, increased

contractility). They are sensitive to both norepinephrine and epinephrine, and are more sensitive than the α1 receptors.

Mechanism of action: Gs protein, stimulation of adenylate cyclase and increase in cAMP.

d. β2 Receptors:
They are located on vascular smooth muscle of skeletal muscle, bronchial smooth muscle and in the walls of the GI tract and bladder. They produce relaxation (e.g., dilation of vascular smooth muscle, dilation of bronchioles, and relaxation of the bladder wall). They are more sensitive to epinephrine than to norepinephrine. They are more sensitive to epinephrine than the α1 receptors.

Mechanism of action: same as for β1 receptors.

2. CHOLINOCEPTORS:

　　a. NICOTINIC RECEPTORS: These are located in the autonomic ganglia of the sympathetic and parasympathetic nervous systems, at the neuromuscular junction (N_M), and in the adrenal medulla (N_N).

　　b. MUSCARINIC RECEPTORS:

　　M1: CNS

　　M2: Heart

　　M3: Glands and Smooth Muscle

SYMPATHETIC ACTIVITY AND PARASYMPATHETIC ACTIVITY:

EFFECTOR	ACTION	RECEPTOR	ACTION	RECEPTOR
heart sa node contractility	tachycardia increase	beta 1 beta1	bradycardia decrease (atria)	m2 m2
blood vessels skin skeletal muscles	constriction dilation	alpha 1 beta2	- -	- -
sweat glands	secretion	alpha 1	-	-
bronchial muscle	relaxation	beta 2	constriction	m
eye radial muscle iris sphincter muscle iris	contraction	alpha 1	contraction	m
git motility secretion sphincters	decrease decrease constricts	alpha 2 beta 2 beta 2 alpha 1	increase increase relaxes	m3 m3 m3
urinary bladder detrusor trigone and sphicters	relaxation contraction	beta 2 alpha 1	contraction relaxation	m3 m3
male sex organs	ejaculation	alpha 1	erection	m

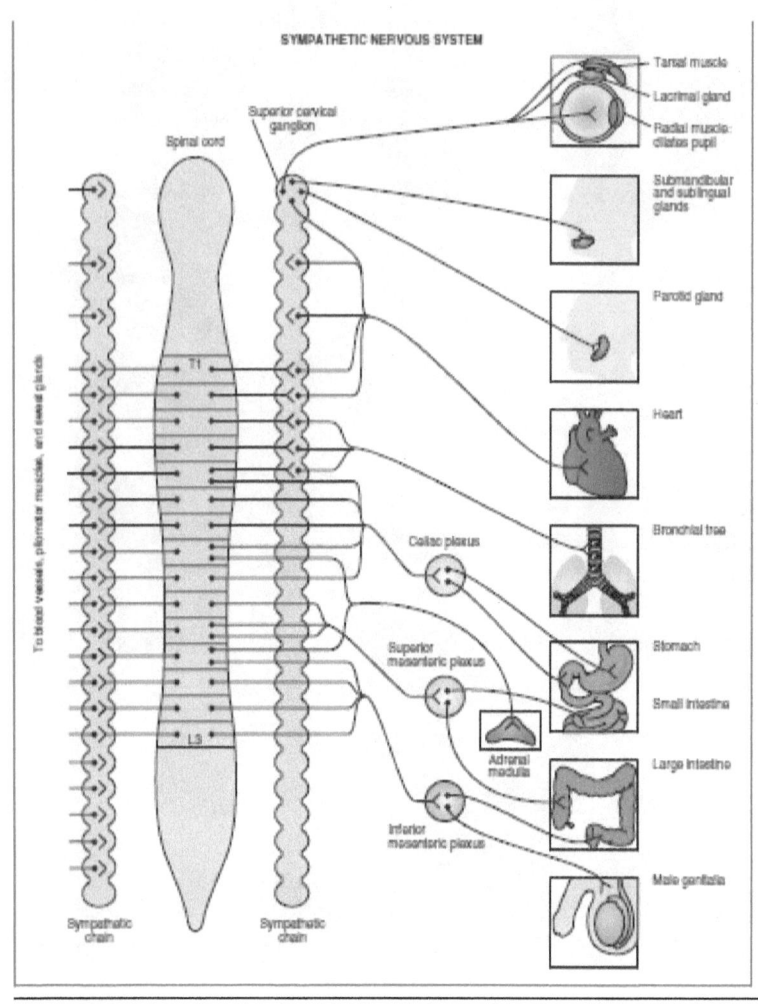

SYMPATHETIC NERVOUS SYSTEM

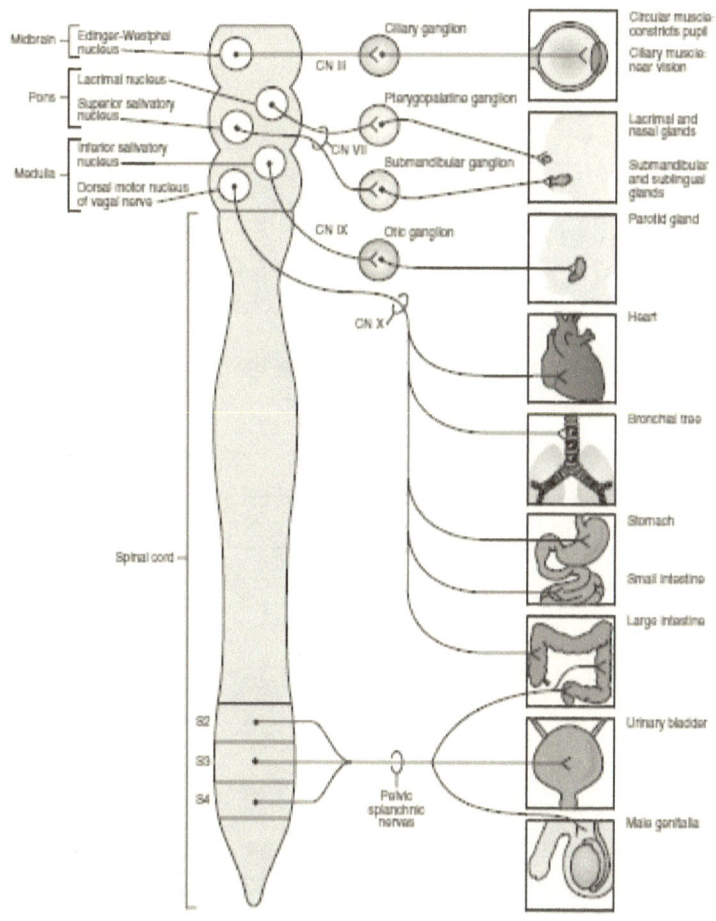

PARASYMPATHETIC NERVOUS SYSTEM

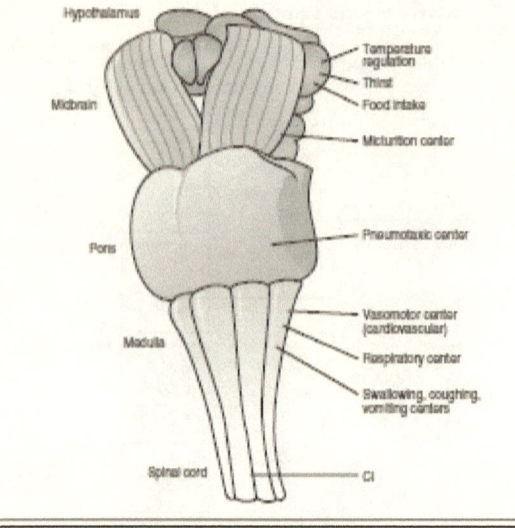

AUTONOMIC CENTERS IN THE BRAIN STEM

BASAL GANGLIA:

Basal ganglia are the deep nuclei of the Telencephalon. The main function is to influence the motor cortex via pathways through the thalamus. The role of basal ganglia is to aid in planning and execution of smooth movements. Almost all areas of cerebral cortex project topographically onto straitum including cortical input from motor cortex. The straitum then communicate with the thalamus and then back to cortex via 2 different pathways.

1. Indirect pathway
2. Direct pathway

Basal ganglia initiate and provide gross control over skeletal muscle movements. The major components of basal ganglia include;

a. Striatum which consists of caudate nucleus and putamen.
b. External and Internal segments of globus pallidus
c. Substantia nigra in midbrain
d. Subthalamic nucleus in Diencephalon.

Together with cerebral cortex and Venterolateral nucleus of Thalamus, these structures are interconnected to form two parallel but antagonistic circuits known as Direct and Indirect basal ganglia pathways. Both pathways are driven by extensive inputs from large areas of cerebral cortex and both project back to motor cortex after a relay in the VL nucleus of thalamus. Both pathways use a process known as"Disinhibition" to mediate their effects, whereby one population of inhibitory neurons inhibits a second population of inhibitory neurons.

DIRECT BASAL GANGLIA PATHWAY:

In the direct pathway, excitatory input from cerebral cortex projects to striatal neurons in the caudate nucleus and putamen. Through disinhibition, activated inhibitory neurons in the striatum, which use (GABA) as their neurotransmitter, project to and inhibit additional GABA neurons in the internal segment of the globus pallidus. The GABA axons of internal segment of the globus pallidus project to the thalamus (VL). Because their input to the thalamus is disinhibited, the thalamic input excites the motor cortex. The net effect of disinhibition in the direct pathway results in an increased level of cortical excitation and promotion of movement.

INDIRECT BASAL GANGLIA PATHWAY:

In the indirect pathway, excitatory input from cerebral cortex also projects to striated neurons in the caudate nucleus and putamen. These inhibitory neurons in the striatum, which also use GABA as their neurotransmitter, project to and inhibit additional GABA neurons in the external segment of the globus pallidus. The GABA axons of external segment of globus pallidus project to the sub thalamic nucleus. Through disinhibition, the subthalamic nucleus excites inhibitory GABA neurons in the internal segment of globus pallidus which inhibits the thalamus. The net effect of disinhibition in indirect pathway results in a decreased level of cortical excitation.

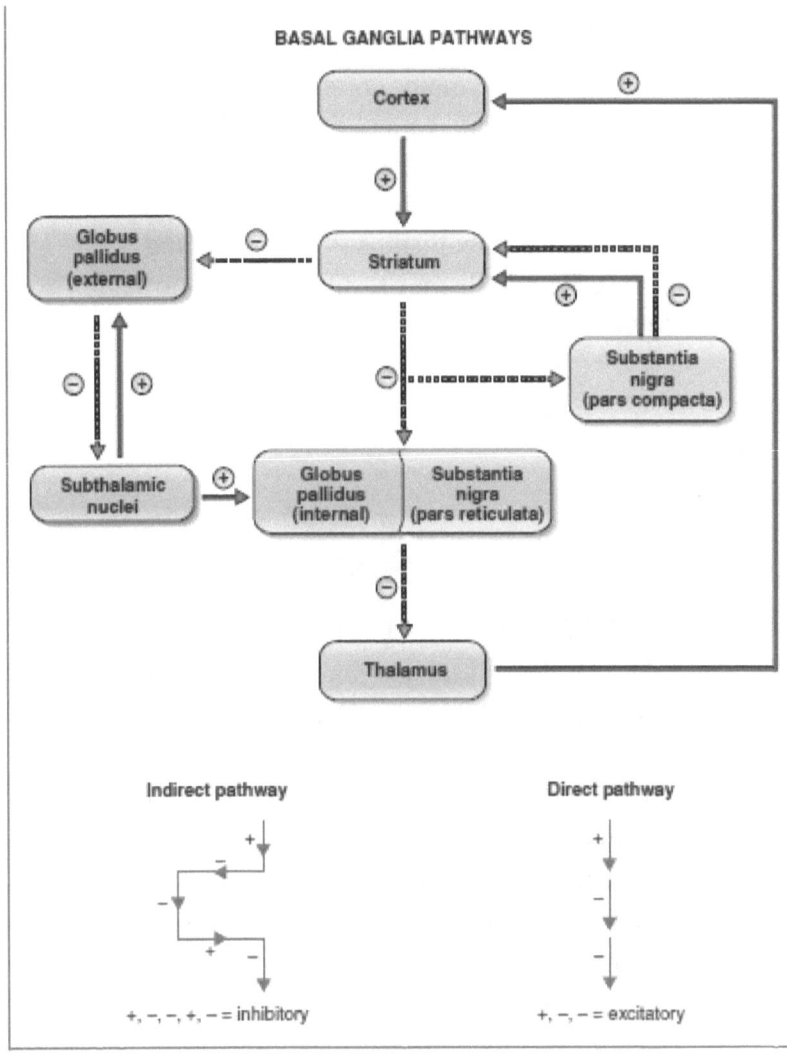

LESIONS OF DIRECT PATHWAY:

Under active cortex which produces hypokinetic motor disturbances. The classic disorder caused by degeneration of dopaminergic neurons of substantia nigra in Parkinson's disease. These patients are characterized by tremor at rest (pill rolling), increased tone, and mask face and hypokinetic movement.

LESIONS OF INDIRECT PATHWAY:

It cause an over active motor cortex. These movements occur spontaneously and cannot be controlled by the patient. Examples of these disorders include chorea (multiple movements), athetosis (slow serpentine movements) and hemiballismus (violent flinging movements). Hemiballismus result from hemorrhagic destruction of contralateral subthalamic nucleus.

FUNCTIONS OF BASAL GANGLIA:

1. CONTROL OF VOLUNTARY MOTOR ACTIVITY: Basal ganglia control the voluntary movements which are initiated by motor cortex.
2. COGNITIVE CONTROL OF MOTOR ACTIVITY: Most of the motor actions occur as a consequence of thoughts generated in mind.
3. TIMING ANDSCALING OF INTENSITY OF MOVEMENTS: Timing of movements: how rapidly the movements should be performed. Scaling of intensity of movement i-e how large the movement should be.
4. SUBCONSCIOUS EXECUTION OF SOME MOVEMENTS: Subconscious execution of some movements during the performance of trained motor activities i-e skilled activities. Examples of movements executed subconsciously at the level of basal ganglia are;
    a. Swinging of arm while walking

b. Crude movement of facial expression that accompany emotions.
c. Movements of limbs while swimming.
d. Control of clutch and brake while driving (constant attention is required during initial stages; however they are carried out by basal ganglia as they become routine.

IMPORTANCE: By subconscious control of activities the basal ganglia relieve cortex from routine so that cortex can be free to plan its actions.

e. CONTROL OF REFLEX MUSCULAR ACTIVITY: The basal ganglia exert inhibitory effect on spinal reflexes and regulate activity of muscles which maintain posture.
f. CONTROL OF MUSCLE TONE: Muscle spindle and gamma motor neurons of spinal cord (which are responsible for maintaining the tone of muscles) are controlled by basal ganglia, esp. substantia nigra. In lesion of basal ganglia muscle tone increases .Rigidity (lead pipe type) is a characteristic feature of Parkinson's disease.
g. ROLE OF AROUSAL MECHANISM: Globus pallidus and red nucleus are involved in arousal mechanism because of their connections with reticular formation .Extensive lesions in globus pallidus are associated with drowsiness, leading to sleep.

SUMMARY OF BASAL GANGLIA:

The basal ganglia play important motor function in starting and stopping voluntary motor functions and inhibiting unwanted movements. It consists of three nuclei masses deep in the cerebrum (caudate nucleus, putamen and globus pallidus), one nucleus in the midbrain (substantia nigra) and subthalamic nucleus in the diencephalon. The striatum combines the caudate nucleus and the putamen while the corpus striatum consists of these two nuclei plus the globus pallidus. There are two parallel circuits (direct and indirect)through basal ganglia .These circuits receive extensive input from the cerebral cortex that project back to the motor cortex after a relay in the VL nucleus of thalamus. Both of these pathways demonstrate disinhibition.

The direct pathway increases the level of cortical excitation and promotes movement. The indirect pathway decreases the level of cortical excitation and stops movement. The striatum is the major input center and globus pallidus is the major output center for pathways through basal ganglia. Critical to proper function of striatum is dopamine production by substantia nigra. Dopamine excites the direct pathway and inhibits the indirect pathway.

BLOOD SUPPLY OF BRAIN:

The cortex is supplied by the two internal carotid arteries and two vertebral arteries. On the base (or inferior surface) of the brain, branches of ICA and basilar artery anastomose to form circle of Willis. The anterior part of the circle lies in front of the optic chiasm, whereby posterior part is situated just below the mammillary bodies. The circle of Willis is formed by the terminal part of internal carotid arteries; the proximal parts of anterior and posterior cerebral arteries and anterior and posterior communicating arteries. The middle, anterior and posterior cerebral arteries which arise from the circle of Willis, supply all of the cerebral cortex, basal ganglia and diencephalon.

The ICA arises from the bifurcation of common carotid and enters the skull through the carotid canal. It enters the subarachnoid space and terminates by dividing into anterior and middle cerebral arteries. Just before splitting into the middle and anterior cerebral arteries, the internal carotid arteries rise to ophthalmic artery. The ophthalmic artery enters the orbit through the optic canal and supplies the eye, including the retina and optic nerve.

The middle cerebral artery is the larger terminal branch of the internal carotid artery. It supplies the bulk of the lateral surface of the hemisphere. Exceptions are superior inch of frontal and parietal lobe which are supplied by the anterior cerebral artery and inferior part of temporal lobe and occipital lobe, which are supplied by posterior cerebral artery. The middle cerebral artery also supplies the genu and posterior limb of internal capsule and basal ganglia.

The anterior cerebral artery is the smaller terminal branch of ICA. It is connected to opposite anterior cerebral artery by anterior communicating artery, completing the anterior part of circle of Willis. The anterior cerebral artery supplies the medial surface of frontal and parietal lobes, which include motor and sensory cortical areas for the pelvis and lower limbs. The anterior cerebral artery also supplies the anterior 4/5th of the corpus callosum and approximately 1 inch of the frontal and parietal cortex on the superior aspect of lateral aspect of hemisphere.

Occlusion of anterior cerebral artery results in spastic paresis of contralateral lower limb and anesthesia of contralateral lower limb. Urinary incontinence may be present, but this usually occurs only with bilateral damage. A trans cortical apraxia of the left limbs may result from involvement of anterior portion of corpus callosum. A trans cortical apraxia occurs because of left hemisphere (language dominant) has been disconnected from motor cortex of right hemisphere. The anterior cerebral artery also supplies the anterior limb of the internal capsule.

The posterior cerebral artery is formed by the terminal bifurcation of the basilar artery. The posterior communicating artery arises near the termination of ICA and passes posteriorly to join the posterior cerebral artery. The posterior communicating arteries complete the circle of Willis by joining the verteberobasilar and carotid circulations. The posterior cerebral artery supplies the occipital and temporal cortex on the inferior and lateral surfaces of the hemisphere, the occipital lobe and posterior 2/3rd of the temporal lobe on the medial surface of hemisphere, and the thalamus and subthalamus.

ANTERIOR CEREBRAL ARTERY: supplies median surface of frontal and parietal lobe, anterior 4/5th of corpus callosum and anterior limb of internal capsule.

MIDDLE CEREBRAL ARTERY: supplies lateral surface of frontal, parietal and upper temporal lobes, posterior limb and genu of internal capsule and basal ganglia.

POSTERIOR CEREBRAL ARTERY: supplies occipital lobe, splenium and lower temporal lobe and midbrain.

SYMPTOMS FOLLOWING OCCLUSION OF CEREBRAL ARTERIES:

POSTERIOR CEREBRAL ARTERY:

Contralateral homonymous hemianopia (usually with macular sparing) occurs.

LEFT SIDE: Alexia without agraphia (cannot read but can write).

MIDDLE CEREBRAL ARTERY:

Contralateral spastic paralysis and anesthesia of arm and face occurs.

ON LEFT SIDE: Aphasia (Brocas, Wernicke, global or conduction)

ON RIGHT SIDE: Inattention and neglect of contralateral side of the body and spatial perception defects.

ANTERIOR CEREBRAL ARTERY:

Contralateral spastic paralysis and anesthesia of lower limbs, urinary incontinence and trans cortical apraxia (cannot move left arm in response to a command).

HUMUNCULUS:

Homunculus of motor and sensory cortex indicates that the upper limb and head are demonstrated on the lateral surface of the cortex. The pelvis and lower limb are represented on the medial surface of the hemisphere. Therefore motor and sensory functions of the lower limb are supplied by anterior cerebral artery while motor and sensory functions of upper limb and head are supplied by middle cerebral artery.

INTERNAL CAPSULE:

It is a large mass of white matter that connects almost all tracts to and from the cerebral cortex. It is divided into anterior limb, genu and posterior limb. The anterior limb is supplied by anterior cerebral artery and genu and posterior limb are supplied by the middle cerebral artery. The primary motor and sensory systems course through the posterior limb and genu.

BRAIN STEM:

Brain stem consists (from below upwards) of the medulla oblongata, pons and midbrain.

MEDULLA OBLONGATA:

It is conical in shape and connects the pons above with the spinal cord below:

FUNCTIONS:

1. Pathway for ascending and descending tracts.
2. House of vital centers.
3. It contains many important centers which control the vital functions of the body.
   a. Respiratory center (inspiratory and expiratory) control the normal rhythmic respiration.
   b. Vasomotor and cardiac centers; control the blood pressure and functions of heart and vascular system.
   c. Swallowing center controls the pharyngeal and esophageal phase of swallowing.
   d. Vomiting center is responsible for inducing disorders of GIT.
   e. Superior and inferior salivatory nuclei located in the medulla control the salivary function.
4. CRANIAL NERVE NUCLEI: located in medulla control following functions.
   a. 12th –movements of tongue.
   b. 11th –control movements of shoulder.
   c. 10th –control functions of important viscera e.g. heart, lungs and GIT.
   d. 8th –controls auditory function.

PONS:

It is situated on the anterior surface of cerebellum below the midbrain and above the medulla oblongata.

FUNCTIONS:

1. It is the connecting pathway between cerebral cortex and cerebellum
2. It is a pathway for ascending and descending tracts of spinal cord and medulla oblongata.
3. It is the joining station for medial leminiscus with fibers of 5th, 7th, 9th and 10th cranial nerves.
4. It contains pneumotaxic and apneustic centers for regulation of respiration.

MIDBRAIN:

It is a narrow part of brain that connects forebrain to hindbrain. The cerebral aqueduct, that connects 3rd and 4th ventricle, passes through the midbrain. The inferior colliculi and superior colliculi are found on the dorsal aspect of midbrain above the cerebral aqueduct. The cerebral peduncles contain corticospinal and corticobulbar fibers. Substantia nigra is the largest nuclei of midbrain. Ascending and descending tracts traverse through the midbrain. It houses the cranial nerve nuclei of 3rd and 4th cranial nerves.

CEREBELLUM:

GENERAL FEATURES:

The cerebellum is derived from the metencephalon and is located dorsal to the pons and the medulla. The fourth ventricle is found between the cerebellum and the dorsal aspect of the pons. The cerebellum functions in the planning and fine tuning of skeletal muscle contractions. It performs these tasks by comparing an intended with an actual performance.

The cerebellum consists of midline vermis and two lateral cerebellar hemispheres. The cerebellar cortex consists of multiple parallel folds that are referred to as folia. The cerebellar cortex contains several maps of the skeletal muscles in the body.

The topographic arrangement of these maps indicates that the vermis controls the axial and proximal musculature of the limbs, the intermediate part of the hemisphere controls distal musculature and the lateral part of the hemisphere is involved in motor planning.

The flocculonodular lobe is involved in control of balance and eye movements.

REGION	FUNCTION	PRINCIPAL INPUT
VERMIS AND INTERMEDIATE ZONES	ONGOING MOTOR EXECUTION	SPINAL CORD
HEMISPHERE	OLANNING /COORDINATION	CEREBRAL CORTEX AND INFERIOR OLIVARY NUCLEI
FLOCCULONODULAR LOBE	BALANCE AND EYE MOVEMENTS	VESTIBULAR NUCLEI (VIII)

Major input to the cerebellum travels in the inferior cerebellar peduncle (ICP) (restiform body) and middle cerebellar peduncle (MCP). Major outflow form the cerebellum travels in the superior peduncle (SCP).

MAJOR AFFERENTS TO THE CEREBELLUM:

name	tract	enter cerebellum via	target and function
mossy fibers	vestibulicerebellar spinocerebellar (cortico)pontocerebellar	icp icp and scp mcp(decussate)	excitatory terminals on granule cells
climbing fibers	olivocerebellar	icp(decussate)	excitatory terminals on purkinje cells

CEREBELLAR CYTOARCHITECTURE:

All afferents and efferent projections of the cerebellum traverse the ICP, MCP or SCP. Most afferent input enters the cerebellum in the ICP and MCP; most efferent outflow leaves in the SCP.

Internally the cerebellum consists of outer cortex and an inner medulla.

The three cell layers of the cortex are the molecular layer, the Purkinje cell layer, and the granule cell layer.

The molecular cell layer is the outer layer and is made up of basket and stellate cells as well as parallel fibers, which are the axons of the granule cells. The extensive dendritic tree of the Purkinje cell extends into the molecular layer.

The Purkinje layer is the middle and most important layer of the cerebellar cortex. All of the inputs to the cerebellum are directed toward influencing the firing of Purkinje cells, and only axons of Purkinje cells leave the cerebellar cortex. A single axon exits from each Purkinje cells and projects to one of the deep cerebellar nuclei or to vestibular nuclei of the brain stem.

The granule cell layer is the innermost layer of cerebellar cortex and contains the Golgi cells, granule cells, and glomeruli. Each glomerulus is surrounded by a glial capsule and contains a granule cell and axons of Golgi cells, which synapse with granule cells. The granule cell is the only excitatory neuron within the cerebellar cortex. All other neurons in the cerebellar cortex, including Purkinje, Golgi, basket, and stellate cells, are inhibitory.

CEREBELLUM; CELL TYPES:

NAME	TARGET (AXON TERMEINATION)	TRANSMITTER	FUNCTION
purkinje cell	deep cerebellar nuclei	gaba	inhibitory
granule cell	purkinje cell	glutamate	excitatory
stellate cell	purkinje cell	gaba	inhibitory
basket cell	purkinje cell	gaba	inhibitory
golgi cell	granule cell	gaba	inhibitory

The internal white matter contains the deep cerebellar nuclei.

From medial to lateral, deep cerebellar nuclei in the internal white matter are the fastigial nucleus, interposed nuclei and dentate nucleus. Two kinds of excitatory input enter the cerebellum in the form of climbing fibers and mossy fibers. Both types influence the firing of deep cerebellar nuclei by axon collaterals.

CLIMBING FIBERS:

These originate exclusively from the inferior olivary complex of nuclei on the contralateral side of the medulla. Climbing fibers provide a direct powerful monosynaptic excitatory input to Purkinje cells.

MOSSY FIBERS:

These represent the axons from all other sources of cerebellar input. Mossy fibers provide an indirect, more diffuse excitatory input to Purkinje cells.

All mossy fibers exert an excitatory effect on granule cells. Each granule cell sends its axons into the molecular layer, where it gives off collateral at 90 degree angle that run parallel to the cortical surface (i-e ,parallel fibers).These granule cell axons stimulate the apical dendrites of the Purkinje cells. Golgi cells receive excitatory input from mossy fibers and from the parallel fibers of the granule cells. The Golgi cell in turn inhibits the granule cell, which activated it in the first place.

The basket and stellate cells, which also receive excitatory input from parallel fibers of granule cells, inhibit Purkinje cells.

CIRCUITORY:

The basic cerebellar circuits begin with Purkinje cells that receive excitatory input directly from climbing fibers and from parallel fibers of granule cells.

Purkinje cell axons project to and inhibit the deep cerebellar nuclei or the vestibular nuclei in an orderly fashion.

Purkinje cells in the flocculonodular lobe project to the lateral vestibular nucleus.

Purkinje cells in the vermis project to the fastigial nuclei

Purkinje cells in the intermediate hemisphere primarily project to the interposed (globose and emboliform) nuclei.

Purkinje cells in the lateral hemisphere project to the dentate nucleus.

DYSFUNCTION:

HEMISPHERE LESION:

Ipsilateral symptoms: intention tremor, dysmetria, dysdiadokokinesia, scanning dysarthria, nystagmus, hypotonia.

VERMAL LESIONS:

Truncal ataxia.

MAJOR PATHWAY:

Purkinje cells –deep cerebellar nucleus; dentate nucleus- contralateral VL- first –degree motor cortex- pontine nuclei-contralateral cerebellar cortex.

MAJOR EFFERENTS FROM THE CEREBELLUM:

CEREBELLAR AREAS	DEEP CEREBELLAR NUCLEUS	EFFERENTS TO	FUNCTION
VESTIBULOCEREBELLUM (FLOCULONODULAR LOBE)	FASTIGIAL NUCLEUS	VESTIBULAR NUCLEUS	ELICIT POSITIONAL CHANGES OF EYES AND TRUNK IN RESPONSE TO MOVEMENT OF THE HEAD.
SPINICEREBELLUM (INTERMEDIATE HEMISPHERE)	INTERPOSITUS NUCLEUS	RED NUCLEUS RETICULAR FORMATION	INFLUENCE LMNS VIA THE RETICULOSPINAL AND RUBROSPINAL TRACTS

			TO ADJUST POSTURE AND EFFECT MOVEMENT
PONTOCEREBELLUM (LATERAL HEMISPHERES)	DENTATE NUCLEUS	THALAMUS(VA,VL) THEN CORTEX	INFLUENCE ON LMNS VIA THE CORTICOSPINAL TRACT, WHICH EFFECT VOLUNTARY MOVEMENTS, ESPECIALLY SEQUENCE AND PRECISION.

Efferents from the deep cerebellar nuclei leave mainly through the SCP and influence all upper motor neurons. In particular, axons from the dentate and interposed nuclei leave through the SCP, cross the midline, and terminate in the Ventrolateral (VL) nucleus of the thalamus.

The VL nucleus of the thalamus projects to motor cortex and influences the firing of corticospinal and corticobulbar neurons.

Axons from other deep cerebellar nuclei influence upper motor neurons in the red nucleus and in the reticular formation and vestibular nuclei.

CEREBELLAR LESIONS:

The hallmark of cerebellar dysfunction is a tremor with intended movement without paralysis or paresis. Symptoms associated with cerebellar lesions are expressed ipsilaterally because the major outflow of the cerebellum projects to the contralateral motor cortex, and then the corticospinal fibers cross on their way to the spinal cord. Thus, unilateral lesions of the cerebellum will result in a patient falling toward the side of the lesion.

LESIONS THAT INCLUDE THE HEMISPHERE:

Lesions that include the hemisphere produce a number of dysfunctions, mostly involving distal musculature.

An intention tremor is seen when voluntary movements are performed. For example, if a patient with a cerebellar lesion is asked to pick up a penny is approached. The tremor is barely noticeable or is absent at rest.

Dysmetria (past pointing) is the inability to stop a movement at the proper place. The patient has difficulty performing the finger –to –nose test.

Dysdiadokokinesia is the reduced ability to perform alternating movements such as pronation and supination of the forearm, at a moderately quick pace.

Scanning dysarthria is caused by asynergy of the muscles responsible for speech. In scanning dysarthria, patients divide words into syllables, thereby disrupting the melody of speech.

Gaze dysfunction occurs when the eyes try to fix on a point. They may pass it or stop too soon and then oscillate a few times before they settle on the target. A nystagmus may be present, particularly with cerebellar damage. The nystagmus is often coarse, with the fast component usually directed towards the involved cerebellar hemisphere.

Hypotonia usually occurs with an acute cerebellar insult that includes the deep cerebellar nuclei. The muscle feel flabby on palpation, and deep tendon reflexes are usually diminished.

LESIONS IN THE VERMAL REGION:

Vermal lesions result in difficulty maintaining posture, gait, or balance (an ataxic gait).Patients with vermal damage may be differentiated from those with a lesion of the dorsal columns by the Romberg sign. In cerebellar lesions, patients will sway or lose their balance with their eyes open; in dorsal column lesions, patients sway with their eyes closed.

SUMMARY:

The cerebellum controls the posture, muscle tone, and learning of repeated motor functions, and coordinates voluntary motor activity. Diseases of the cerebellum result in disturbances of gait, posture, and coordinated motor actions, but there is no paralysis or inability to start or stop movement.

The cerebellum is functionally divided into (1) the vermis and intermediate zone (2) the hemisphere, and (3) the flocculonodular lobe.

Each of these 3 areas receives afferent fibers mainly from the spinal cord, cortex and inferior olivary nucleus, and vestibular nuclei, respectively. These afferents fibers (mossy and climbing) reach the cerebellum via the inferior and middle cerebellar peduncles, which connect the cerebellum with the brain stem. The afferent fibers are excitatory and project directly or indirectly via granule cells to the Purkinje cells of the cerebellar cortex. The axons of the Purkinje cells are inhibitory and are the only outflow from the cerebellar cortex. They project to and inhibit the deep cerebellar nuclei (dentate, interposed, and fastigial nuclei) in the medulla. From the deep nuclei, efferents project mainly through the superior cerebellar peduncle and drive the upper motor neurons of the motor cortex. The efferents from the hemisphere project through the dentate nucleus, to the contralateral ventral lateral/ ventral anterior nuclei of the thalamus, to reach the contralateral gyrus. These influence contralateral lower motor neurons via the corticospinal tract.

Symptoms associated with cerebellar lesions are expressed ipsilaterally. Unilateral lesions of the cerebellum will result in a patient falling toward the side of the lesion. Hallmarks of cerebellar dysfunction include ataxia, intention tremor, dysmetria and dysdiadokokinesia.

CORTICAL AREAS AND THEIR FUNCTIONS:
1. FRONTAL LOBE:
   A. PRECENTRAL CORTEX:
      (I) PRIMARY MOTOR AREA :(4) Concerned with initiation of voluntary movements of contralateral half of the body and initiation of speech.
      (II) PREMOTOR AREA:
         a. (6) Gives rise to pyramidal tracts.
         b. (8) Frontal eye field- concerned with control of eye movements.
         c. (44, 45) Motor speech area- concerned with movements of those structures which are responsible for production of voice and articulation of speech.
   B. PREFRONTAL CORTEX: (9-14,23,24,29,32,44-47)
      Center for planned actions,
      Center for higher intelligence,
      Seat of intelligence and
      Control of intellectual activities: To plan the future; allows person to concentrate on central theme of thought; allows to consider the consequences of motor functions before their performance.
2. PARIETAL LOBE:
   A. PRIMARY SENSORY AREA: (3, 1, 2) receives input from the opposite side of the body.

B. **SECONDARY SENSORY AREA AND SENSORY ASSOCIATION AREA:** (5,7) receives input from primary sensory area.
3. **TEMPORAL LOBE:**
   A. **PRIMARY AUDITORY AREA:** (41, 42) perceives the nerve impulses as sound i-e auditory information such as loudness, pitch, source and direction of sound.
   B. **AUDITORY ASSOCIATION AREA:** (22,21,20)
      (I) (22) Wernicke's speech area –concerned with interpretation of meaning of what is heard and comprehension of spoken language and formation of ideas that are to be articulated in speech.
      (II) (21, 20) receives impulses from primary area and are concerned with interpretation of auditory impulses.
4. **OCCIPITAL LOBE:**
   A. **PRIMARY VISUAL CORTEX:** (17) Perception of visual impulses
   B. **VISUAL ASSOCIATION AREA:** (18) interpretation of visual impulses
   C. **OCCIPITAL EYE FIELD**: (19) Movements of eyeball

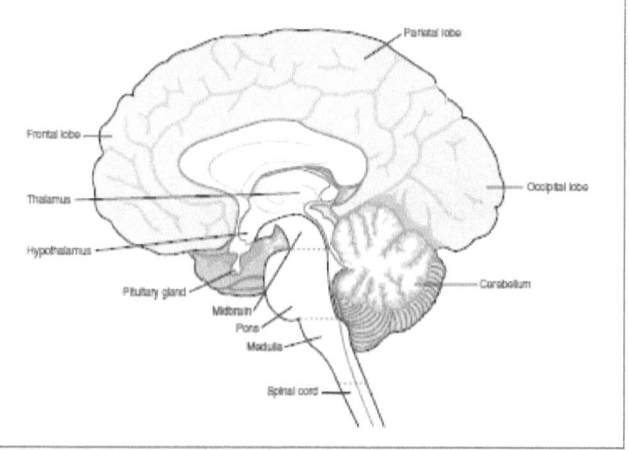

MID SAGITTAL SECTION OF THE BRAIN

CORTICOSPINAL TRACT:

The primary motor cortex, located in the precentral gyrus of the frontal lobe and the premotor area, located immediately anterior to the primary motor cortex, give rise to about 60% of the fibers of corticospinal tract. Primary and secondary somatosensory cortical areas located in the parietal lobe give rise to about 40% of the fibers of the corticospinal tract.

Fibers in the corticospinal tract leave the cerebral cortex in the internal capsule, which carries all axons in and out of cortex. Corticospinal fibers then descend through the length of the brain stem in the ventral portion of the midbrain, pons and medulla.

In the lower medulla, 80-90% of corticospinal fibers cross the decussation of the pyramids and continue in the contralateral spinal cord as the lateral corticospinal tract. The lateral corticospinal tract descends the full length of the cord in the lateral part of the white matter. As it descends, axons leave the tract and enter the gray matter of the ventral horn to synapse on lower motor neurons.

LESIONS OF CORTICOSPINAL TRACT:

The crossing or decussation of the corticospinal tract at the medulla/spinal cord junction has significant clinical implications. If lesions of the corticospinal tract occur above the pyramidal decussation, a weakness is seen in muscles on the contralateral side of the body; lesions below this level produce an ipsilateral muscle weakness. In contrast to upper motor neurons, the cell bodies of lower motor neurons are ipsilateral to the skeletal muscles that their axons innervate. A lesion to any part of a lower motor neuron will result in an ipsilateral muscle weakness at the level of the lesion.

CSF DISTRIBUTION, SECRETION AND CIRCULATION:

CSF fills the subarachnoid space and the ventricles of the brain. The average adult has 90-150 ml of total CSF, although 400-500 ml is produced daily. Only 25 ml of CSF is found in the ventricles themselves.

Approximately 70% of the CSF is secreted by the choroid plexus which consists of glomerular tufts of capillaries covered by ependymal cells that project into the ventricles (the remaining 30 % represents metabolic water production). The choroid plexus is located in parts of each lateral ventricle, the third ventricle and the fourth ventricle.

CSF from the lateral ventricles passes through the interventricular foramina of Monro into the third ventricle. From there, the CSF flows through the aqueduct of Sylvius into the fourth ventricle. The only sites where CSF can leave the ventricles and enter the subarachnoid space outside the CNS are through the openings in the fourth ventricle, two lateral foramina of lushka and the median foramen of magendie. Within the subarachnoid space, CSF also flows up over the convexity of the brain and around the spinal cord. Almost all CSF returns to the venous system by draining through arachnoid granulations into the superior sagittal dural venous sinus.

Normal CSF is a clear fluid, isotonic with serum (290-295 mosmol/l)

The pH of CSF is 7.33 (arterial blood pH, 7.40, venous blood pH, 7.36)

Sodium ion (Na) concentration is equal in serum and CSF (=138 mEq/l)

CSF has a higher concentration of chloride (Cl) and magnesium (Mg) ions than serum.

CSF has a lower concentration of potassium (K), calcium (Ca) and bicarbonate (HCO3) ions, as well as glucose, than serum.

The concentration of protein C (including all immunoglobulins) is much lower in the CSF as compared with serum.

Normal CSF contains 0-4 lymphocytes or mononuclear cells per cubic millimeter. Although the presence of a few monocytes or lymphocytes is normal, the presence of polymorphonuclear leukocytes is always abnormal, as in bacterial meningitis.

Red blood cells (RBC) are not normally found in the CSF but may be present after traumatic spinal tap or subarachnoid hemorrhage.

Increased protein levels may indicate a CNS tumor.

Tumor cells may be present in the CSF in cases with meningeal involvement.

FUNCTIONS OF CSF:

1. It cushions and protects CNS from trauma.
2. It provides mechanical buoyancy and support for the brain.
3. It serves as a reservoir and assists in the regulation of the contents of the skull
4. It nourishes the CNS.
5. It removes metabolites from the CNS.

6. It serves as a pathway for pineal secretion to reach pituitary.

CLINICAL CORRELATE:

CSF ABNORMALITIES:

Hydrocephalus is caused by an excess volume or pressure of CSF, producing ventricular dilatation.

COMMUNICATING HYDROCEPHALUS:

It is caused by over secretion of CSF without obstruction in the ventricles or obstruction in the ventricles or by CSF circulation or absorption problems from the subarachnoid space. Choroid plexus papilloma is a possible cause of over secretion, a tumor in the subarachnoid space limits circulation, or meningitis may limit absorption into superior sagittal sinus.

NONCOMMUNICATING HYDROCEPHALUS:

It is caused by obstruction to the CSF flow inside the ventricular system at a foramen Monro, in the cerebral aqueduct, or in the fourth ventricle. CSF is prevented from exiting through foramina of Magendie or Lushka in the fourth ventricle into the subarachnoid space.

NORMAL PRESSURE HYDROCEPHALUS:

It results when CSF is not absorbed by arachnoid villi and the ventricles are enlarged, pressing the cortex against the skull. Patients present with confusion, gait, apraxia and urinary incontinence.

HEADACHE:

Headaches which are new, severe or acute are more likely due to intracranial disorders then are chronic headaches.

Chronic headaches are divided into:

   a. **PRIMARY:**
      (I)   <u>MIGRAINE</u>: They are pulsatile headaches usually unilateral associated with nausea and vomiting, photophobia is common accompanied by an aura of transient neurologic symptoms may present due to neurovascular dysfunction. Headaches occur due to dilation of blood vessels innervated by trigeminal nerve caused by release of neuropeptides from parasympathetic nerve fibers approximating these blood vessels.

      (II)   <u>TENSION HEADACHE</u>: It is a common type of headache. Patients complain of pericranial tenderness, poor concentration. These are not pulsatile but like a tight band across the head. Headaches are exacerbated by emotions, fatigue, noise and glare. Not associated with focal neurological deficit. Treatment is massage, hot baths and biofeedback.

      (III) <u>CLUSTER HEADACHE</u>: It may be due to activation of cells in the ipsilateral hypothalamus, triggering the trigeminal autonomic vascular system. Unilateral periorbital pain daily for several weeks accompanied by one of the following; nasal congestion, rhinorrhea, lacrimation, redness of eye 15mm-3 hours. Spontaneous remission may occur,

b. **SECONDARY:**
- (i) <u>POST TRAUMATIC HEADACHE:</u> Headache often appears within a day or so following injury, may worsen over the weeks and then gradually subsides. It can be localized, generalized, dull aching or throbbing.
- (ii) <u>HEADACHE DUE TO INTRACRANIAL MASS LESION:</u> Headache occurs due to displacement of vascular and other pain sensitive structures.
- (iii) <u>MEDICATION OVERUSE:</u> (Analgesic rebound) headache: Half of all the patients with chronic daily headaches, medication over use is responsible. Patients have severe pain unresponsive to medications.
- (iv) <u>HEADACHE DUE TO LUMBER PUNCTURE:</u> Dull or throbbing headache is a frequent sequel of L.P, may last for several days. It is aggravated by erect posture and alleviated by recumbency.
- (v) <u>WHEN TO REFER:</u>
  - a. Headache of acute onset "worst headache of my life"
  - b. Increased headache not responsive to simple measures.
  - c. History of trauma, hypertension, fever and visual changes.
  - d. Presence of neurologic signs or scalp tenderness.

LEARNING:

It is the neural mechanisms by which an individual changes his or her behavior on the basis of past experiences.

1. REFLEX LEARNING: Learning is associated with immediate behavioral changes.
2. INCIDENTAL LEARNING: Behavioral changes are not immediately apparent. The individual acquire information about the world while attending incidentally to sensory inputs and thereby develop the potential to behave differently.

Two classes of reflex learning are there:

a. NON ASSOCIATIVE LEARNING: The subject learns about the properties of a single stimulus. It results when an animal or a person is repeatedly exposed to a single type of stimulus.
   (1) HABITUATION: It refers to decrease in response to a benign stimulus when the stimulus is presented repeatedly. When the stimulus is presented for the first time it is novel and evokes a reaction. This response is called "orientation reflex" or "what is it" response. Hence due to habituation, lesser and lesser response is evoked on repeated stimulation. Eventually the subject totally ignores the stimulus and thus gets habituated to it. So a repeated stimulus causes a response, but that response gradually diminishes as it is "learned" that the stimulus is not important. For example New Yorker first coming to New York may be awakened by street noises, but eventually the

noises will be ignored as it is learned that they are not relevant.
(2) SENSITIZATION: It is opposite to habituation, where a stimulus results in greater probability of a subsequent response when it is learned that the stimulus is important. Thus repeated application of a distinctly pleasant or unpleasant (strong) stimulus produces greater and greater response. Learning occurs in sensitization, in a direction opposite to that seen in habituation.

b. ASSOCIATIVE LEARNING: In associative learning, the subject learns about the relationship between two stimuli or between a stimulus and a behavior.

There are two types of associative learning:

(1) CLASSICAL CONDITIONING: It refers to learning a relationship between two stimuli. A conditioned reflex is reflex response to stimulus that acquired by repeatedly pairing the stimulus with another stimulus that normally does produce the response. It depends for its appearance on the formation of new functional connections in CNS.

RE-INFORCEMENT: A process of following a conditioned stimulus (CS) with the basic unconditioned stimulus (US) is must for retaining a conditioned reflex otherwise it will be extinct.

PAVLOV'S EXPERIMENT TO DEMONSTRATE CLASSICAL CONDITIONED REFLEX IS:

a. When food i-e an unconditioned stimulus (US) is presented to an hungry dog, it

produces salivation (an unconditioned response) or,
b. If a bell a conditioned stimulus (CS) just before the food (US) is presented, the dog learns to associate the bell (CS) with the food (US).
c. Eventually, ringing the bell (CS) alone causes salivation.
d.

(2) OPERANT CONDITIONING:
Also called instrumental conditioning, type 2 conditioning, type R conditioning or trial and error conditioning.

OPERANT CONDITIONING IS OF TWO TYPES:
1. REWARD CONDITIONING: In it a naturally occurring response is strengthened by positive reinforcement (reward).
2. ADVERSE CONDITIONING: In it a naturally occurring (innate) response is weakened by a negative reinforcement (punishment).

EXPERIMENT TO DEMONSTRATE OPERANT CONDITIONING:

A hungry animal (e.g. rat) is placed in a cage with a lever (bars) projecting in the cage. Because of naturally occurring (innate) response, the rat will randomly press the lever.

If the pressing of the lever is not associated with any event the pressing of the lever will be at a random rate. If the pressing of the lever is associated with a positive reinforcement i-e reward (e.g. food) the rate of pressing the lever will be much more than the random rate (reward conditioning). If the pressing of the lever is associated with a negative reinforcement i-e punishment (e.g. electric shock), the lever pressing rate will be much less than the random rate (aversive conditioning).

MEMORY: It refers to acquisition, storage and retrieval of sensory information. Learning is the change in behavior based on the sensory information stored in the brain.

TYPES OF MEMORY:

It is classified in two ways:

Physiologically on the basis of how information is stored and recalled, memory can be classified into:

a. IMPLICIT MEMORY: Also called non-declarative or reflexive memory refers to information about how to perform something. It is not associated with awareness and does not involve processing in the hippocampus in most instances. Examples of implicit memory include:
   (i) Motor skills
   (ii) Behavioral reflexes
   (iii) Learning of certain types of procedures and rules.
   All of which once acquired, becomes unconscious and automatic.
b. EXPLICIT MEMORY: Also called declarative or recognition memory, refers to

factual knowledge of people, places and things and what these facts mean. This is called declarative conscious effort. Explicit memory is highly flexible and involves association of multiple bits and pieces of information. In contrast, implicit memory is more rigid and tightly connected to the original stimulus conditions under which the learning occurred.

Explicit memory: It can be further classified as:

(A) SEMANTIC MEMORY: A memory of facts. It is that form of long term explicit memory that embraces knowledge of objects, facts and concepts as well as words and their meaning. It includes the naming of objects, the definition of spoken words and verbal fluency. It is stored in a distributed fashion in different association cortices.

(B) EPISODIC MEMORY: It refers to memory of events and personal experiences. It is stored in association areas of prefrontal cortex. These prefrontal areas work with other areas of neocortex to allow recollection of when and where a past event occurred.

DEPENDING UPON PERMEANCY OF STORAGE MEMORY:

a. SHORT TERM MEMORY: Example of this is the memory of a new telephone number after calling the operator or after looking into directory. Most of times the number is forgotten after short period of time. It may contain 7 or less piece of information and is easily disrupted with distraction; may last from seconds to minutes.

b. <u>INTERMEDIATE MEMORY:</u> It is also called secondary memory. It lasts for days to weeks but is eventually lost.

c. <u>LONG TERM MEMORY:</u> It is also called tertiary memory which once stored, can be recalled years later or for a long time. It includes explicit information about facts for e.g. distant personal or public memories, reciting the helping verbs.

<u>MOLECULAR BASIS OF MEMORY:</u>

Input to the brain is processed into short term memory before it is transferred through one or more stages (intermediate, long term) into permanent long term storage.

<u>MECHANISM OFSHORT TERM IMPLICIT MEMEORY:</u> The mechanism for short forms of learning result from changes in the effectiveness of synaptic transmission.

<u>MECHANISM OF LONG TERM STORAGE OF IMPLICIT MEMORY:</u> The process by which transient short term memory is converted into stable long term memory is called CONSOLIDATION.

Consolidation of long term implicit memory for simple forms of learning involves three processes:

a. Gene expression
b. New protein synthesis
c. Growth (or pruning) of synaptic connections.

HIPPOCAMPUS AND DECLARATIVE MEMORIES: It is involved in consolidation into long term memory. It stores long term memory for short periods and transfer them to other cortical sites for more permanent storage. The role in declarative memories (involves consciousness recall)-What memories of specific people, places and objects facts and events that often result after only one experience)

CEREBELLUM AND PROCEDURAL MEMORIES: It is "how to" procedural memories involving motor skills gained through repetitive training, such as memorizing a particular dance routine and procedural memories are brought forth without conscious effort.

PREFRONTAL CORTEX AND WORKING MEMORY: Prefrontal cortex is associated with working memory. Temporary storage site for holding relevant data online and is largely responsible for the so-called executive functions involving manipulations and integration of this information for planning ,juggling ,competing priorities, problem solving, making choices, organizing activities and inhibiting impulses. Executive functions allow a person to decide what to do instead of just reacting to the situation at hand.

ANTEROGRADE AMNESIA: inability to retain new information through conversion of short term memories to long term memories. It occurs in the lesions of medial portions of temporal lobes which are areas of consolidation.

RETROGRADE AMNESIA: It is the inability to recall events occurring before the onset of amnesia; may be temporally graded (i-e distant events are easier to recall than more recent ones). It is the Inability to recall recent past events. It occurs in stroke, traumatic event (short term memory is erased).

CONSOLIDATION: It refers to conversion of short term memory to long term memory.

REMEMBERING: It is the process of retrieving specific information from memory stores.

FORGETTING: It is the inability to retrieve stored information.

WORKING MEMORY: It temporarily holds and inter relates various pieces of information relevant to a current mental task. It is briefly held and processing of data occurs for intermediate use.

LIMBIC SYSTEM:

COMPONENTS OF LIMBIC SYSTEM:

The term limbic system is applied for those parts of the cortex (limbic cortex or limbic lobe) and subcortical structures that form a ring around the brain stem. The components are:

Limbic cortex is composed of:

    a. Orbitofrontal cortex
    b. Subcallosal gyrus
    c. Cingulate gyrus
    d. Parahippocampal gyrus
    e. Uncus.

Subcortical structures included in the limbic system are:

    a. Hypothalamus
    b. Septum
    c. Paraolfactory area
    d. Anterior nuclei of thalamus
    e. Amygdala
    f. Portions of basal ganglia
    g. Hippocampus

PAPEZ CIRCUIT:

Refers to a closed circuit formed by connections between cingulate gyrus (located in the parietal lobe), hippocampus, mammillary bodies and anterior nucleus of thalamus. This circuit is responsible for resting EEG, and for those emotions and aspects of behavior that are related to preservation of individual and species.

FUNCTIONS OF LIMBIC SYSTEM:

1. AUTONOMIC FUNCTIONS: Stimulation of many parts of the limbic system especially amygdala produces autonomic responses such as changes in cardiovascular, respiratory and gastrointestinal system through hypothalamus. Such changes are also observed during emotional stress.
2. REGULATION OF FEEDING BEHAVIOR: Limbic system regulates feeding behavior mainly through hypothalamus and amygdala.
3. MATERNAL BEHAVIOR: Maternal behavior is the function of cingulate gyrus and retrosplenial portion of the limbic cortex. In general, the maternal behavior is concerned with the nursing (breastfeeding) and protection of the offspring by the mother.
4. EMOTIONAL BEHAVIOR: Emotional behavior is one of the most important functions of limbic system. Hypothalamus has been considered the main seat of emotions.
   Areas of Hypothalamus associated with behavioral control functions are:
   a. Increased level of general activity leading to rage and aggression. It occurs when lateral hypothalamus is stimulated.
   b. Feeling of reward, tranquility and pleasure are appreciated when reward center is stimulated.
   c. Fearing, feeling of punishment and aversion are felt when punishment center is stimulated.
   d. Lesions of Hypothalamus are associated with:

Extreme passivity and loss of drive, rage and violent behavior and excessive eating and drinking are seen.

ROLE OF AMYGDALA: Amygdala coordinates the affective component of emotions (functions of cerebral cortex) with the autonomic response to emotions (function of hypothalamus) through the ventral amygdalofugal pathway and stria terminalis.

5. MOTIVATIONAL BEHAVIOR: Motivation is that component of behavior which is responsible for accomplishing a particular task.

MENINGES OF THE BRAIN:

The brain is enclosed within the cranial cavity by three concentric tissue layers; pia mater, arachnoid mater and dura mater, which constitutes the meninges of the brain.

PIA MATER: Pia mater covers closely and continuously the external surface of the brain, and is a thin and highly vascular membrane. Folds of the pia mater enclose tufts of capillaries called choroid plexus to form tela choroidea in relation to ventricles of the brain.

ARACHNOID MATER: Arachnoid is connected to pia mater by many filamentous fibers. Subarachnoid between these two layers is filled with CSF.

DURA MATER: It is composed of two layers; outer endosteal layer and inner meningeal layer. These are fused except where folds form (falx cereberi) or venous sinuses (e.g. superior sagittal sinus) are enclosed between them.

SUBDURAL SPACE: This space separates dura mater from arachnoid mater. The arachnoid mater has minute protrusions (arachnoid villi) which pass through fenestra in dura mater and project into venous sinuses to allow escape of CSF into venous sinuses.

CLASSIFICATION OF NERVE FIBER:

FIBER TYPE	CONDUCTION VELOCITY	FIBER DIAMETER	FUNCTION	MYELIN
A FIBERS A ALPHA	70-120M/SEC	12-20 μm	MOTOR AND SKELETAL MUSCLE	YES
A BETA	40-70	5-12	SENSORY TOUCH PRESSURE AND VIBRATION	YES
A GAMMA	10-50	3-6	MUSCLE SPINDLE	YES
A DELTA	6-30	2-5	PAIN (SHARP LOCALIZED)TEMPERATURE TOUCH	YES
B FIBERS	3-15	<3	PREGANGLIONIC AUTONOMIC	YES
C FIBERS	0.5-2.0	0.4-1.2	PAIN (DIFFUSE,DEEP) TEMPERATURE POST GANGLIONICAUTONOMIC	NO

CLASSIFICATION ACCORDING TO SUSCEPTIBILITY:

EFFECT	MOST SUSCEPTIBLE	INTERMEDIATE	LEAST
BLOCKED BY HYPOXIA	B	A	C
BLOCKED BY PRESSURE	A	B	C
BLOCKED BY LOCAL ANESTHESIA	C	B	A

GLIAL AND SUPPORTING CELLS IN THE CNS AND PNS:

The supporting cells or glial cells of the CNS are small cells which are different from neurons. Supporting cells have only one kind of process and do not form chemical synapses. Supporting cells readily divide and proliferate; gliomas are the most common type of primary tumor of the CNS.

ASTROCYTES:

They are the most numerous glial cells in the CNS and have large number of radiating processes. They provide structural support for the CNS and contain large bundles of intermediate filaments that consist of glial fibrillary acidic protein (GFAP). They have uptake systems that remove neurotransmitters glutamate and K ions from extracellular space. They have foot processes that contribute to the blood brain barrier by forming glial limiting membrane. Astrocytes hypertrophy and proliferate after an injury to the CNS, fill up the extra cellular space left by degenerating neurons by forming astroglial scar.

Radial glia are precursors of astrocytes that guide neuroblast migration during CNS development.

MICROGLIAL CELLS:

They are the smallest cells in the CNS. It is derived from bone marrow monocytes and enters cells after birth. They provide a link between the cells of CNS and the immune system. Microglia proliferates and migrates to the site of a CNS injury and phagocytose the neuronal debris after injury. Pericytes are microglial cells that contribute to blood brain barrier. CNS microglia that becomes phagocytic in response to neuronal tissue damage may secrete toxic free radicals. Accumulation of free radicals, such as superoxide may lead to disruption of calcium homeostasis of neurons. Microglia determine the chances of a survival of a CNS tissue graft and are the cells in the CNS that are targeted by the HIV-1 virus in patients with AIDS. The targeted microglia may produce cytokines that are toxic to neurons.

OLIGODENDROCYTES:

It forms myelin for axons in the CNS. Each of the processes of the oligodendrocytes can myelinate individual segments of many axons. Unmyelinated axons in the CNS are not ensheathed by the oligodendrocytes cytoplasm.

SCHWANN CELLS:

They are the supporting cells of the peripheral nervous system (PNS) and are derived from neural crest cells. It forms the myelin for axons and processes in the PNS. Each Schwann cells forms myelin for only a single internodal segment of a single axon. Unmyelinated axons in the PNS are enveloped by the cytoplasmic processes of a Schwann cell. Schwann cells act as phagocytes and remove neuronal debris in the PNS after injury. A node of ranvier is the region between adjacent myelinated segments of axons in the CNS and PNS.

In all myelinated axons, nodes of ranvier are sites that permit action potential to jump from node to node (saltatory conduction). Saltatory conduction dramatically increases the conduction velocity of impulses in myelinated axons.

EPENDYMAL CELLS:

They line the ventricles in the adult brain. Some ependymal cells differentiate into choroid epithelial cells forming part of the choroid plexus, which produces CSF. Ependymal cells are ciliated, ciliary action helps circulate the CSF.

TANYCYTES:

These are specialized ependymal cells that have basal cytoplasmic processed in contact with blood vessels, these processes may transport substances between a blood vessel and a ventricle.

NEURONS:

These are signal transmitting cells of the nervous system which are permanent in nature and do not divide in adulthood (and have no progenitor stem cells population). Also called as signal relaying cells with dendrites (receive input), cell bodies and axons (send output). The cell bodies and dendrites can be stained via Nissl substance (stains RER). RER is not present in the axon.

If an axon is injured, it undergoes Wallerian degeneration – degeneration distal to the injury and axonal retraction proximally, allows for potential regeneration of the axon (if in PNS).

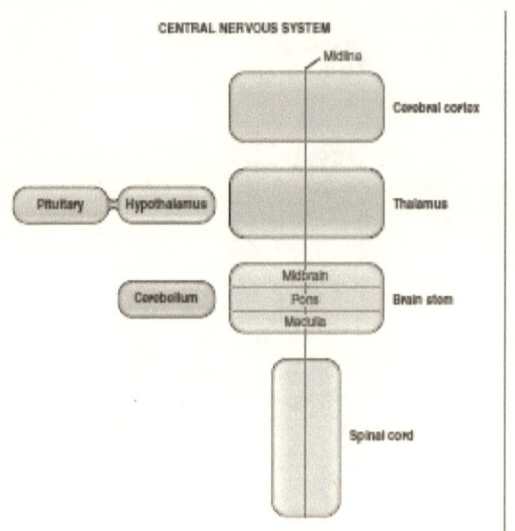

SCHEMATIC REPRESENTATION OF CNS

PAIN PHYSIOLOGY:

Unpleasant sensory and emotional experience associated with actual or potential tissue damage.

1. It makes one aware of a harmful agent in close contact with the body and body gives preferential treatment to this information.
2. It causes the individual to react to remove from the pain stimulus to prevent further damage to the tissues.
3. Pain receptors are non-adapting receptors; therefore they keep the person apprised of damaging stimulus as long as it persists. Thus pain sensation has a protective function.

NOCICEPTORS:

These are receptors of pain that respond to noxious stimuli. The noxious stimuli can be:

   a. Damaging
   b. Mechanical
   c. Chemical
   d. Thermal

Nociceptors are special type of free nerve endings of:

1. A delta myelinated nerve fibers
2. C unmyelinated nerve fibers.

TYPES:

SOMATIC NOCICEPTORS: Free nerve endings of A delta and C fibers

VISCERAL NOCICEPTORS: Visceral pain is not produced by many tissue damaging stimuli such as localized cutting, clamping or burning. Widespread inflammation, ischemia, mesenteric stretching, spasm or dilation of viscera produces pain.

PAIN STIMULI:

Pain receptors are activated by three types of noxious stimuli:

Mechanical and Thermal stimuli: tend to elicit fast pain. Fast pain is felt when a needle is struck in to the skin, when the skin is cut with a knife or when the skin is acutely burned. It is also felt when the skin is subjected to electric shock. Fast, sharp pain is not felt in the deeper tissues. Mechanical and thermal stimuli however can elicit slow pain.

Chemical stimuli: Damaged tissue releases certain chemicals which act on Nociceptors and cause pain sensations.

Chemical mediators of pain include:

a. K, ATP and ADP are released following cell death.
b. Bradykinin is formed by reaction of certain circulating globulins with proteolytic enzymes released by dying cells. It is most powerful in causing tissue damage pain.
c. Leukotrienes are released from the mast cells.
d. Serotonin is released from platelets.
e. Histamine is released from mast cells.
f. Accumulation of lactic acid in tissues due to anaerobic mechanism during ischemia.
g. Prostaglandins.

h. Substance P

QUALITATIVE TYPE OF PAIN SENSATIONS:

FAST PAIN: Fast pain is sharp, well localized, pricking sensation that results from the activation of the Nociceptors on the A delta fibers. The fast pain sensations travel faster and thus appear within 0.1 millisecond after the application of the stimulus.

ACCOMPANIMENTS OF FAST PAIN:

a. WITHDRAWAL REFLEX: This causes the individual to move the involved body part away from the source of painful stimulus.
b. SYMPATHETIC RESPONSE: This results in increased blood pressure, tachycardia and mobilization of body energy supply.

SLOW PAIN: Slow pain is poorly localized, dull, throbbing, burning sensation that results from activation of Nociceptors on the C fibers. It appears after one second or more following the application of stimulus.

ACCOMPANIMENTS OF SLOW PAIN:

a. EMOTIONAL PERCEPTION: This occurs in the form of unpleasant ness, and in long standing cases, irritation, frustration and depression.
b. AUTONOMIC SYMPTOMS: This occurs in the form of nausea, profuse sweating, vomiting and lowering of blood pressure.
c. GENERALIZED REDUCTION IN MUSCLE TONE:

CLINICAL TYPES OF PAIN:

a. **SOMATIC PAIN:** Somatic pain as the name indicates arises from the tissues of the body other than the viscera. It is of two types:

i. **SUPERFICIAL SOMATIC PAIN:** arises from the skin and superficial tissues. Its features are usually similar to fast pain.

ii. **DEEP SOMATIC PAIN:** pain arises from the muscles, joints, bones, and fascia. Usually the features are similar to slow pain.

CLINICAL CONDITIONS ASSOCIATED WITH SOMATIC PAIN:

a. Injuries
b. Tissue ischemia
c. Inflammation
d. Muscle spasm

b. **REFERRED PAIN:** It originates due to irritation of a visceral organ and is felt not in the organ but in some other somatic structure (usually skin) supplied by the same neural segment.

CHARACTERISTIC FEATURES OF REFERRED PAIN ARE:

1. Such a pain is referred to a second structure For example:
   a. In myocardial ischemia, the pain is referred to the left shoulder and arm.
   b. Pain due to stone in the lower part of the ureter is usually referred to the corresponding testes and inner thigh.

c. Inflammation of the diaphragm secondary to pleurisy or severe cholecystitis produces pain at the tip of the shoulder.
2. Because the skin is topographically mapped and the viscera are not, the pain is identified as originating on the skin and not within the viscera.
3. Pain is usually referred to a structure with common embryonic origin and hence is innervated by a common neural segment. This principle is called the dermatomal rule. For example, embryologically the heart and the left arm have the same segmental origin. Similarly the testis and the kidney originate from the same urogenital ridge.
4. THEORIES OF REFFERED PAIN ARE:
   A. CONVERGENCE THEORY: According to this theory when the first order neurons carrying pain sensation from a somatic area and a visceral organ converge on a common second order neuron, the brain is unable to identify the source of pain. Since somatic pain is far more common, the brain interprets all pain as somatic pain even when the source is actually visceral.
   B. FACILITATION THEORY: According to this theory the visceral irritation is inadequate for producing pain by itself. However, it facilitates pain fibers from somatic structures so that even minor somatic irritation produces perceptible pain.

c. <u>PROJECTED PAIN:</u> When the sensory fibers carrying pain sensations are stimulated anywhere in their course to the sensory cortex, the pain sensations evoked are projected to the area where receptors are located. This is called projected pain. Examples of projected pain are:
1. After amputation of the limb sometimes the patient complains of intense pain in the absent limb (phantom limb).The pain sensations are produced due to irritation of Nociceptors fibers at the stump but are projected to the area where the receptors used to be located.
2. Striking the elbow causes pain to be projected to the hand.

d. <u>VISCERAL PAIN:</u>
FEATURES OF VISCERAL PAIN ARE:
1. Poorly localized, because pain receptors in viscera are comparatively few.
2. Unpleasant because of emotional perception.
3. Autonomic symptoms in the form of nausea, vomiting, profuse sweating and lowering of blood pressure.
4. Reflex contraction of skeletal muscle of abdominal wall, clinically known as guarding, is a common association especially when the inflammation of viscera involves the peritoneum. It is a protective reflex which helps to protect the underlying inflamed structures from unintentional injury.
5. Radiates or is referred to other site.
COMMINCAUSES OF VISCERAL PAIN ARE:

- (i) Inflammation
- (ii) Over distension of hollow viscera
- (iii) Spasm of hollow viscus
- (iv) Chemical stimuli
- (v) Ischemia.

NEURAL PATHWAY:

Visceral pain sensations is carried by unmyelinated type C fibers in the sympathetics (from most of the viscera) and in the parasympathetics (from many pelvic viscera) nerves. Their cell bodies are located in the dorsal roots and the homologous cranial nerve ganglion.

In the central nervous system, visceral pain fibers travel along the somatic pain fibers in the spinothalamic tract and medial leminiscus.

e. RADIATING PAIN: Sometimes visceral pain is experienced both locally and also at a distant site (referred pain). In fact pain seems to spread from the local area to the distant site. This is called radiating pain. The examples of radiating pain are: <u>In appendicitis pain starts from the right iliac fossa and radiates towards the center of the abdomen.</u>

f. HYPERALGESIA: It refers to enhanced painful response to a stimulus. It is of two types:
   - (i) PRIMARY HYPERALGESIA: In it the noxious stimulus produces more severe pain than expected. It occurs over an area of tissue damage. The pain threshold is lowered, so that even non –noxious stimuli produces pain(eg.touch)

(ii) **SECONDARY HYPERALGESIA:** It refers to occurrence of far more severe pain than expected in response to noxious stimulus applied to the normal healthy skin. In this condition there is no lowering of pain threshold. It has been explained to the phenomena of subliminal fringe.

g. **CAUSALGIA:** It is a condition in which a spontaneous burning pain sensation occurs after a long time in the area of even trivial injuries. It is also accompanied by hyperalgesia and reflex sympathetic dystrophy.

REFLEX SYMPATHETIC DYSTROPHY:
Mean sympathetic discharge reflexly causes pain in the injured skin area. The exact cause is not known, but research in the animals reveals that:
In the affected area the skin becomes thin, hair growth increases and nerve injuries lead to sprouting of sympathetic nerve fibers.

PATHWAY FOR SLOW PAIN:

IN THE PERIPHERAL NERVES: The slow pain impulses are carried by slow conducting unmyelinated fibers at velocities ranging from 0.5-2 m/sec to dorsal root ganglion and then enter the spinal cord at dorsal root of spinal nerve.

IN THE SPINAL CORD: C fibers terminate in the laminae II and III of dorsal horn. Axon impulses from C fibers cross the midline near their level of origin from the Paleospinothalamic tract which passes upwards to the brain in the anterolateral column along with the fibers of fast pain.

IN THE BRAIN STEM: These fibers terminate very widely in the reticular formation, superior colliculus and periaqueductal grey region.

PAIN SUPPRESSION SYSTEMS IN THE CNS:

The degree of reaction to pain stimuli varies from individual to individual, mainly because of pain suppression system in the CNS.

1. Spinal pain suppression system: Pain inhibitory complex in the dorsal horn of spinal cord which blocks the pain signals at the initial entry point to the spinal cord.

2. Supraspinal pain suppression system

GATE CONTROL HYPOTHESIS:

The dorsal grey horn acts as a gate for transmission of pain sensations and this gate can be partly or completely closed by:

a. Segmental suppression: Activation of large myelinated touch fibers (Ab) reduces pain. Ab fibers give collaterals which causes presynaptic inhibition of pain carrying (both Adelta and C fibers), where they synapse in the dorsal horn. Although poorly understood, such circuitry probably explains the relief of pain achieved by following maneuvers.
   - (i) Rubbing or massage or pressure in the vicinity of painful area.
   - (ii) Local application of warmth and cold.
   - (iii) Local application of counter irritants, i-e stimulation of skin.

(iv) Acupuncture
(v) Trans cutaneous electric nerve stimulation (TENS) in which pain site or the nerves leading from it are stimulated by electrodes placed on the surface of skin.

b. Supraspinal suppression:
There exist three different supra spinal descending pain modulation pathways.

(i) Descending serotonergic and opioid inhibitory system.
Components of this system are:
a. Raphe magnus nucleus: The serotonergic neurons of RMN project down the dorsolateral column to influence the neurons in dorsal horn of spinal cord, which are excited by primary nociceptive afferents. The serotonergic fibers are believed to exert their effect by post synaptic inhibition.
b. Periaqueductal grey region (PAG) area in the midbrain: It inhibits pain by stimulating the raphe magnus nucleus .Neurons of PAG have opioid receptors on their surface membranes. When opioid receptors are stimulated by exogenously administered opioid compounds(analgesia)or by endogenous administered opioid neurotransmitters (endorphins or enkephalins)found in the brain, the pain reducing circuitry system are activated and this leads to reduced pain perception.

CONDITIONS UNDER WHICH DESCENDING SEROTONERGIC PAIN INHIBITORY SYSTEM IS STIMULATED ARE:

(A) WHEN THE LIMBIC SYSTEM IS STIMULATED: Limbic system is the seat of emotions. Fibers from the limbic system supply the PAG. This explains why a soldier wounded in the battle may feel no pain during the heat of battle.

(B) AUTOFEEDBACK: When the spinothalamic tract is stimulated, the collaterals from it stimulate the descending inhibitory pathways.

(ii) Descending purinergic inhibitory system: It comprises specifically of adenosine. Adenosine exhibits both pre and post synaptic actions and produces anti nociception by indirect interaction with excitatory amino acid release.

(iii) Descending adrenergic inhibitory system: Fibers from this system originate from locus ceruleus and medullary reticular formation and descend in dorsolateral fasciculus. Environmental factors such as stress may activate this descending inhibitory mechanism.

PATHWAY FOR FAST PAIN:

IN PERIPHERAL NERVES: Fast pain signals are transmitted in the A delta fibers at velocities 6 and 30 m/sec to dorsal root ganglion and then enter the spinal cord at dorsal root of spinal nerve(formed by axons of cells of dorsal root ganglion).

IN THE SPINAL CORD: A delta fibers ascend or descend for one or two segments. These neurons give rise to fibers which immediately cross to the opposite side of the cord through anterior white commissure and then pass upwards to the brain in the anterolateral columns as neospinothalamic tract.

IN THE BRAIN STEM: A few fibers from the neospinothalamic tract terminate in the reticular formation, but most of them pass upwards to the thalamus.

IN THE THALAMUS: Most of the fibers project to the ventral posterolateral nucleus (VPL). From here, thalamic neurons project to the primary sensory cortex.

This system is primarily used in the localization of pain stimuli when tactile receptors are also stimulated along with fast pain fibers; localization of fast pain is exact. If only pain receptors are stimulated, localization is poor.

Receptors are classified by the type of stimulus that activates them. The five types of receptors are mechanoreceptors, photoreceptors, chemoreceptors, thermoreceptors, and nociceptors.

TYPES AND EXAMPLES OF SENSORY RECEPTORS:

TYPE OF RECEPTOR	MODALITY	RECEPTOR	LOCATION
MECHANORECEPTORS	TOUCH AUDITION VESTIBULAR	PACINIAN HAIR CELL HAIR CELL	SKIN ORGAN OF CORTI MACULA, SEMICIRCULAR CANAL
PHOTORECEPTORS	VISION	RODS AND CONES	RETINA
CHEMORECEPTORS	OLFACTION TASTE ARTERIAL PO2 pH of CSF	OLFACTORY RECEPTOR TASTE BUDS	OLFACTORY MUCOSA TONGUE CAROTID AND AORTIC BODIES VENTROLATERAL MEDULLA
THERMORECEPTORS	TEMPERATURE	COLD RECEPTORS WARM RECEPTORS	SKIN SKIN
NOCICEPTOR	EXTREM	THERMA	SKIN

S	ES OF PAIN AND TEMPERATURE	L NOCICEPTORS POLYMODAL NOCICEPTORS	SKIN

1. <u>MECHANORECEPTORS:</u>
Mechanoreceptors are subdivided into different types of receptors, depending on which kind of pressure or proprioceptive quality they encode. Some types of mechanoreceptors are found in nonhairy skin and other types in hairy skin. Mechanoreceptors are described in Table 1 according to their location in the skin or muscle, the type of adaptation they exhibit, and the sensation they encode. An important characteristic of each receptor is the type of adaptation that it exhibits. Among the various mechanoreceptors, adaptation varies from "very rapidly adapting" (e.g., pacinian corpuscle), to "rapidly adapting" (e.g., Meissner's corpuscle and hair follicles), to "slowly adapting" (e.g., Ruffini's corpuscle, Merkel' receptors, and tactile discs). Very rapidly and rapidly adapting receptors detect changes in the stimulus and, therefore, detect changes in velocity. Slowly adapting receptors respond to intensity and duration of the stimulus.
    a. <u>Pacinian corpuscle</u>: Pacinian corpuscles are encapsulated receptors found in the subcutaneous layers of nonhairy and hairy skin and in muscle. They are the most rapidly adapting of all mechanoreceptors. Because of their very rapid on-off response, they can detect changes in stimulus velocity and encode the sensation of vibration.

b. <u>Meissner's corpuscle</u>: Meissner's corpuscles are also encapsulated receptors found in the dermis of nonhairy skin, most prominently on the fingertips, lips, and other locations where tactile discrimination is especially good. They have small receptive fields and can be used for two-point discrimination. Meissner's corpuscles are rapidly adapting receptors that encode point discrimination, precise location, tapping, and flutter.
c. <u>Hair follicle:</u> Hair-follicle receptors are arrays of nerve fibers surrounding hair follicles in hairy skin. When the hair is displaced, it excites the hair-follicle receptors. These receptors are also rapidly adapting and detect velocity and direction of movement across the skin.
d. <u>Ruffini's corpuscle</u>. Ruffini's corpuscles are located in the dermis of non - hairy and hairy skin and in joint capsules. These receptors have large receptive fields and are stimulated when the skin is stretched. The stimulus may be located some distance from the receptors it activates. Ruffini's corpuscles are slowly adapting receptors. When the skin is stretched, the receptors fire rapidly, then slowly adapt to a new level of firing that corresponds to stimulus intensity. Ruffini's corpuscles detect stretch and joint rotation.
e. <u>Merkel's receptors and tactile discs</u>.

Merkel's receptors are slowly adapting receptors found in Non-hairy skin and have very small receptive fields. These receptors detect vertical indentations of the skin, and their response is proportional to stimulus intensity. Tactile discs are similar to Merkel's receptors but are found in hairy, rather than nonhairy skin.

TYPE OF MECHANORECEPTOR	LOCATION	ADAPTATION	SENSATION ENCODED
PACINIAN COPUSCLE	S/C,I/M	VERY RAPIDLY	VIBRATION AND TAPPING
MEISSNER'S CORPUSCLES	NON HAIRY SKIN	RAPIDLY	POINT DISCRIMINATION TAPPING AND FLUTTER
HAIR FOLLICLES	HAIRY SKIN	RAPIDLY	VELOCITY, DIRECTION OF MOVEMENT
RUFFINI'S CORPUSCLES	HAIRY SKIN	SLOWLY	STRETCH AND JOINT ROTATION
MERKLE'S DISCS	NON-HAIRY SKIN	SLOWLY	VERTICAL INDENTATION OF SKIN
TACTILE DISC'S	HAIRY SKIN	SLOWLY	VERTICAL INDENTATION OF SKIN

2. <u>THERMORECEPTORS:</u>

Thermoreceptors are slowly adapting receptors that detect changes in skin temperature. The two classes of thermoreceptors are cold receptors and warm receptors (Fig.) Each type of receptor functions over a broad range of temperatures, with some overlap in the moderate temperature range (e.g., at 36°C, both receptors are active). When the skin is warmed above 36°C, the cold receptors become quiescent, and when the skin is cooled below 36°C, the warm receptors become quiescent.

If skin temperature rises to damaging levels (above 45°C), warm receptors become inactive; thus, warm receptors do not signal pain from extreme heat. At temperatures above

45°C, polymodal nociceptors will be activated. Likewise, extremely cold (freezing) temperatures also activate nociceptors.

NOCICEPTORS: Nociceptors respond to noxious stimuli that can produce tissue damage. There are two major classes of nociceptors: thermal or mechanical nociceptors and polymodal nociceptors.
  a. **Thermal or mechanical nociceptors** (TRPV or TRPM8 channels) are supplied by finely myelinated A-delta afferent nerve fibers and respond to mechanical stimuli such as sharp, pricking pain.
  b. **Polymodal nociceptors** are supplied by unmyelinated C fibers and respond to high-intensity mechanical or chemical stimuli and hot and cold stimuli. Damaged skin releases a variety of chemicals including bradykinin, prostaglandins, substance P, K+, and H+, which initiate the **inflammatory response.** The blood vessels become permeable, and, as a result, there is local edema and redness of the skin. Mast cells near the site of injury release histamine, which directly activates nociceptors. In addition, axons of the nociceptors release substances that sensitize the nociceptors to stimuli that were not previously noxious or painful. This sensitization process, called **hyperalgesia,** is the basis for various phenomena including reduced threshold for pain.

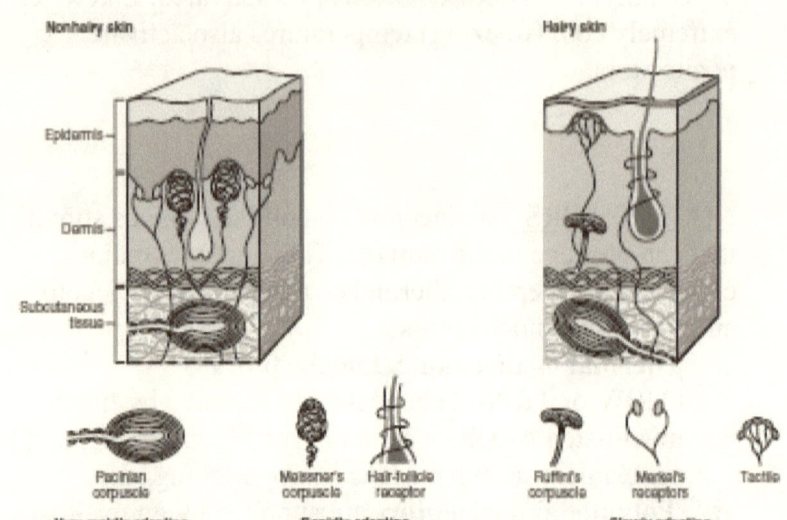

TYPES OF MECHANORECEPTORS FOUND IN HAIRY AND NON HAIRY SKIN

RETICULAR ACTIVATING SYSTEM:

Reticular formation refers to complex network of neurons and nerve fibers which occupy midventral portions of brain stem around the central cavity. The brainstem reticular formation (RF) can be considered to comprise medullary RF, pontine RF, and midbrain RF.

Reticular activating system is a complex polysynaptic pathway that projects diffusely from the brain stem reticular formation to the cerebral cortex.

COLLATERALS to RAS funnel through following sources:

1. Long ascending sensory pathway such as spinothalamic tract which are the important sources of collaterals to RAS. The fibers of the tracts conveying slow pain send the richest collateral connections to the RAS.
2. In addition to the long ascending pathways, collaterals to the RAS also funnel from the trigeminal, auditory, visual and olfactory pathway systems.

EFFERERENT PROJECTIONS:

1. Majority of the RAS fibers end in the nonspecific thalamic nuclei and from there project diffusely to the whole neocortex.
2. Another part of the RAS bypasses the thalamus to project diffusely to the cortex.

STIMULATION OF RAS:

It is stimulated by impulses funneled into it through the collaterals as described. Thus RAS is a nonspecific system that can be excited by any sensation.

FUNCTIONS OF RETICULAR FORMATION:

1. **SLEEP WAKEFULNESS:** The RAS of reticular formation is the neural substrate for the consciousness.
   a. RAS sends strong facilatatory drive to the central neurons, raising their background excitability and increasing their responsiveness to specific stimuli. Thus, when RAS is stimulated, there is wakefulness and alertness of the subject and the subject becomes fully conscious. Conversely when RAS is inhibited, the subject is asleep.
   b. Lesions of RAS produce prolonged sleep in humans.
   c. Many agents producing sedation, hypnosis, and anesthesia (e.g benzodiazepines and barbiturates) act by preventing synaptic transmission in RAS and thus inhibit the RAS.
2. **CONDITIONING AND LEARNING:** Reticular formation is an integral part of the neural substance for conditioning and learning.
3. **CONTROL OF MUSCLE TONE AND REGULATION OF POSTURAL REFLEX CHANGES:** Reticular formation modulates the tone of extensor (antigravity) muscles.
4. **AUTONOMIC FUNCTIONS:** The visceral regulating centers are an integral part of the

reticular formation. The influence of higher neurons over the viscera and autonomic functions are mediated through the visceral centers in reticular formation.
5. MODULATION OF PAIN: By affecting the transmission of the pain impulses through the substantia gelatinosa of the spinal cord, the serotonergic neurons modulate the perception of pain.
6. CONTROL OF NEUROENDOCRINE SYSTEM: The reticular formation projections play a role in the control of neuroendocrine systems in the hypothalamus.

ELECTROENCEPHALOGRAM:

EEG refers to record of spontaneous electric activity of the brain taken from the surface of the scalp. The spontaneous electric activity of the brain is due largely to graded or summated postsynaptic potentials in the many hundreds or thousands of brain neurons that underlie the recording electrode at the surface of the scalp.

NORMAL ELECTROENCEPHALOGRAM: Different waves recorded in a normal person, depending on their frequency are classified as alpha, beta, theta and delta waves.

WAVES OF EEG:
ALPHA WAVES:

These are the most prominent component of EEG obtained from adult humans who are awake but quiet and at rest with the eyes closed. Alpha waves are said to result from spontaneous activity of non specific thalamocortical system. Frequency is 8-13 Hz. These are most marked in the parieto occipital area of the scalp. They disappear during sleep.

CAUSES OF DECREASED FREQUENCY OF ALPHA WAVES ARE:

1. Old age, due to decreased cerebral perfusion leading to decreased cerebral metabolism.
2. Low blood glucose level.
3. Low body temperature
4. Low levels of adrenal glucocorticoids.
5. High arterial pressure of CO_2
6. Sleep.

CAUSES OF INCREASED FREQUENCY OF ALPHA WAVES:

1. High blood glucose level.
2. Rise in body temperature.
3. Low arterial pCO_2
4. High levels of adrenal glucocorticoids
5. Alerting states.

ALPHA BLOCK:

It refers to a phenomenon in which alpha waves attenuates and are replaced by the fast, irregular waves of low amplitude. Alpha block occurs when:

A. The person opens their eyes.
B. When the individual engage in conscious mental activity such as doing math calculations
C. When any form of stimulation is applied.
D. The term aroused or alerting response is also used to denote alpha block, since it is correlated with arousal or alerting response.

BETA WAVES:

The frequency is usually between 14-30 cycles/sec. They are frequently recorded from the parietal and frontal region. They are seen in the following conditions:

A. Tension and CNS activation
B. Arousal response(in alpha block)
C. Infants have fast beta like activity in EEG and occipital rhythm is slow 0.5-2/sec patterns.

THETA WAVES:

CHARACTERISTICS FEATURES OF THETA WAVES ARE:

The frequency is between 4-7 Hz. They are recorded from the temporal and parietal region in children.

DELTA WAVES:

Delta waves do not occur in normal waking individuals. They are seen in the following conditions:

a. Deep sleep (stage III AND IV of NON REM sleep)
b. Infancy
c. Serious brain damage.

CHARACTERISTIC FEATURES ARE:

The frequency is less than 4 HZ. It can be produced by over breathing.

ABNORMAL EEG PATTERNS:

1. **EPILEPSY:** The wave forms of epilepsy include idiopathic abnormal waves such as a spike, sharp wave and spike and slow wave complex.
2. **CONSCIOUS DYSFUNCTION:** A slow wave appears in case of conscious dysfunction.
    A. **COMA:** It refers to permanent state of sleep which is characterized by a loss of consciousness from which arousal cannot be elicited.
    B. **SYNCOPE:** It refers to transient pathologic loss of consciousness.

C. STUPOR: It is a more persistent loss of consciousness from which arousal can be obtained.
3. ORGANIC BRAIN DYSFUCNTION: An abnormal wave appears when in brain functional trouble occurs due to cerebral tumor, brain blood vessel trouble (bleeding ,clogging, artery/vein leakage, hardened brain artery etc.) or brain injury caused by an external wound of the head.
4. BRAIN DEATH: The criteria for labeling brain death are important because of the desire to obtain organs for transplant operations and the desire to remove the heroic life supports. An individual is declared dead when brain cells stop activity; the EEG waveforms become flat in all channels and finally disappear.

WAKEFULLNESS AND SLEEP:

WAKEFULLNESS:

The reticular activating system of the reticular formation is the neural substrate of the consciousness and sleep waking cycle. RAS is a complex polysynaptic pathway that projects diffusely from the brain stem reticular formation to the cerebral cortex both directly as well as via thalamus.

NEURAL SUBSTRATES FOR WAKEFULLNESS:

1. RETICULAR ACTIVATING SYSTEM: It is mainly responsible for the tonic maintenance of the cortical activation and behavioral arousal of the wakefulness.

2. **THALAMUS:** The non specific thalamic system is involved in the activation of entire cerebral cortex. These nuclei get tonic drive from the reticular formation and in turn project diffusely to cerebral cortex.
3. **HYPOTHALAMUS AND SUBTHALAMUS:** The ascending impulses from midbrain reticular formation also relay to cerebral cortex through posterior hypothalamus also acts as waking center, as its stimulation causes wakefulness. Conversely, lesions of posterior hypothalamus result in coma.
4. **BASAL FOREBRAIN:** The basal forebrain receives input from the reticular formation and in turn project to the cerebral cortex for cortical activation of wakefulness.

CHEMICAL MEDIATORS OF WAKEFULNESS:

Chemical mediators of wakefulness include:

1. Neurotransmitters: The main neurotransmitters which are responsible for wakefulness are:
   a. Catecholamines,
   b. Acetylcholine
   c. Histamine
   d. Glutamate
2. CSF borne peptides: Some of the CSF born peptides which have been known to produce wakefulness include:
   a. Substance P
   b. Hypothalamic releasing factors
   c. Vasoactive intestinal peptide.
3. Blood borne peptides: Blood borne peptides that act as wakefulness promoting factors are:

a. Epinephrine
   b. Histamine

SLEEP:

It refers to a state of unconsciousness from which the individual can be aroused by sensory or other stimuli. When asleep an individual is not aware of the environment and is unable to perform activities that require consciousness.

SLEEP WAKE CYCLE AND FACTORS AFFECTING SLEEP:

Sleep and wakefulness have circadian rhythms of about 24 hours .Ina normal adult the sleep wake cycle consists of 7-8 hours of sleep and 16-17 hours of wakefulness. A newborn infant has many cycles of sleep and wakefulness in 24 hours, but after the age of 2 years, a single sleep wake cycle is established.

FACTORS AFFECTING SLEEP:

The factors which favor the onset of natural sleep are:

1. Darkened room
2. Comfortable surrounding temperature
3. Silence
4. Physical and mental relaxation
5. Consumption of basic urge such as hunger or sex
6. Low frequency stimulation, such as by patting or rocking in a cradle or sitting in a moving vehicle.

TYPES AND STAGES OF SLEEP:

Sleep is of two types: non-REM sleep and REM sleep, which alternate in a sleep cycle.

Non-REM sleep:

Non-REM sleep i-e non rapid eye movement sleep is also known as slow wave sleep (SWS), because in this type of sleep brain waves are very slow. In normal adults, sleep mostly begins with non-REM sleep.

It is rest type of sleep which a person experiences during first hour of sleep after having been kept awake for many hours.

STAGES AND EEG PATTERNS OF NON-REM SLEEP:

STATE OF QUIET AWAKE REST WITH EYES CLOSED: State of quiet awake rest with eyes closed is the period in between the stage of wakefulness and stage of sleep characterized by alpha waves which are highly synchronized.

STATE OF NON-REM SLEEP:

When an individual from the state of quiet rest with eyes closed enters the state of non-REM sleep the consciousness is reduced. The non-REM sleep progresses in an orderly way from light to deep sleep in four stages.

STAGE 1 OF NON-REM SLEEP: STAGE OF VERY LIGHT SLEEP: EEG pattern in this stage is characterized by low amplitude mixed frequency activity.

STAGE 2 OF NON REM SLEEP: also called LIGHT SLEEP is characterized by appearance of sleep spindles. These are burst of alpha like waves which periodically interrupt the alpha rhythm.

STAGE 3 OF NON REM SLEEP: also called stage of MODERATE SLEEP is characterized by an EEG that display high amplitude slow waves called delta waves.

STAGE 4 OF NON –REM SLEEP: or stage of DEEP SLEEP produces an EEG pattern dome like very slow, large waves called delta waves.

PHYSIOLOGICAL CHANGES DURING NON-REM SLEEP:

1. Muscle tone decreases progressively
2. Heart rate and blood pressure are decreased.
3. Respiration rate is also decreased.
4. Eyes begin slow rolling movement until they finally stop in stage 4 (deep sleep) with eyes turned upwards.
5. Body metabolism is lowered.
6. Pituitary shows pulsatile release of growth hormone and gonadotropins.

REM SLEEP:

It is also called "rapid eye movement" sleep or fast wave sleep or "paradoxixal sleep" or "dream sleep". In adults the REM sleep follows non-REM sleep.

EEG PATTERN OF REM SLEEP: During REM sleep EEG is characterized by a high frequency and low amplitude pattern (beta rhythm),i-e some desynchronized pattern that is seen in the waking state. Because the EEG pattern is of wakefulness, the REM sleep is also called "paradoxical sleep". Dreaming occurs during REM sleep so it is also called "dream sleep".

PHYSIOLOGICAL CHANGES DURING REM SLEEP:

Rapid eye movements are hallmark of this state of sleep and that is why the name REM sleep. Rapid eye movements are burst of small jerky movements that bring the eye from one fixation point to another to allow a swapping of visual images of dream.

1. Heart rate and respiration rate become irregular
2. Muscle tone is reduced
3. Penile erection in males and engorgement of clitoris in females may occur during REM sleep, and
4. Teeth grinding (bruxism) may be seen in children.

SLEEP CYCLE:

In a normal adult individual the average sleep period of about 7-8 hours is divided into about 5 cycles during which non-REM sleep and REM sleep alternate with each other. There is an orderly progression of sleep states and stages during a typical sleep cycle.

GENESIS OF SLEEP:

The sleep state does not result from the passive withdrawal of arousal due to fatigue of reticular activating system (RAS) as thought earlier. Now it is established that the sleep is produced by an active process which is different for non-REM sleep and REM sleep.

GENESIS OF NON-REM SLEEP:

The non-REM sleep is generated by interaction of neurons which are grouped as:

a. Diencephalic sleep zone: A sleep facilatatory center is considered to be located in anterior hypothalamus, as its stimulation causes sleep. Posterior hypothalamus acts as a waking center, as its stimulation causes wakefulness. The diencephalic sleep zone must be stimulated at low frequency to produce sleep.
b. Medullary synchronizing zone is present in the reticular formation of the medulla oblongata at the level of the nucleus of tractus solitarius produces sleep when stimulated at low frequency.
c. Basal forebrain sleep zone includes preoptic area and the diagonal band of broca. Unlike the other two zones, stimulation of this zone at low as well as high frequency produces sleep.

GENESIS OF REM SLEEP:

Rapid eye movements sleep is generated by the interaction of neurons in the caudal midbrain and pons with neurons in the medulla and forebrain.

PHYSIOLOGICAL SIGNIFICANCE OF SLEEP:

Sleep is an indispensible phenomenon. Its physiological significance is highlighted.

a. Sleep may serve as a period of body's rest and metabolic restoration
b. Sleep is necessary for certain forms of learning.
c. REM sleep is necessary for mental well-being.

d. REM sleep plays important role in homeostatic mechanism.

SLEEP DISORDERS:

A. <u>INSOMNIA:</u> it refers to an inability to have sufficient or restful sleep despite an adequate opportunity for sleep.
B. <u>NARCOLEPSY:</u> It refers to an irresistible urge to sleep. In narcolepsy, REM sleep is entered directly from the waking states. Narcolepsy may manifests as episodes of sudden sleep. The individuals go to sleep while performing day time tasks.
C. <u>SLEEP WALKING (SOMNAMBULISM):</u> Episodes of sleep walking are more common in children than in adults and can occur predominantly in males. Such individuals walk with their eyes open and avoid obstacles, but when awakened, they cannot recall the episode.
D. <u>BED WETTING:</u> (Nocturnal enuresis)i-e involuntary voiding of urine ,occurs in children during slow wave sleep.

LANGUAGE:

It refers to that faculty of nervous system which enables humans to understand the spoken and printed words, and to express ideas in the form of speech and writing.

TWO ASPECTS OF COMMUNICATION:

Language input: sensory aspect through visual, auditory and proprioceptive impulses.

Language output: motor aspect through mechanisms concerned with expression of spoken language and written language.

SPEECH: Is of two types:

a. **SPOKEN SPEECH:** Understanding of spoken words as well as expressing ideas in the form of spoken words.
b. **WRITTEN SPEECH:** Understanding of written words as well as expression of ideas in the form of written words.

Mechanisms of speech involve co-ordinated activities of central speech apparatus (cortical and sub-cortical structures) and peripheral speech apparatus (larynx, pharynx, mouth, nasal cavities, tongue and lips).

UNDERSTANDING OF SPOKEN SPEECH:

1. **HEARING OF SPOKEN WORDS:** It requires intact auditory pathways from ears to primary auditory areas.

PRIMARY AUDITORY AREA: (41, 42) perceives auditory information such as loudness, pitch, source and direction of sound.
2. RECOGNITION AND UNDERSTANDING OF SPOKEN WORDS:
AUDITORY ASSOCIATION AREAS: (21, 20) receives input from primary area and are concerned with interpretation and integration of auditory impulses.
3. INTERPRETATION AND COMPREHENSION OF SPEECH: WERNICKE'S SPEECH AREA
It is involved in:
   a. Interpretation of meaning of what is heard
   b. Comprehension of spoken language and formation of ideas that are to be articulated in speech.

UNDERSTANDING OF WRITTEN SPEECH:

1. PERCEPTION OF WRITTEN WORDS: It requires an intact visual pathway from eyes to primary visual cortex (17)
2. INTERPRETATION OF WRITTEN SPEECH: Visual association areas (18,19) It is concerned with interpretation of written words and involved in recognition and identification of written words in the light of past experience.
3. GENERATION OFTHOUGHTS/IDEAS IN RESPONSE TO WRITTEN SPEECH: DEJERINE AREA (38) Generation of thoughts/ideas in response to written speech, also called VISUAL SPEECH CENTER.

EXPRESSIONOF SPEECH (MOTOR ASPECT OF COMMMUNICATION):

Expression of speech in response to both spoken speech and written speech can be in the form of spoken speech or written speech or both. It involves the activities of motor speech centers which include BROCA'S AREA (area 44) and EXNER'S AREA.

1. **EXPRESSION IN THE FORM OF SPOKEN SPEECH:** It involves activities in the motor speech area (Broca's area-44)It processes the information receiving from sensory speech centers(Wernicke's area and Djerine area) into a detailed and co-ordinated pattern for vocalizing which is then projected to motor cortex for implementation. Thus it is concerned with movements of those structures which are responsible for production of voice and articulation of speech.
2. **EXPRESSION IN THE FORM OF WRITTENSPEECH:** Function of Exner's area (Motor writing center).It processes the information received from Broca's area into detailed and co-ordinated pattern and then along with motor cortex (area 4) initiates the appropriate muscle movements of hand and fingers to produce written speech.

SPEECH DISORDERS:

DYSARTHRIA:

It is a disorder of speech in which articulation of words is impaired but the comprehension of spoken and written speech is not affected.

APHASIA:

It refers to inability to understand spoken and written speech or inability in expressing the spoken or written speech in the absence of mental confusion or motor deficit. The aphasia may be:

    a. <u>Sensory aphasia:</u> result in lesion of Wernicke's area.
        (i) Difficulty in understanding of meaning of speech
        (ii) Motor speech is intact and patients talk very fluently that is why it is called FLUENT APHASIA, but the speech does not make sense.
        (iii) Impairment in reading and writing: Since the patient cannot comprehend the written words (word blindness), he/she is unable to read aloud or copy print into writing.
        (iv) Lesion in the area 22 in temporal lobe and 39 or 40 in the parietal lobe produces a fluent, receptive or Wernicke's aphasia. The patient cannot comprehend spoken language and may or may not be able to read (alexia) depending on the extent of lesion. The deficit is characterized by fluent verbalization but lacks meaning. Patients are paraphasic ,often misusing words as if speaking using a "word salad"
        (v) They are generally unaware of their deficit and show no distress as a result of their condition.

b. <u>Motor aphasia:</u> Broca's aphasia results from lesions involving Broca's motor speech area (44) in frontal lobe.
   (i) Comprehension of written or spoken speech is good.
   (ii) Difficulty in speaking.
   (iii) Speech is non-fluent, non fluent aphasia or expressive aphasia
   (iv) Inability to write(agraphia)
   (v) Broca's area is just anterior to motor cortex region that provides upper motor neuron innervation of cranial nerve motor nuclei. This area in the left or dominant hemisphere is the center for motor speech and corresponds to Broad man's area 44 and 45.
   (vi) Damage to Broca's area produces a motor, non fluent or expressive aphasia that reflects a difficulty in piecing together words to produce expressive speech. Patients with this lesion can understand written and spoken language but normally say almost nothing. The ability to write is also affected in a similar way (agraphia) in all aphasias, although the hand used for writing can be used normally in all other tasks. Patients are keenly aware and frustrated by an expressive aphasia, because of their lack of ability to verbalize their thoughts orally or in writing.
c. <u>Conduction aphasia</u>: there is a large fiber bundle connecting areas 22,39 and 40 with Broca's area in the frontal lobe known as superior longitudinal fasciculus (or arcuate fasciculus).A lesion affecting

this fiber bundle results in a conduction aphasia. In this patient, verbal output is fluent, but there are many paraphrases, word finding pauses. Both verbal and visual language comprehension is also normal, but if asked to, the patient cannot repeat words or execute verbal commands by an examiner (such as count backwards beginning at 100) and also demonstrates poor object naming. This is an example of a disconnect syndrome in which the deficit represents an inability to send information from one cortical area to another .Like an expressive aphasia the patient is aware of deficit and is frustrated by their inability to execute a verbal command that they fully understand.

d. <u>Global:</u> Total inability to use language communication. Loss of both Wernicke's and Broca's area.

SPINAL CORD:

Spinal cord is divided into 31 segments that give rise to 31 pairs of spinal nerves. 8 cervical, 12 thoracic, 5 lumbar, 5 sacral and 1 coccygeal. Each segment is divided into inner gray matter containing neuron cell bodies. Each segment is divided into inner grey matter containing neuron cell bodies .The ventral horn of grey matter contains alpha and gamma motor neurons, the intermediate horn contains preganglionic neurons and clarke's nucleus while dorsal horn contains sensory neurons. The outer covering of the spinal cord is the white matter containing ascending and descending axons that form the tracts.

MOTOR PATHWAY:

Corticospinal tract is involved in voluntary contraction of skeletal muscles, esp in the distal extremeties. This tract consists of two neurons, an upper motor neuron and a lower motor neuron. Most of the upper motor neurons have their cell bodies in the primary motor cortex and premotor cortex of the frontal lobe. These axons leave the cerebral hemispheres through the posterior limb of internal capsule and descend medially through the midbrain, pons and medulla. In the medulla, 80-90% of these fibers decussates at the pyramids and then descends in the spinal cord as the lateral corticospinal tract in the lateral funiculus of white matter. These enter the ventral horn of the grey matter at each cord segment and synapse upon the lower motor neurons. Axons of the lower motor neurons leave via the ventral root of the spinal nerves and innervate the skeletal muscles.

Lesions above the decussation (in the brain stem or cortex) produce contralateral deficits and lesions below the decussation (in the spinal cord) produce ipsilateral findings.

Patients with upper motor neuron lesions present with spastic paralysis, hyperrelexia, hypertonia and a positive Babinski's sign. Lower motor neuron lesions present with flaccid paralysis, areflexia, atonia, muscle atrophy and fasciculation.

SENSORY PATHWAYS:

Most sensory systems use three neurons to project sensory modalities to the cerebral cortex. The first neuron (primary afferent neuron) has its cell body in the dorsal root ganglion of spinal nerve. This axon enters the spinal cord and either synapse in the spinal cord or brain stem. The second order neuron will decussate and project to the thalamus. The third order neuron then projects from the thalamus to the somatosensory cortex of the parietal lobe.

DORSAL COLUMN MEDIAL LEMINISCAL SYSTEM:

This pathway conducts sensory information for touch, proprioception, vibration and pressure. The primary afferent neurons of this pathway have their cell bodies in the dorsal root ganglia. Their axons enter the spinal cord and ascend in the dorsal columns of white matter as the fasciculus cuneatus (from upper limb) and fasciculus gracilus(from the lower limb). They synapse with the second order neuron in the same named nuclei in the lower medulla. Axons of the second order neuron decussate (internal arcuate fibers) and ascend the midline of the brain stem in the medial leminiscus to teach the VPL nucleus of the thalamus. The third order neuron then projects through the posterior limb of the internal capsule to the somatosensory cortex.

Lesions above the decussation (in the brain stem or cortex) produce contralateral loss of joint position, vibration and touch, whereas lesions below decussation (in the spinal cord) produce ipsilateral deficits below the level of lesion. A positive Romberg test indicates lesions of dorsal column.

ANTEROLATERAL SPINOTHALAMIC TRACT:

The spinothalamic tract carries pain and temperature sensations. The first order neuron enters the spinal cord and synapse in the dorsal horn with second order neuron. The first order neuron often ascends or descends one or two segments of the spinal cord before they synapse. The second order neuron axons then decussate (ventral white commissure) and ascend the spinal cord as the spinothalamic tract in the lateral funiculus of the white matter. The spinothalamic tract ascends the lateral aspect of brainstem and synapse in the VPL nucleus of the thalamus where the third order neuron projects to the cortex. All lesions of the spinothalamic tract in the spinal cord, brainstem or cortex produce contralateral loss of pain and temperature below the lesion. Note, that a central cord lesion at spinal cord (syringomyelia) produces bilateral loss of pain and temperature at the level of the lesion.

SPINAL CORD LESIONS:

1. ## POLIO:
   Selective destruction of lower motor neurons in the ventral horn by the polio virus occurs. Flaccid paralysis of muscles with accompanying hyporeflexia and hypotonicity result. Some patients may recover most function, whereas others progress to muscle atrophy and permanent disability.

2. **AMYOTROPHIC LATERAL SCLEROSIS:**

   This is a pure motor system disease that affects both upper and lower motor neurons. It begins at cervical level of the cord and progresses either up or down the cord. Patients present with bilateral flaccid weakness of upper limbs and bilateral spastic weakness of the lower limbs. Lower motor neurons of the brain stem nuclei may be involved later.

3. **ANTERIOR CORD SYNDROME:**

   Occlusion of anterior spinal artery interrupts blood supply to the Ventrolateral parts of the cord, including the corticospinal tracts and spinothalamic tracts. Below the level of lesion, the patient exhibits bilateral spastic paresis and bilateral loss of pain and temperature.

4. **SYRINGOMYELIA:**
   There is progressive cavitation of the central canal, usually in the cervical spinal cord. Early in the disease, there is a bilateral loss of pain and temperature sensation in the hands and forearms as a result of destruction of the spinothalamic fibers crossing in the anterior white commissure. When the cavitation expands, lower motor neurons in the ventral horns are compressed, resulting in bilateral flaccid paralysis of upper limb muscles. A late manifestation of cavitation is Horner's syndrome, which occurs as a result of involvement of descending hypothalamic fibers innervating preganglionic sympathetic neurons in T1 through

T4 cord segments. Horner syndrome consists of miosis, ptosis and anhidrosis.

5. **TABES DORSALIS:**
   It is a possible manifestation of neurosyphilis. It is caused by bilateral degeneration of dorsal roots and secondary degeneration of dorsal columns. There may be impaired vibration and position sense, astereognosis, paroxysmal pains and ataxia, as well diminished stretch reflexes or incontinence. Owing to the loss of proprioception pathways, patients are unsure of where the ground is and walk with a characteristic and almost diagnostic "high stepping gait".

6. **SUBACUTE COMBINED DEGENERATION OF THE CORD:**
   It is most commonly seen in cases of Vitamin B12 deficiency. It is characterized by patchy loss of myelin in the dorsal columns and lateral corticospinal tracts, resulting in a bilateral spastic paresis and a bilateral alteration of touch, vibration, pressure sensations below the lesion sites. Myelin of CNS and PNS is affected.

7. **BROWN SEQUARD SYNDROME:**
   Hemi section of the cord results in a lesion of each of the three main neural pathways; the principal upper motor neurons pathway of corticospinal tracts, one or both dorsal columns and spinothalamic tracts. The hallmark of a lesion of these three long tracts is that the patient presents with 2 ipsilateral signs and 1 contralateral sign. Lesion of the corticospinal tract results in an

ipsilateral spastic paresis below the level of the lesion. Lesion to the fasciculus gracilus or cuneatus results in ipsilateral loss of joint position sense, tactile discrimination and vibratory sensations below the lesion. Lesion of the spinothalamic tract results in a contralateral loss of pain and temperature sensations starting 1 or 2 segments below the level of the lesion. At the level of lesion there will be an ipsilateral loss of all sensations including touch modalities as well as pain and temperature and an ipsilateral flaccid paralysis in muscles supplied by the injured spinal cord segments.

MUSCLE SENSORS: refer to proprioceptors present in the muscles, tendons of muscles, joints, ligaments and fasciae.

PROPRIOCEPTION: gives information about the change in position of different parts of body in space esp. joints or tendons of muscles at any given movement.

TYPES OF MUSCLE SENSORS:

    a. Muscle spindles
    b. Golgi tendon organs
    c. Pacinian corpuscles
    d. Free nerve endings.

MUSCLE SPINDLES: Stretch receptors in skeletal muscles meant for proprioception .For precise movements, the muscle spindles are required which are less in back muscles.

STRUCTURE: Each muscle spindle consists of 3-10 small muscle fibers (called intrafusal fibers), present in between or parallel to extrafusal fibers. Either end of muscle spindles is attached to endomysium of extrafusal fibers.

INTRAFUSAL MUSCLE FIBERS: They have a central non-contractile portion which does not contain ACTIN AND MYOSIN FILAMENTS and has no striations. Portions on either side of the central part are contractile (contain actin and myosin) called as striated poles.

INTRAFUSAL FIBERS ARE OF TWO TYPES:

NUCLEAR BAG FIBERS: Each spindle has 2-5 nuclear bag fibers and the nuclei are concentrated into an expanded bag in the central portion.

NUCLEAR CHAIN FIBERS: Nuclei are arranged in a single file in the central part in the form of a chain and 6-10 nuclear chain fibers exist in each typical spindle.

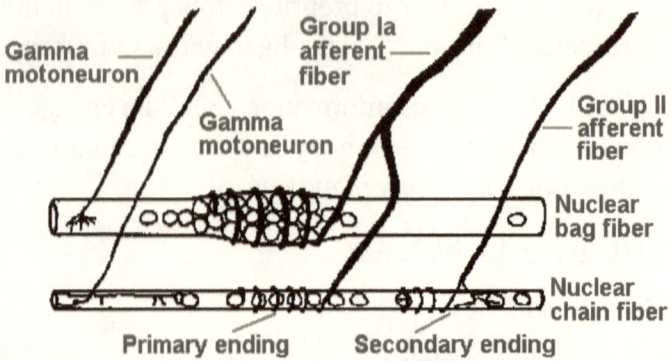

NERVE SUPPLY OF MUSCLE SPINDLE: Both motor and sensory nerve supply

SENSORY NERVE SUPPLY: Central non contractile portion of each intrafusal fibers is the receptor portion. Sensory fibers supply this area. There are two types of sensory fibers:

    a. GROUP IA FIBERS: also called primary sensory endings, supplying central receptor portions of both nuclear bag and nuclear chain fibers. They are known as Annulospiral endings.

DYNAMIC RESPONSE: is shown by the nerve endings supplying nuclear bag fibers.

STATIC RESPONSE: is shown by nerve endings supplying the nuclear chain fibers.

    b. TYPE II FIBERS: They are also known as secondary sensory endings that innervate the receptor portions of mainly nuclear chain fibers on one side of primary endings. They are also called

Flower spray endings that respond to sustained stretch therefore measure muscle length.

MOTOR SUPPLY: The efferent fibers to muscle spindles are called gamma efferent fibers because their axons belong to A gamma group of fibers.

THERE ARE TWO TYPES OF GAMMA FIBERS:

a. DYNAMIC GAMMA FIBERS: Innervate the striated poles of nuclear bag fibers where they end as motor end plate hence called plate endings. These fibers increase the sensitivity of Ia afferent fibers to stretch.

b. STATIC GAMMA FIBERS: Primarily innervate the striated poles of nuclear chain fibers where they end as a network of branches called as trail endings. They increase the tonic activity in the Ia afferent fibers at any given muscle length.

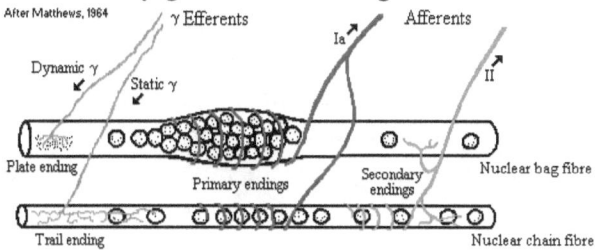

FUNCTION OF MUSCLE SPINDLES:

Function of Muscle Spindles
Muscle spindles are **stretch receptors** whose function is to correct for changes in muscle length when extrafusal muscle fibers are either shortened (by contraction) or lengthened (by stretch). Thus, muscle spindle reflexes operate to return muscle to its resting length after it has been shortened or lengthened. To illustrate the function of

the muscle spindle reflex, consider the events that occur when a muscle is stretched.
1. When a muscle is stretched, the extrafusal muscle fibers are lengthened. Because of their parallel arrangement in the muscle, the intrafusal muscle fibers also are lengthened.
2. The increase in length of the intrafusal fibers is detected by the sensory afferent fibers innervating them. The **group Ia afferent fibers** (innervating the central region of nuclear bag and nuclear chain fibers) detect the *velocity* of length change, and the **group II afferent fibers** (innervating the nuclear chain fibers) detect the *length* of the muscle fiber. Thus, when the muscle is stretched, the increase in the length of the intrafusal fibers activates both group Ia and group II sensory afferent fibers.
3. Activation of the group Ia afferent fibers stimulates α motor neurons in the spinal cord. These α motor neurons innervate extrafusal fibers in the homonymous (same) muscle and, when activated, cause the muscle to contract (i.e., to shorten). Thus, the original stretch (lengthening) is opposed when the reflex causes the muscle to contract and shorten. γ Motor neurons are coactivated with the α motor neurons, ensuring that the muscle spindle will remain sensitive to changes in muscle length even during the contraction.

Spinal Cord Reflexes

Spinal cord reflexes are **stereotypical** motor responses to specific kinds of stimuli, such as stretch of the muscle. The neuronal circuit that directs this motor response is called the **reflex arc.** The reflex arc includes the sensory receptors; the sensory afferent nerves, which carry information to the spinal cord; the interneurons in the spinal cord; and the motor neurons, which direct the muscle to contract or relax.

The stretch reflex is the simplest of all spinal cord reflexes, having only one synapse between sensory afferent nerves and motor efferent nerves. The Golgi tendon reflex is of intermediate complexity and has two synapses. The most complex of the spinal cord reflexes is the flexor-withdrawal reflex, which has multiple synapses.

Characteristics of the three types of spinal cord reflexes are summarized in Table 1

TYPE OF REFLEX	NUMBER OF SYNAPSE	STIMULUS FOR REFLEX	SENSORY AFFERENT FIBERS	RESPONSES
Stretch reflex(knee jerk)	One	Stretch (lengthening of muscle)	Ia	Contraction of muscle
Golgi tendon reflex(clasp knife)	Two	Contraction(shortening of muscle)	Ib	Relaxation of the muscle
Flexor Withdrawal reflex(touching a hot stove)	Many	Pain and temperature	II,III and IV	Contraction of ipsilateral muscles and Extension of contralateral muscles.

Stretch Reflex:

113

The stretch (**myotatic**) reflex is exemplified by the knee-jerk reflex (Fig.1) The following steps occur in the stretch reflex, which has only one synapse between the sensory afferent nerves (group Ia afferents) and the motor efferent nerves (α motor neurons):

1. When the muscle is stretched, group Ia afferent fibers in the muscle spindle are activated and their firing rate increases. These group Ia afferents enter the spinal cord and synapse directly on and activate
α motor neurons. This pool of α motor neurons innervates the homonymous muscle.

2. When these α motor neurons are activated, they cause contraction of the muscle that was originally stretched (the homonymous muscle). When the muscle contracts, it shortens, thereby decreasing stretch on the muscle spindle. The muscle spindle returns to its original length, and the firing rate of the group Ia afferents returns to baseline.

3. Simultaneously, information is sent from the spinal cord to cause contraction of synergistic muscles and relaxation of antagonistic muscles. The stretch reflex is illustrated by the **knee-jerk reflex,** which is initiated by tapping the patellar tendon, causing the quadriceps muscle to stretch. When the quadriceps and its muscle spindles are stretched, group Ia afferent fibers are stimulated. These group Ia afferent fibers synapse on and activate α motor neurons in the spinal cord. These α motor neurons innervate and cause contraction of the quadriceps (the muscle that originally was stretched). As the quadriceps muscle contracts and shortens, it forces the lower leg to extend in the characteristic knee-jerk reflex.

STRETCH REFLEX

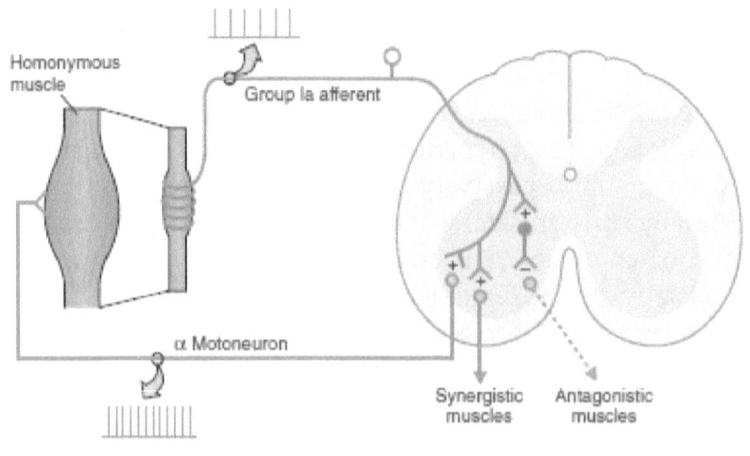

Golgi Tendon Reflex:
The Golgi tendon reflex is a disynaptic spinal cord reflex, which is also called the **inverse myotatic reflex** (inverse or opposite of the stretch reflex). The **Golgi tendon organ** is a stretch receptor found in tendons, which senses contraction (shortening) of muscle and activates group Ib afferent nerves. Golgi tendon organs are arranged in series with the extrafusal muscle fibers (contrasting the parallel arrangement of muscle spindles in the stretch reflex). The steps in the
Golgi tendon reflex are shown and described as follows:
1. When the muscle contracts, the extrafusal muscle fibers shorten, activating the Golgi tendon organs attached to them. In turn, the group Ib afferent fibers that synapse on inhibitory interneurons in the
spinal cord are activated. These inhibitory interneurons synapse on the motoneurons.
2. When the inhibitory interneurons are activated (i.e., activated to inhibit), they inhibit firing of the α motor neurons, producing relaxation of the homonymous muscle (the muscle that originally was contracted).

3. As the homonymous muscle relaxes, the reflex also causes synergistic muscles to relax and antagonistic muscles to contract. An exaggerated form of the Golgi tendon reflex is illustrated by the **clasp-knife reflex.** This reflex is abnormal and occurs when there is an increase in muscle tone (e.g., hypertonicity or spasticity of muscle). When a joint is passively flexed, the opposing muscles initially resist this passive movement. However, if the flexion continues, tension increases in the opposing muscle and activates the Golgi tendon reflex, which then causes the opposing muscles to relax and the joint to close rapidly. The initial resistance to flexion followed by a rapid flexion is similar to the way a pocket knife closes: At first the knife closes slowly against high resistance, and then it quickly snaps shut.

Golgi Tendon Organ

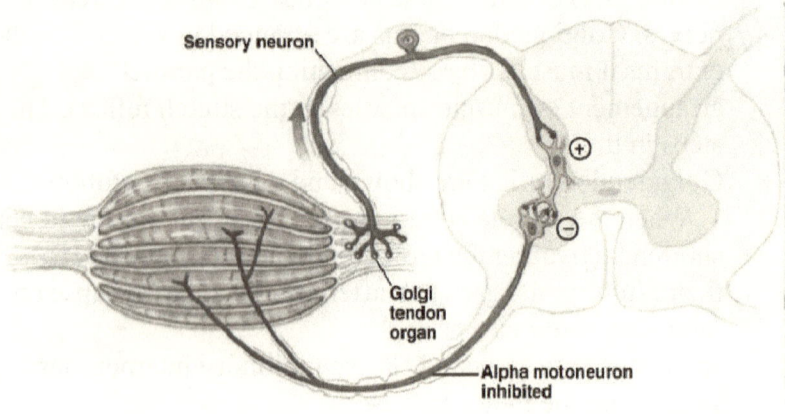

Flexor-Withdrawal Reflex:
The flexor-withdrawal reflex is a polysynaptic reflex that occurs in response to tactile, painful, or noxious stimulus. Somatosensory and pain afferent fibers initiate a flexion reflex that causes withdrawal of the
affected part of the body from the painful or noxious stimulus (e.g., touching a hand to a hot stove and then rapidly withdrawing the hand). The reflex produces **flexion** on the ipsilateral side (i.e., side of the stimulus) and **extension** on the contralateral side . The steps involved in the flexor-withdrawal reflex are explained as follows:
1. When a limb touches a painful stimulus (e.g., hand touches a hot stove), flexor reflex afferent fibers (groups II, III, and IV) are activated. These afferent fibers synapse on multiple interneurons in the spinal cord (i.e., polysynaptic reflex).
2. On the ipsilateral side of the pain stimulus, reflexes are activated that cause flexor muscles to contract and extensor muscles to relax. This portion of the reflex produces flexion on the ipsilateral side (e.g.
withdrawal of the hand from the hot stove).
3. On the contralateral side of the pain stimulus, reflexes are activated that cause extensor muscles to contract and flexor muscles to relax. This portion of the reflex produces extension on the contralateral side and is called the **crossed-extension reflex.** Thus, if the painful stimulus occurs on the left side, the left arm and leg will flex or withdraw and the right arm and leg will extend to maintain balance.
4. A persistent neural discharge, called an **afterdischarge,** occurs in the polysynaptic reflex circuits. As a result of the after discharge, the contracted muscles remain contracted for a period of time after the reflex is activated.

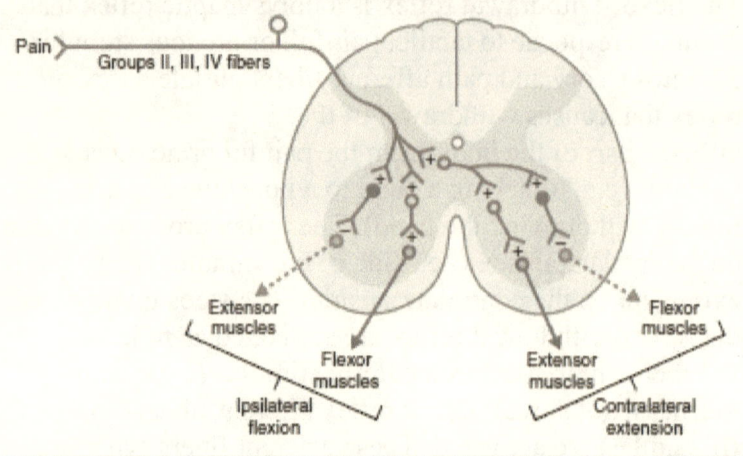

VOLUNTARY INNERVATION OF THE SKELETAL MUSCLE:

UPPER AND LOWERMOTOR NEURONS:

Two motor neurons, an upper motor neuron and a lower motor neuron, together form the basic neural circuit involved in the voluntary contraction of skeletal muscle everywhere in the body. The lower motor neurons are found in the ventral horn of the spinal cord and in the cranial nerve nuclei in the brain stem. Axons of lower motor neurons of spinal nerves exit the ventral root, and then join the spinal nerve to course in one of its branches to reach and synapse directly at a neuromuscular junction in skeletal muscle. Axons of lower motor neurons in the brain stem exit in a cranial nerve.

To initiate a voluntary contraction of skeletal muscle, lower motor neuron must be innervated by an upper motor neuron. The cells bodies of upper motor neurons are found in the brain stem and cerebral cortex and their axons descend into the spinal cord in a tract to reach and synapse on lower motor neurons, or on interneurons, which then synapse on lower motor neurons. At a minimum, therefore, to initiate a voluntary contraction of skeletal muscle, two motor neurons an upper and a lower motor neuron innervates the skeletal muscle.

The cell bodies of upper motor neurons are found in the red nucleus, reticular formation, and the lateral vestibular nuclei of the brain stem, but the most important location of upper motor neurons is in the cerebral cortex. Axons of these cortical neurons course in the corticospinal tract.

UPPER MOTOR NEURON VERSUS LOWER MOTOR NEURON LESIONS:

A fundamental requirement of interpreting the cause of motor weakness in neuroscience is the ability to distinguish between a lesion of an upper versus a lower motor neuron. Because a lesion to either an upper or a lower motor neuron produces a weakness in the ability to voluntary contract skeletal muscles, the key to distinguishing an upper from a lower motor neuron lesion will be in the condition of reflexes of the affected muscles.

A lesion in any part of a lower motor neuron will result in hypoactive muscle stretch reflexes and a reduction in muscle tone (hypotonicity) because lower motor neurons form the motor component of the reflex. Therefore, lower motor neuron lesions result in a paresis combined with suppressed or absent muscle stretch reflexes. An early sign of a lower motor neuron lesion is muscle fasciculation, which are twitches or contractions of a group of muscle fibers that may produce movement visible on the skin. Later, lower motor neuron lesions produce fibrillations, which are invisible 1-5ms potentials, detected with electromyography. Muscles denervated by a lower motor neuron lesion undergo pronounced wasting and atrophy. The constellation of lower motor neuron lesion signs combining paresis with suppressed or absent reflexes, fasciculation, and atrophy is known as a flaccid paralysis. With few exceptions, lower motor neuron lesion produce a flaccid paralysis ipsilateral and at the level of the lesion.

Neurologically, upper motor neurons including the corticospinal tract have a net overall inhibitory effect on the muscle stretch reflexes. As a result, upper motor neuron lesions combine paresis of skeletal muscle with muscle stretch or deep tendon reflexes that are hyperactive or hyper tonic. The hypertonia may be seen as decorticate rigidity (i-e postural flexion of the arm and extension of the leg) or decerebrate rigidity (i-e postural extension of the arm and leg) depending on the location of the lesion. Lesions above the midbrain produce decorticate rigidity; lesions below the midbrain decerebrate rigidity. Upper motor neuron lesions result in atrophy of weakened muscles only as a result of disuse, because these muscles can still be contracted by stimulating muscle stretch reflex.

Upper motor neuron lesions are also accompanied by reversal of cutaneous reflexes, which normally yield a flexor motor response. The best known of the altered flexor reflexes is the Babinski's reflex. The test for the Babinski's reflex is performed by stroking the lateral surface of the sole of the foot with a slightly painful stimulus. Normally, there is plantar flexion of the big toe. With a lesion of the corticospinal tract, the Babinski's reflex is present, which is characterized by extension of the big toe and fanning of other toes. Two other flexor reflexes, the abdominal and cremasteric, are also lost in the upper motor neurons. The constellation of upper motor neuron lesion signs combing paresis with increases of hyperactive reflexes, disuse atrophy, disuse atrophy of skeletal muscles, and altered cutaneous reflexes is known as spastic paresis.

In contrast to lower motor neurons, lesions of upper motor neurons result in a spastic paresis that is ipsilateral or contralateral and below the site of the lesion. Upper motor neuron lesions anywhere in the spinal cord will result in an ipsilateral spastic paresis below the level of the lesion. Upper motor neuron lesions between the cerebral cortex and the medulla above the decussation of the pyramids will result in a contralateral spastic paresis below the level of the lesion.

UPPER VERSUS AND LOWER MOTOR NEURON LESIONS:

UMN	LMN
SPASTIC PARALYSIS	FLACCID PARALYSIS
HYPERRELFEXIA	AREFLEXIA
BABINSKI SIGN PRESENT	NO BABINSKI
INCREASED MUSCLE TONE	FASCICULATION
MUSLCE WEAKNESS	DECREASED MUSLCE TONE
DISUSE ATROPHY OF MUSCLE	ATROPHY OF MUSCLE(S)
DECREASED SPEED OF VOLUNATARY MOVEMENT LARGE AREA OF THE BODY INVOLVED	LOSS OF VOLUNTARY MOVEMENTS SMALL AREA OF THE BODY AFFECTED

FUNCTIONAL AND STRUCTURAL ORGANIZATION OF GIT

FUNCTIONAL ORGANIZATION OF GIT:

Two groups of organs compose the digestive system the gastrointestinal (GI) tract and the accessory digestive organs.

A. The **gastrointestinal (GI) tract,** or **alimentary canal** (*alimentary_* nourishment), is a continuous tube that extends from the mouth to the anus through the thoracic and abdomino pelvic cavities. Organs of the gastrointestinal tract include the

a. **Mouth:** (receives food, starts digestion of starch)

b. **Pharynx:** (median passage common to GIT and Respiration)

c. **Esophagus:** Passageway (25cm long, has Upper Esophageal Sphincter in pharyngeal region and Lower Esophageal Sphincter in stomach region)

d. **Stomach:** (Storage of food, acidity kills bacteria; gastric glands release gastric juices, starts digestion of protein)

e. **Small intestine:** –Duodenum –first part-25cm, Jejunum- middle part-25 meters, Ileum- last part-3.5 meters. (Digestion of all foods and absorption of nutrients)

f. **Large intestine:** consists of Colon, Appendix, Cecum, Rectum and Anal canal.(Absorption of water, storage of indigestible remains)

The length of the GI tract is about 5–7 meters (16.5–23 ft) in a living person.

B. The **accessory digestive organs** include the teeth, tongue, salivary glands, liver, gallbladder, and pancreas.
Teeth aid in the physical breakdown of food.
Tongue assists in taste, chewing and swallowing.
Salivary glands, Liver and Exocrine part of pancreas.
Secretions from the salivary glands, pancreas, and liver add fluid, electrolytes, enzymes, and mucus to the lumen of the gastrointestinal tract. These secretions further aid in digestion and absorption.

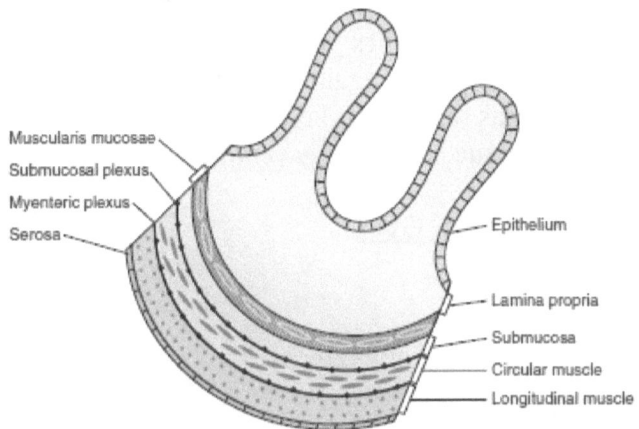

STRUCTURAL ORGANIZATION OF GIT:

1. Mucosa (mucous membrane layer) A layer of epithelium supported by connective tissue and smooth muscle lines the **lumen** (central cavity). This layer contains glandular epithelial cells that secrete digestive enzymes and goblet cells that secrete mucus.

2. Submucosa (submucosal layer) A broad band of loose connective tissue that contains blood vessels lies beneath the mucosa. Lymph nodules, called Peyer patches, are in the submucosa. Like the tonsils, they help protect us from disease.

It has Messiner's plexus for secretory activity of GIT.

3. Muscularis (smooth muscle layer): Two layers of smooth muscle make up this section. The inner, circular layer encircles the gut; the outer, longitudinal layer lies in the same direction as the gut. (The stomach also has oblique muscles.).

Myenteric plexus is present between the two layers and is for the motility of GIT.

4. Serosa (serous membrane layer) Most of the alimentary canal has a serosa, a very thin, outermost layer of squamous epithelium supported by connective tissue.

The serosa secretes a serous fluid that keeps the outer surface of the intestines moist so that the organs of the abdominal cavity slide against one another. The esophagus has an outer layer composed only of loose connective tissue called the *adventitia*.

FUNCTIONS OF GIT:

INGESTION:

Taking food into the mouth.

SECRETION:

Release of water, acid, buffers and enzymes into lumen of GIT.

MIXING AND PROPULSION:

Churning and propulsion of food through the GI tract.

DIGESTION:

Mechanical and chemical breakdown of food.

ABSORPTION:

Passage of digested products from GI tract into blood and lymph.

Innervation of the GI tract
The autonomic nervous system (ANS) of the GI tract comprises both extrinsic and intrinsic
nervous systems.
1. Extrinsic innervation (parasympathetic and sympathetic nervous systems)
 Efferent fibers carry information from the brain stem and spinal cord to the GI tract. Afferent fibers carry sensory

information from chemoreceptors and mechanoreceptors in the GI tract to the brain stem and spinal cord.

a. Parasympathetic nervous system

It is usually excitatory on the functions of the GI tract. It is carried via the vagus and pelvic nerves.

The Preganglionic parasympathetic fibers synapse in the myenteric and submucosal plexuses. The Cell bodies in the ganglia of the plexuses then send information to the smooth muscle, secretory cells, and endocrine cells of the GI tract.

(1) The vagus nerve innervates the esophagus, stomach, pancreas, and upper large intestine.

The Reflexes in which both afferent and efferent pathways are contained in the vagus nerve are called vagovagal reflexes.

(2) The pelvic nerve innervates the lower large intestine, rectum, and anus.

b. Sympathetic nervous system

It is usually inhibitory on the functions of the GI tract. The Fibers originate in the spinal cord between T-8 and L-2. The Preganglionic sympathetic cholinergic fibers synapse in the prevertebral ganglia. The Postganglionic sympathetic adrenergic fibers leave the prevertebral ganglia and synapse in the myenteric and submucosal plexuses. Direct postganglionic adrenergic innervation of blood vessels and some smooth muscle cells also occurs. The Cell bodies in the ganglia of the plexuses then send information to the smooth muscle, secretory cells, and endocrine cells of the GI tract.

2. Intrinsic innervation (enteric nervous system)

It coordinates and relays information from the parasympathetic and sympathetic nervous
systems to the GI tract. It uses local reflexes to relay information within the GI tract.

It controls most functions of the GI tract, especially motility and secretion, even in the
absence of extrinsic innervation.

a. Myenteric plexus (Auerbach's plexus)

It primarily controls the motility of the GI smooth muscle.
b. Submucosal plexus (Meissner's plexus)
It primarily controls secretion and blood flow.
It receives sensory information from chemoreceptors and mechanoreceptors

PHYSIOLOGY OF MASTICATION:

Mastication or chewing refers to the process by which food placed in the mouth is cut and grounded into smaller pieces. It involves:

1. Movements of jaws
2. Action of teeth- incisors provide strong cutting actions whereas the molars have a grinding action.
3. Co-ordinated movements of tongue and muscles of oral cavity.

FUNCTIONS OF MASTICATION:

1. It mixes food with saliva, lubricating it to facilitate swallowing.
2. It reduces the size of food particles, which facilitates swallowing.
3. It mixes ingested carbohydrates with salivary amylase to begin carbohydrate digestion.

CHEWING REFLEX AND REGULATION:

When the mouth is opened to place food inside it, the muscles of the jaw are stretched which leads to their contraction due to stretch reflex, thereby raising the jaw to closure of the mouth.

When mouth is closed, the food comes into contact with buccal receptors which cause reflex inhibition of the muscles of mastication and also initiates a reflex contraction of digastric and lateral pterygoid muscles, causing the mouth to open.

This cycle of opening and closing of the jaw leads to mastication. The tongue contributes to grinding process by positioning the food between the upper and lower teeth.

MUSCLES OF MASTICATION:

- A. MASSETER: raises the mandible, clenches the teeth and help protect the mandible.
- B. TEMPORALIS: raises the mandible, helps to retract the mandible after protraction.
- C. MEDIAL AND LATERAL PTERYGOID: protrude the mandible, depresses the chin and help in opening the mouth.
- D. BUCCINATOR: prevents accumulation of food between cheek and teeth.

NET EFFECT OF MASTICATION:

The bolus of food becomes homogenized mixture of small food particles, saliva and mucus, which is easy to swallow and digest.

Swallowing refers to passage of food from the oral cavity into the stomach. It comprises of three phases:

1. Oral phase (voluntary)
2. Pharyngeal (involuntary)
3. Esophageal (involuntary)

ORAL PHASE:

This is the first stage of swallowing: it is a voluntary phase. During this phase the bolus of food formed after mastication is put over the dorsum of the tongue. The tongue forces the bolus into oropharynx by pushing up and back against the hard palate.

PHARYNGEAL STAGE:

Events which take place during movement of bolus from pharynx into esophagus occur in the following sequence:

a. Oral cavity is shut off from pharynx by approximation of posterior pillars of fauces.
b. Nasopharynx is closed by upward movement of soft palate.
c. Palatopharyngeal folds are pulled medially.
d. Vocal cords approximate strongly, stopping the breathing temporarily (deglutition apnea)
e. Larynx is pulled upward and anteriorly by neck muscles enlarging the opening of esophagus.
f. All this guides the food towards the esophagus and prevents its entry into trachea.
g. Upper esophageal sphincter opens up and allows bolus of food to be pushed into upper part of esophagus.

h. Once the bolus of food has passed into esophagus ,cricopharyngeus contracts, vocal cords open up allowing normal breathing to resume and upper esophageal sphincter goes once again into tonic contraction.

ESOPHAGEAL PHASE:

The food is propelled from the upper part of esophagus to the stomach by the esophageal peristalsis and aided by gravity.

SWALLOWING REFLEX AND ITS REGULATION:

STIMULUS	FOOD
RECEPTORS	SWWALLOWING RECEPTOR AREAS OF PHARYNX
AFFERENTS	TRIGEMINAL ,GLOSSOPHARYNGEAL AND VAGUS NERVES
CENTER	SWALLOWING CENTER IN THE MEDULLA AND LOWER PONS
EFFERENTS	1. MOTOR IMPULSES CARRIED BY $5^{TH}, 9^{TH}, 10^{TH}, 12^{TH}$ NERVES TO SERIAL PHARYNGEAL MUSCLE CONTRACTIONS 2. RESPIRATORY CENTER- DEGLUTITION APNEA
EFFECT AND RESPONSE	THE PROCESS IN 1-2 SEC:
	1. SOFT PALATE CLOSES THE NASAL CAVITIES
	2. FOOD PASSES TO

	PHARYNX 3. VOCAL CORDS COMECLOSE- LARYNX CLOSED 4. LARYNX PULLED UPWARD AND FORWARD. 5. UES RELAXED 6. RAPID PERISTALTIC WAVE

SALIVA:

Saliva is formed by three major salivary glands-the parotid, submandibular and sublingual glands. Each gland is composed of acinus and branching duct system. The acinus is lined with acinar cells and secretes initial saliva. A branching duct system is lined with columnar epithelial cells, which modify the initial saliva. When myoepithelial cells which line acinus contracts, the saliva is ejected into the mouth.

ACINUS:

It produces an initial saliva with a composition similar to plasma (isotonic) and has the same Na, K, Cl and HCO_3 concentrations as plasma.

THE DUCTS:

It modifies the initial saliva by the following processes:

1. Reabsorption of Na and Cl
2. Secretion of K and HCO_3
3. Hypotonic as ducts are impermeable to water.

EFFECT OF ALDOSTERONE:

Aldosterone acts on ductal cells to increase the reabsorption of Na and the secretion of K.

EFFECT OF FLOW RATE:

It depends on the contact time available for reabsorption and secretion processes to occur in the ducts. At high flow rates, saliva is most like the initial secretion from the acinus: it has the highest Na and Cl concentrations and lowest K concentration. At low flow rates, it has lowest Na and Cl concentrations and highest K concentrations. HCO3 secretion is selectively stimulated when saliva secretion is stimulated.

FUNCTIONS AND COMPOSITION OF SALIVA:

FUNCTIONS OF SALIVA:

1. Initial starch digestion by α amylase (ptyalin) and initial triglycerides digestion by lingual lipase.
2. Lubrication of ingested food by mucus.
3. Protection of the mouth and esophagus by dilution and buffering of ingested foods.

COMPOSITION OF SALIVA:

Saliva is characterized by:

1. High volume
2. High K and HCO3 concentrations
3. Low Na and Cl concentrations
4. Hypotonicity
5. Presence of α amylase, lingual lipase and kallikrein.

At low flow rates saliva has the lowest osmolarity and lowest Na, Cl and HCO3 concentrations but has highest K concentrations.

At highest flow rates (up to 4ml/min), the composition of saliva is closest to plasma.

REGULATION OF SALIVA PRODUCTION:

Saliva production is controlled by parasympathetic and sympathetic nervous system (not by GI hormones). Saliva production is unique in that it is increased by both parasympathetic and sympathetic activity.

PARASYMPATHETIC STIMULATION:

Increase saliva production by increasing transport processes in the acinar and ductal cells and by causing vasodilation.

SYMPATHETIC STIMULATION:

Increase the production of saliva and the growth of salivary glands, although the effects are smaller than those of parasympathetic stimulation.

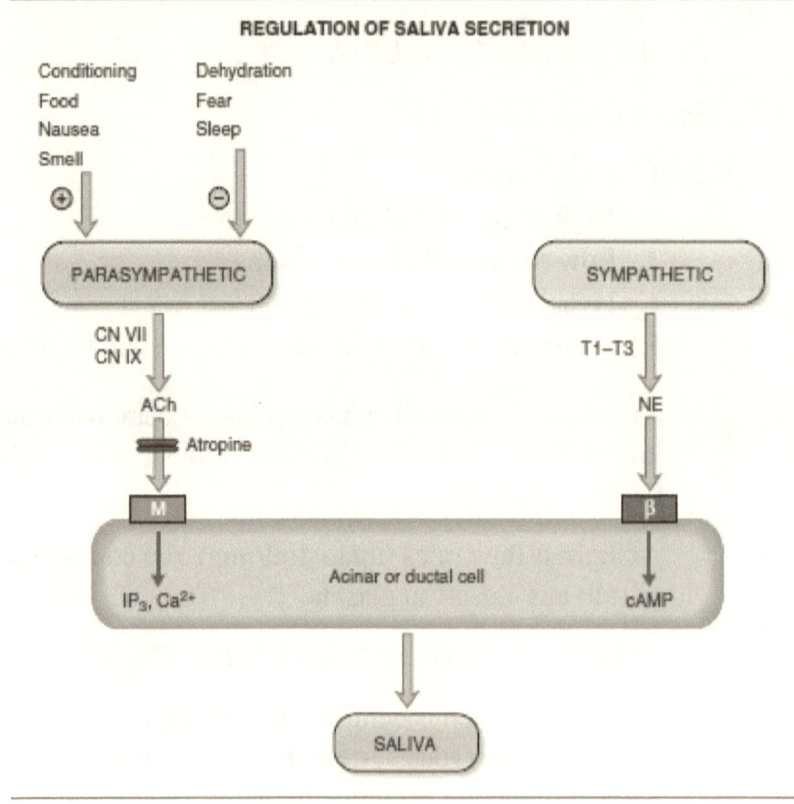

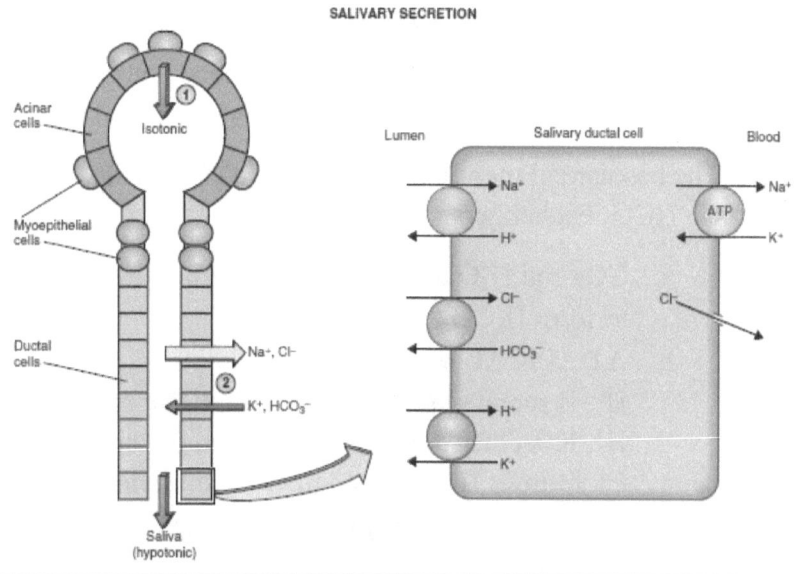

SALIVA PRODUCTION:

It is increased (via activation of the parasympathetic nervous system) by food in the mouth, smells, conditioned reflexes and nausea.

It is decreased (via inhibition of parasympathetic nervous system) by sleep, dehydration, fear and anticholinergic drugs.

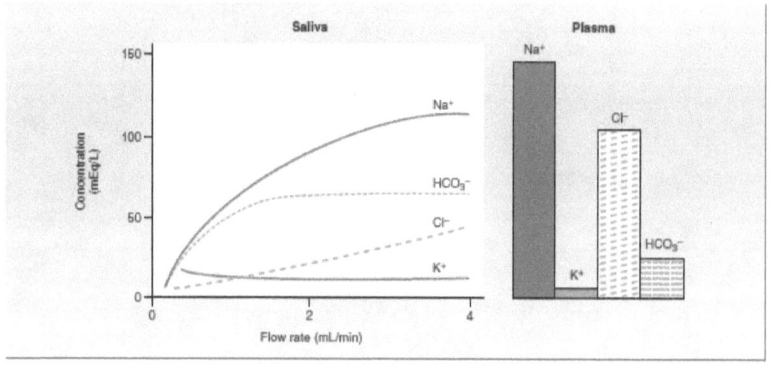

GASTRIC ACID SECRETION:

The apical membrane of the gastric parietal cell contains H^+, K^+ ATPase and Cl^- channels.

The basolateral membrane contains Na^+, K^+, ATPase and Cl^- HCO_3 exchangers.

a. CO_2 and H_2O are catalyzed by carbonic anhydrase to form H_2CO_3.
b. AT APICAL MEMBRANE:
   H^+ is secreted into the lumen of the stomach (via H^+, K^+ ATPase) which is inhibited by omeprazole.
c. Cl^- follows H^+ into the lumen by diffusing through Cl^- channels in the apical membrane.
d. AT BASOLATERAL MEMBRANE:
   HCO3 is absorbed from cells into the blood via Cl-HCO3 exchanger. The absorbed HCO3 is responsible for the alkaline tide (high pH) observed in gastric venous blood after a meal. HCO3 will be secreted into GIT in pancreatic secretion.

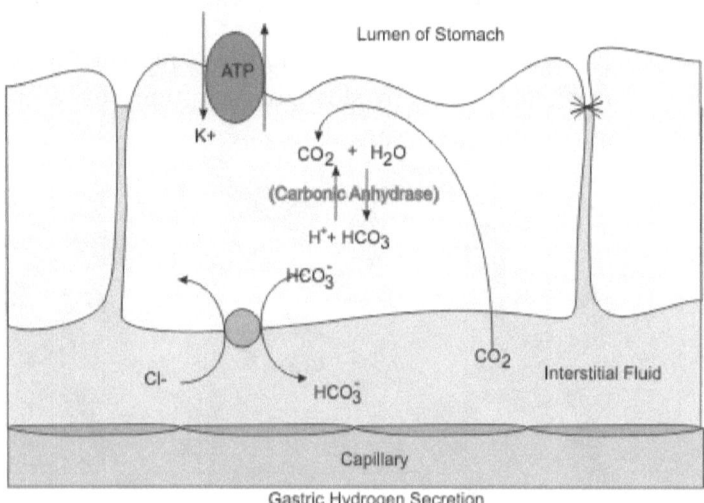

Gastric Hydrogen Secretion

Frank Boumphrey M.D.
2009

STIMULATION OF GASTRIC H+SECRETION:
a. Vagal stimulation
b. Gastrin
c. Histamine

INHIBITION OF GAASTRIC H+SECRETION:

a. Low pH(<3.0) in the stomach
b. Somatostatin
c. Prostaglandins.

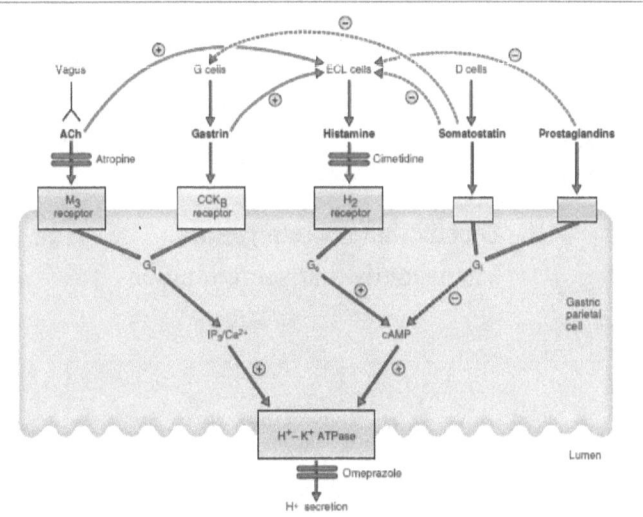

MAJOR COMPONENTS OF GASTRIC JUICE:

1. HCl
2. Pepsinogen
3. Intrinsic factor
4. Mucus.

OXYNTIC GLANDS: Are present in the body of the stomach and has:

1. Mucus neck cells
2. Parietal (oxyntic) cells secrete HCl and intrinsic factor
3. Chief (peptic) cells secrete pepsinogen.

PYLORIC GLANDS: Are present in the antrum of the stomach and has:

1. G cells that secrete gastrin
2. Mucus cells that secrete mucus.

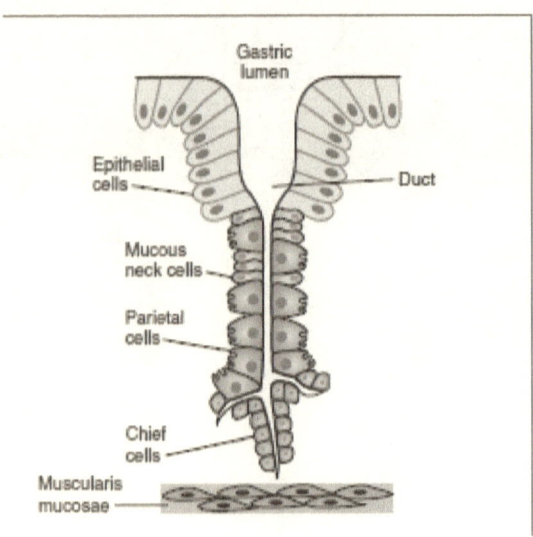

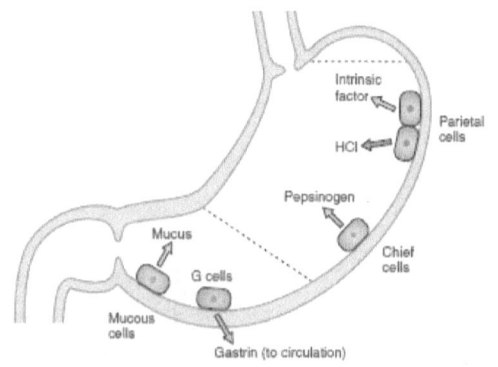

DIFFERENT PHASES OF GASTRIC ACID SECRETION:

PHASE	% OF HCL SECRETION	STIMULI	MECHANISMS
CEPHALIC	30%	Smell Taste Conditioning	Vagus nerve stimulates parietal cells. Vagus nerve stimulation gastrin release that acts on parietal cells.
GASTRIC(OCCURS IN RESPONSE TO A MEAL)	60%	Distension	Vagus nerve stimulates parietal cells. Vagus nerve stimulates gastrin release that acts on parietal cells.
		Distension	Local

		of antrum	reflexes that release gastrin that act on the parietal cells
		Amino acids and peptides	Gastrin that acts on the parietal cells.
INTESTINAL PHASE	10%	Products of protein digestion Hydrogen ion and lipids in duodenum	Vagus nerve Local reflexes Secretin and CCK decreases the gastric secretion.

REGULATION OF HCl SECRETION

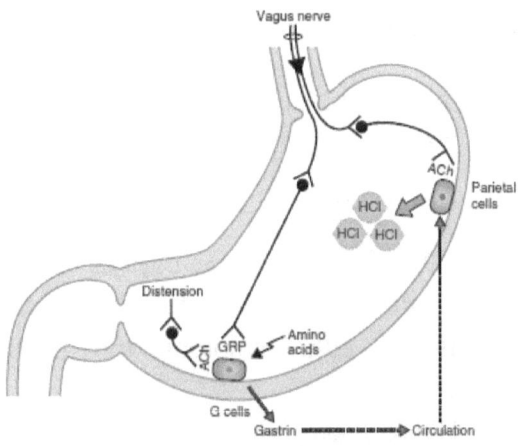

Phase	% of HCl Secretion	Stimuli	Mechanisms
Cephalic	30%	Smell, taste, conditioning	Vagus ⟶ parietal cell Vagus ⟶ gastrin ⟶ parietal cell
Gastric	60%	Distension	Vagus ⟶ parietal cell Vagus ⟶ gastrin ⟶ parietal cell
		Distension of antrum	Local reflex ⟶ gastrin ⟶ parietal cell
		Amino acids, small peptides	Gastrin ⟶ parietal cell

GASTRIC EMPTYING:

The process by which, the chyme is pushed from stomach into duodenum.

FACTORS REGULATING GASTRIC EMPTYING:

1. FLUIDITY OF CHYME: Liquids empty more rapidly than solids. Isotonic fluids empty more rapidly than either hypotonic or hypertonic contents.
2. GASTRIC FACTORS:
   a. VOLUME OF FOOD IN STOMACH: Greater the volume of food in stomach, greater the stretching of stomach wall leads to peristaltic waves and increased rate of gastric emptying.
   b. TYPE OF FOOD INGESTED:
      (i) Carbohydrate rich food causes rapid gastric emptying.
      (ii) Proteins rich food causes slow gastric emptying.
      (iii) Fat rich food causes slowest gastric emptying.
   c. GASTRIN: It promotes gastric emptying.
3. DUODENAL FACTORS: Inhibit gastric emptying.
   a. ENTEROGASTRIC REFLEX: Stimulation of receptors in the duodenal mucosa leads to this reflex.
      IMPORTANT STIMULI ARE:
      (i) Distention of duodenum.
      (ii) Acid in duodenum (pH<4)
      (iii) High or low osmolarity of chyme.

- (iv) Presence of fat or protein digestion products.
b. ENTEROGASTRIC HORMONES: Cholecystokinin, Secretin and GIP inhibit gastric contractions.
c. OTHER FACTORS AFFECTING GASTRIC EMPTYING: Emotions, anger and aggression increases gastric emptying.
d. VAGOTOMY: It slows emptying.

FUNCTIONAL ANATOMY OF SMALL INTESTINE:

GROSS ANATOMICAL CONSIDERATIONS:

The small intestine is a convoluted tube which extends from the pylorus to the ileocecal valve, where it joins the cecum, the first part of large intestine. It is about 6-7 meters long in length. It is divided into three parts: the duodenum, the jejunum and the ileum.

DUODENUM: The first and the shortest part of the small intestine, is also the widest and most fixed part. It is C shaped and for descriptive purposes, divided into four parts; superior (1st), descending (2nd) part, horizontal (3rd) part, and ascending (4th) part. The bile and pancreatic ducts open by a common hepatopancreatic ampulla of Vater on the posteromedial wall of descending (2nd) part of duodenum.

JEJUNUM AND ILEUM:

Jejunum and ileum form respectively, the proximal $2/5^{th}$ and distal $3/5^{th}$ of the remaining part of the small intestine. There is no sharp demarcation between jejunum and ileum.

STRUCTURAL CHARACTERISTICS OF SMALL INTESTINE:

Histologically the wall of small intestine is made up of four layers, which from within to outwards consist of mucosa, submucosa, muscle coat and serosa.

Although the small intestine is about 6v meters long, it has an absorptive area of 250 square meters. This large surface is created by:

a. Numerous folds of intestinal mucosa called PLICA CIRCULARIS.
b. Villi which line the entire mucosal surface
c. Microvilli which protrude from the surface of intestinal cells and the presence of numerous depressions (crypts of liberkuhn) that invade the lamina propria.

SMALL INTESTINAL SECRETIONS:

COMPOSITION AND FORMATION:

The intestinal juice also called SUCCUS ENTERICUS comprises of intestinal secretions which include:

a. Aqueous component (water and electrolytes)
b. Intestinal enzymes and
c. Mucus.

AQUEOUS COMPONENT (WATER AND ELECTROLYTES):

It is water and electrolytes secreted by the epithelial cells of small intestine especially those present in the crypts of Liberkuhn. About 2 liters of secretion is produced per day by these cells, whose chemical composition is similar to extra cellular fluid except that it is more alkaline.

INTESTINAL ENZYMES:

Brush border of epithelial cells covering the villi contains a large number of intracellular digestive enzymes. The enzymes are:

a. Peptidases (proteolytic enzymes)
b. Disaccharidases such as sucrose, maltase and lactase.

c. Intestinal lipases
   d. Enterokinase.

MUCUS:

Mucus in the small intestine is secreted by:

   a. BRUNNER'S GLANDS: which secrete thick alkaline mucoid secretion that serves a protective role, preventing HCl and chyme from damaging the duodenal mucosa.
   b. GOBLET CELLS: also secrete lot of mucus which protects the intestinal mucosa and lubricates the chyme.

REGULATION OF SMALL INTESTINAL SECRETIONS:

1. LOCAL STIMULI: Mechanical distension of intestinal mucosa by the food or irritation by chemicals, via local myenteric reflexes, increase the volume and total enzyme output of the small intestine, that is why, the greater is the chyme, greater is the secretion of intestinal secretion.
2. ROLE OF VASOACTIVE INTESTINAL PEPTIDE ;(VIP) through the secretion of the crypts of Liberkuhn is mainly regulated by local stimuli, but the local hormone VIP is also reported to increase its secretion.
3. SECRETIONS OF BRUNNER'S GLANDS IS INCREASED BY:
   A. Vagal stimulation
   B. Direct tactile stimulation or irritation of duodenal mucosa and
   C. Secretin.

MOTILITY OF SMALL INTESTINE:

1. DURING INTERDIGESTIVE PERIOD:

MIGRATING MOTOR COMPLEX:

MMC begins in the esophagus and travels through the entire gastrointestinal tract during interdigestive period. It sweeps out the chyme remaining in the small intestine. It occurs every 60-90 minutes and last for about 10 minutes.

2. DURING DIGESTIVE PERIOD:
A. **MIXING MOVEMENTS:** The mixing movements are responsible for proper mixing of chyme with digestive juices like pancreatic juice, bile juice and intestinal juice. These are also called SEGMENTATION CONTRACTIONS. There is back and forth a movement of chyme produced by segmentation contractions causes thorough mixing without any net forward movement of chyme.
B. **PROPULSIVE MOVEMENTS:** It helps to propel the intestinal contents aborally and also help in digestion and absorption of the food particles, because different types of nutrients are digested and absorbed in different segments of the small intestine.
LAW OF INTESTINE: The peristaltic waves always travel from the oral end towards the aboral end of the intestine.
CONTROL OF PERISTALTIC CONTRACTIONS:

It is dependent on the integrity of enteric nervous system. The usual stimulus for peristalsis is distension. This response to stretch is called MYENTERIC REFLEX. The local stretch releases serotonin, which activates sensory neurons that stimulate the myenteric plexus.

a. NEURAL CONTROL:
   (i) Parasympathetic stimulation increases intestinal motility through vagus as seen during strong emotions.
   (ii) Sympathetic stimulation decreases intestinal movements as seen during anger and pain.
b. HORMONAL CONTROL:
   (i) Intestinal motility is enhanced by gastrin, CCK, 5HT, thyroxine and insulin.
   (ii) Intestinal motility is decreased by secretin and glucagon.

FUNCTIONS OF SMALL INTESTINE:

1. **MECHANICAL FUNCTIONS**: The mixing and propulsive movements of the small intestine help in thorough mixing of chyme with the digestive juices and propel it through the large intestine.
2. **DIGESTIVE FUNCTIONS**: This is carried out by enzymes present in the succus entericus, pancreatic enzymes and bile.
3. **ABSORPTIVE FUNCTIONS**: This is accomplished by huge surface area created by the presence of plicae circularis, villi and microvilli.

4. ACTIVATOR FUNCTIONS: The enzyme enterokinase secreted by the small intestine activates trypsinogen into trypsin which in turn activates other enzymes.
5. PROTECTIVE FUNCTIONS: The mucus secreted into the succus entericus protects the intestinal wall from the gastric acid chyme.
6. HORMONAL FUNCTIONS: The small intestine secretes certain hormones which exert their effect on the secretion and motility of gastrointestinal tract. These hormones are enterogastrone, secretin and cholecystokinin.

LARGE INTESTINE:

GROSS ANATOMICAL CONSIDERATIONS:

The large intestine is a tube about 6 cm in diameter and 100 cm in length. It normally arches around and encloses the coils of small intestine and tends to be more fixed than the small intestine. It is divided into following parts:

a. CECUM: It is a blind ended sac into which opens the lower end of ileum. The ileocecal junction is guarded by a ileocecal valve which allows inflow and prevents backflow of intestinal contents.
b. APPENDIX: It is a vestigial organ in humans and arises from the medial side of the cecum.
c. ASCENDING COLON: It extends upwards from the cecum along the right side of abdomen up to the liver. On reaching the liver it bends to the left, forming the right hepatic flexure.
d. TRANSVERSE COLON: It extends from the hepatic flexure to the left splenic flexure.
e. DESCENDING COLON: It extends from the left splenic flexure to the pelvic inlet below.
f. SIGMOID COLON: It begins at the pelvic outlet as continuation of the descending colon and joins the rectum in front of the sacrum.
g. RECTUM: It descends in front of the sacrum to leave the pelvis by piercing the pelvic floor. Here it becomes continuous with anal canal in the perineum.
h. ANAL CANAL: It opens to the exterior through the anus to the opening which is guarded bytwo sphincters.

STRUCTURAL CHARACTERISTICS:

Histologically it is similar to the rest of the intestine except for some special characteristics:

Mucosa of the small intestine is characterized by:

    a. Absence of plica circularis and villi.
    b. A large number of simple tubular glands (crypts of Liberkuhn) lined by simple columnar epithelial cells with large number of goblet cells which secrete mucus.

LARGE INTESTINAL SECRETIONS AND BACTERIAL ACTIVITY:

LARGE INTESTINAL SECRETIONS:

The large intestinal secretions mainly comprise mucus secreted by the goblet cells and some water and lot of HCO_3 are secreted by glands of Liberkuhn.

The mucus lubricates the fecal matter and also protects the mucous membrane of large intestine by preventing the damage caused by mechanical injury or chemical substances. The alkaline nature (pH 8.0) of the mucoid secretion of the large intestine is due to the presence of HCO_3. It serves to neutralize the acids formed by the bacterial action on the fecal matter.

Large quantities of water and electrolytes are secreted by mucosa of large intestine only when it is intensely irritated.

INTESTINAL BACTERIAL ACTIVITY:

BACTERIAL FLORA:

At birth, the colon is sterile, but the colonic bacterial flora becomes established early in life and includes:

a. Harmless bacteria such as E.coli and Enterobacter areogenosa.
b. Potentially dangerous bacteria such as Bacteroides fragilis, various types of cocci and gas gangrene bacilli. These bacteria can cause serious disease in tissues outside colon.

INTESTINAL BACTERIAL ACTIVITIES CAN BE GROUPED AS:

1. BENEFICIAL BACTERIAL ACTIVITIES:
   A. Synthesis of vitamins such as vitamin C, a number of B-complex vitamins and folic acid.
   B. Trophic effects on colonic mucosa: Unabsorbed carbohydrates are converted to short chain fatty acids by colonic bacteria. Some of the short chain fatty acids have trophic effects on colonic mucosa.
   C. Play a role in cholesterol metabolism by decreasing plasma cholesterol and LDL levels.
2. INDIFFERENT BACTERIAL ACTIVITIES:
   A. Production of intestinal gases; about 7-10 liters of gas is produced every day that contributes to flatus. The gas is produced through breakdown of undigested nutrients that reach the colon.
   B. Organic acids formed by the colonic bacteria from carbohydrates are responsible for slight acidic reaction of stool.
   C. Pigments formed by the colonic bacteria from the bile pigments are responsible for known color of feces.
3. DETRIMENTAL BACTERIAL ACTIVITIES:

A. CONSUMPTION OF NUTRIENTS like vitamin C, vitamin B12 and choline by some bacteria may lead to deficiency symptoms unless these are supplemented in adequate amounts in the diet.
B. PRODUCTION OF AMMONIA: Colonic bacteria also produce ammonia, which is absorbed by blood and is normally detoxified quickly by the liver. However in liver dysfunction, hyperammonemia results, producing neurological symptoms (hepatic encephalopathy)

MOTILITY OF LARGE INTESTINE:

FUNCTIONS:

The principal functions of colon are absorption of water and electrolytes from the chyme and storage of fecal matter until it can be expelled. The proximal half of colon is concerned principally with absorption and distal half is concerned with storage. The contractile activity of the large intestine serves two main functions:

a. It increases the efficiency of colon for water and electrolyte absorption.
b. Promotes excretion of fecal matter remaining in the colon.

TYPES OF MOVEMENTS:

1. HAUSTRAL CONTRACTIONS: They are similar to the segmentation contractions of small intestine and vigorously mix the contents of colon and by exposing more of the contents to mucosa (facilitate absorption)

2. PERISTALSIS: They propel the contents towards rectum very slowly (5cm/hr.). It can take up to 48 hours for the chyme to traverse the colon.
3. MASS MOVEMENTS: The mass movements are special type of peristaltic contractions which are observed in the colon only. These occur 3-4 times a day generally after meals and each contraction lasts for about 3 minutes. They force the fecal material rapidly in mass down the colon. They also move material into the rectum and rectal distension initiates the defecation reflex.

FUNCTIONS OF LARGE INTESTINE:

1. SECRETORY FUNCTION: The large intestinal secretion mainly comprises mucin which helps to lubricate the fecal matter. The alkaline nature (pH-8) of the secretion serves to neutralize the acids formed by bacterial action on the fecal matter.
2. SYNTHESIS FUNCTIONS: The bacterial floras of the large intestine synthesize folic acid, vitamin B12 and vitamin K.
3. ABSORPTIVE FUNCTIONS: Absorption of water and electrolytes is the chief function of proximal part of the colon. Organic substances like glucose, alcohol, some drugs like anesthetic agents, sedatives and steroids can be also be absorbed in large intestine. The vitamin K and a number of B Complex vitamins which are synthesized in colon by bacterial flora are also absorbed in the large intestine.

4. EXCRETORY FUNCTIONS: Heavy metals like mercury, lead, bismuth and arsenic are excreted by large intestine through the feces.

DEFEACATION:

The process of excretion of fecal material involves both voluntary and reflex activity.

1. DISTENSTION OF RECTUM: Usually once or twice a day gastrocolic reflex drives the feces into the rectum which increases the intra rectal pressure passively.
2. DEFEACATION REFLEX: As the rectum starts filling, the resultant rise in the intra rectal pressure stimulates stretch receptors, sets up defecation reflex and produce an urge to defecate (when intra-rectal pressure) rises above 18 mm Hg.)
A. INTRINSIC REFLEX: It is mediated by intrinsic nerve plexus. Distension

BILE:

Bile is necessary for digestion and absorption of lipids in the small intestine. Bile is a mixture of bile salts, bile pigments and cholesterol. Bile is produced and secreted by liver, stored in the gallbladder and ejected in the lumen of small intestine, when the gallbladder is stimulated to contract. In the lumen of the small intestine, bile salts emulsify lipids to prepare them for digestion and then solubilize the products of lipid digestion in packets called MICELLES.

COMPOSITION AND FUNCTION OF BILE:

Bile contains bile salts, phospholipids, and cholesterol and bile pigments (bilirubin).

BILE SALTS:

They are amphipathic molecules because they have both hydrophilic and hydrophobic portions. In aqueous solution, bile salts orient themselves around the lipids and keep the lipid droplets dispersed (emulsification). They aid in the internal digestion and absorption of lipids by emulsifying and solubilizing them in micelles.

FORMATION OF BILE:

Bile is produced continuously by hepatocytes. Bile drains into the hepatic ducts and is stored in the gallbladder for subsequent release. Choleretic agents increase the formation of bile.

Bile is formed by the following processes.

a. <u>PRIMARY BILE ACIDS</u>: (Cholic andchenodeoxycholic acid) are synthesized from cholesterol by hepatocytes.
b. <u>SECONDARY BILE ACIDS</u>: In the small intestine, bacteria convert a portion of each of the primary bile acids to secondary bile acids(deoxycholic acid and lithocolic acid).

Synthesis of new bile acids occurs, as needed, to replace bile acids that are excreted in the feces. The bile acids are conjugated with glycine and taurine to form their respective bile salts, which are named for the parent bile acid (e.g. taurocholic acid is cholic acid conjugated with taurine). Electrolytes and water are added to bile.

During the interdigestive period, the gallbladder is relaxed, sphincter of oddi is closed, and the gallbladder as a result of isosmotic absorption of solutes and water.

FUNCTIONS OF GALLBLADDER:
1. Stores bile
2. Concentrate bile
3. Ejects bile in the lumen of the small intestine in response to CCK which causes contraction of gallbladder and relaxation of sphincter of oddi.

<u>ENTEROHEPATIC CIRCULATION OF BILE SALTS:</u>

The terminal ileum contains a Na-bile co transporter, which is secondary active transporter that recirculates bile acids to liver. Because bile acids are not recirculated until they reach the terminal ileum, bile acids are present for maximal absorption of lipids throughout the upper small intestine.

After ileal resection, bile acids are not recirculated to the liver but are excreted in feces. The bile acid pool is thereby depleted, and fat absorption is impaired, resulting in steatorrhea.

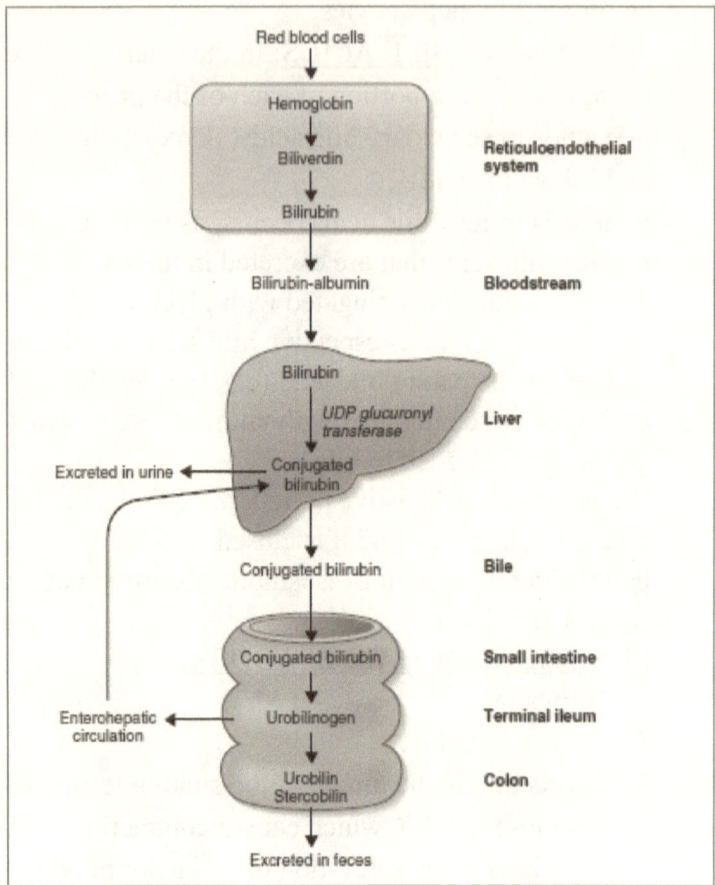

The cellular mechanisms for the hepatic uptake, conjugation and secretion of bile salts and bilirubin.

BILIRUBIN PRODUCTION AND EXCRETION:

Hemoglobin is degraded to bilirubin by the reticuloendothelial system. Bilirubin is carried in the circulation bound to albumin. In the liver, bilirubin is conjugated with glucoronic acid via the enzyme UDP glucoronyl transferase. A portion of the conjugated bilirubin is excreted in the urine, and a portion is secreted into the bile. In the intestine, conjugated bilirubin is converted to urobolinogen, whichis returned to the liver via enterohepatic circulation and urobilin and stercobilin, which is excreted in the feces.

Bile, whether from liver or gallbladder, contains;

1. Water
2. Bile salts
3. Bilirubin
4. Cholesterol
5. Fatty acids
6. Lecithin
7. Sodium
8. Potassium
9. Calcium
10. Chloride
11. Bicarbonate

Liver bile has higher concentration of water, sodium, chloride and bicarbonate. Gallbladder has higher concentration of bile salts, bilirubin, cholesterol and lecithin.

Liver is secreting bile, up to 1 liter in 24 hours period, but most of it is stored in the gallbladder. Gallbladder can hold 50-60 ml of bile and is able to store the large quantities of bile from liver by concentrating it. The gallbladder reabsorbs water, sodium, chloride and other electrolytes through the lining. The other constitutes of bile like bile salts, cholesterol, lectithin and bilirubin stays in the gallbladder.

LIVER PHYSIOLOGY:
The liver is located in the abdominal cavity and receives portal blood from the stomach, small and large intestines, pancreas, and spleen. The functions of the liver include processing of absorbed substances; synthesis and secretion of bile acids; bilirubin production and excretion; participation in metabolism of key nutrients including carbohydrates, proteins, and lipids; and detoxification and excretion of waste products. The majority of the liver's blood supply is venous blood from the gastrointestinal tract (spleen, stomach, small and large intestines, and pancreas), which is delivered to the liver via the portal vein. Therefore, the liver is ideally located to receive absorbed nutrients and to detoxify absorbed substances that may be harmful such as drugs and toxins.

Bile Formation and Secretion

Bile acids are synthesized from cholesterol by the hepatocytes, transported into the bile, stored and concentrated in the gallbladder, and secreted into the intestinal lumen to aid in the digestion and absorption of dietary lipids. Bile acids are then recirculated from the ileum back to the liver via the enterohepatic circulation.

Bilirubin Production and Excretion

The reticuloendothelial system (RES) processes senescent red blood cells. When hemoglobin is degraded by the RES, one of the byproducts is biliverdin (green-colored), which is converted to bilirubin (yellow-colored). Bilirubin is then bound to albumin in the circulation and carried to the liver, where it is taken up by the hepatocytes. In hepatic microsomes, bilirubin is conjugated with glucuronic acid via the enzyme UDP glucuronyl transferase. (Because UDP glucoronyl transferase is synthesized slowly after birth, some newborn babies develop "newborn jaundice.") Conjugated bilirubin is water soluble, and a portion of it is excreted in the urine. The remainder of the conjugated bilirubin is secreted into bile and then, via bile, into the small intestine. The conjugated bilirubin travels down to the terminal ileum and colon, where it is deconjugated by bacterial enzymes and metabolized to urobilinogen, some of which is absorbed via the enterohepatic circulation and delivered back to the liver; the remainder is converted to urobilin and stercobilin, which are excreted in the feces. Jaundice is a yellow discoloration of the skin and sclera of the eyes due to accumulation of either free or conjugated bilirubin. Jaundice can occur when there is increased destruction of red blood cells that results in increased production of unconjugated bilirubin. Jaundice also occurs with obstruction of bile ducts or with liver disease; in these cases, conjugated bilirubin cannot be excreted in the bile and thus is absorbed into the circulation. In obstructive jaundice, the urine is dark, owing to the high urinary concentration of conjugated bilirubin, and the stool is light ("clay-colored"), owing to the decreased amount of fecal stercobilin.

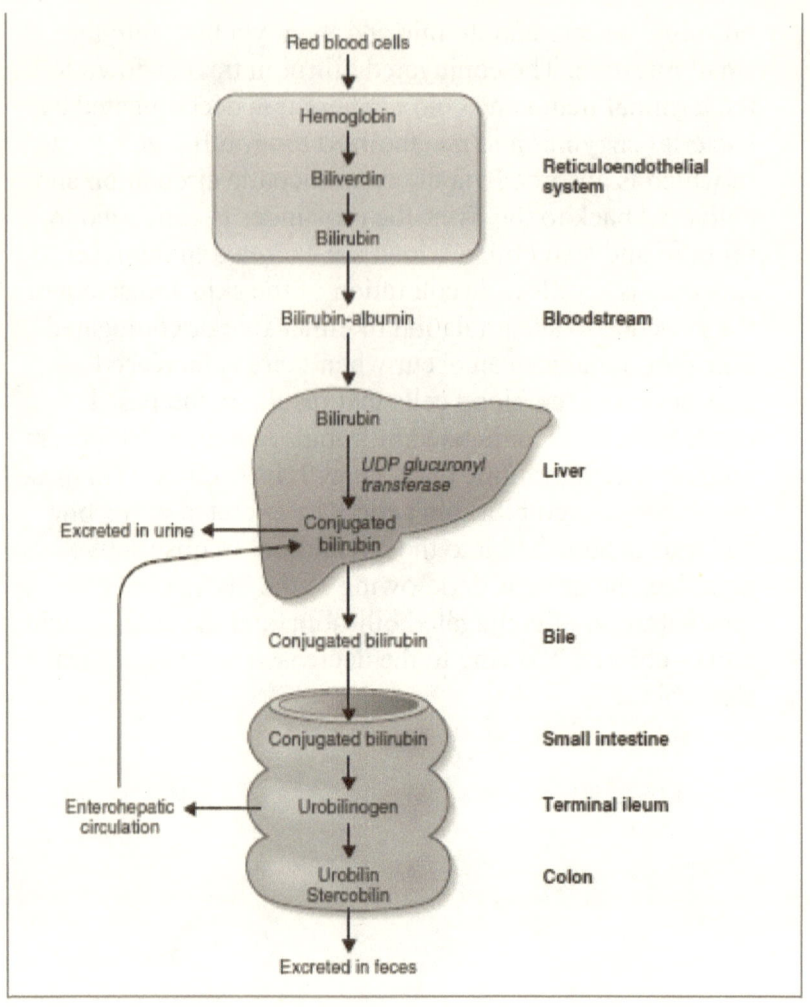

Metabolic Functions of the Liver

The liver participates in the metabolism of carbohydrates, proteins, and lipids. In carbohydrate metabolism, the liver performs gluconeogenesis, stores glucose as glycogen, and releases stored glucose into the bloodstream, when needed. In protein metabolism, the liver synthesizes the nonessential amino acids and modifies amino acids so that they may enter biosynthetic pathways for carbohydrates.

The liver also synthesizes almost all plasma proteins including albumin and the clotting factors. Persons with liver failure develop hypoalbuminemia (which may lead to edema due to loss of plasma protein oncotic pressure) and clotting disorders. The liver also converts ammonia, a byproduct of protein catabolism, to urea, which is then excreted in the urine. In lipid metabolism, the liver participates in fatty acid oxidation and synthesizes lipoproteins, cholesterol, and phospholipids. As previously described, the liver converts a portion of the cholesterol to bile acids, which participate in lipid digestion and absorption.

Detoxification of Substances
The liver protects the body from potentially toxic substances that are absorbed from the GI tract. These substances are presented to the liver via the portal circulation, and the liver modifies them in so-called "first pass metabolism," ensuring that little or none of the substances make it into the systemic circulation.
For example, bacteria absorbed from the colon are phagocytized by hepatic Kupffer cells and thus never enter the systemic circulation. In another example, liver enzymes modify both endogenous and exogenous toxins to render them water soluble and thus capable of being excreted in either bile or urine. Phase I reactions, which are catalyzed by cytochrome P-450 enzymes, are followed by phase II reactions that conjugate the substances with glucuronide, sulfate, amino acids, or glutathione.

PANCREATIC PHYSIOLOGY:
The exocrine pancreas secretes approximately 1 L of fluid per day into the lumen of the duodenum. The secretion consists of an aqueous component that is high in HCO3 – and an enzymatic component. The
HCO3 –-containing aqueous portion functions to neutralize the H+ delivered to the duodenum from the stomach. The enzymatic portion functions to digest carbohydrates, proteins, and lipids into absorbable molecules.

Structure of the Pancreatic Exocrine Glands
The exocrine pancreas constitutes approximately 90% of the pancreas. The rest of the pancreatic tissue is the endocrine pancreas (2%), blood vessels, and the exocrine pancreas secretes approximately 1 L of
fluid per day into the lumen of the duodenum. The secretion consists of an aqueous component that is high in HCO3– and an enzymatic component. The HCO3–-containing aqueous portion functions to neutralize the H+ delivered to the duodenum from the stomach. The enzymatic portion functions to digest carbohydrates, proteins, and lipids into absorbable molecules.

Structure of the Pancreatic Exocrine Glands
The exocrine pancreas constitutes approximately 90% of the pancreas. The rest of the pancreatic tissue is the endocrine pancreas (2%), blood vessels, and Enzymatic component of pancreatic secretion (acinar cells). Most of the enzymes required for digestion of carbohydrates, proteins, and lipids are secreted by the pancreas. Pancreatic amylase and lipases are secreted as active enzymes. Pancreatic proteases are secreted in inactive forms and converted to their active forms in the lumen of the duodenum; for example, the pancreas secretes trypsinogen, which is converted in the intestinal lumen to its active form, trypsin. The pancreatic enzymes are synthesized on the rough endoplasmic reticulum of the acinar cells. They are transferred to the Golgi complex and then to

condensing vacuoles, where they are concentrated in zymogen granules. The enzymes are stored in the zymogen granules until a stimulus (e.g., parasympathetic activity or CCK) triggers their secretion. Aqueous component of pancreatic secretion (Centro acinar and ductal cells). Pancreatic juice is an isotonic solution containing Na^+, Cl^-, K^+, and HCO_3^- (in addition to the enzymes). The Na^+ and K^+ concentrations are the same as their concentrations in plasma, but the Cl^- and HCO_3^- concentrations vary with pancreatic flow rate. Centroacinar and ductal cells produce the initial aqueous secretion, which is isotonic and contains Na^+, K^+, Cl^-, and HCO_3^-. This initial secretion is then modified by transport processes in the ductal epithelial cells as follows: The apical membrane of ductal cells contains a Cl^--HCO_3^- exchanger, and the basolateral membrane contains Na^+-K^+ ATPase and an Na^+-H^+ exchanger. In the presence of carbonic anhydrase, CO_2 and H_2O combine in the cells to form H_2CO_3. H_2CO_3 dissociates into H^+ and HCO_3 The HCO_3^- is secreted into pancreatic juice by the Cl^--HCO_3^- exchanger in the apical membrane. The H^+ is transported into the blood by the Na^+-H^+ exchanger in the basolateral membrane. The net result, or sum, of these transport processes is net
secretion of HCO_3^- into pancreatic ductal juice and net absorption of H^+; absorption of H^+ causes acidification of pancreatic venous blood.

Effect of Flow Rate on Composition of Pancreatic Juice
When the pancreatic flow rate changes, the Na^+ and K^+ concentrations in pancreatic juice remain constant, whereas the concentrations of HCO_3^- and Cl^- change (Fig. 8-22). (Recall that a similar, but not identical, relationship is observed between saliva composition and salivary flow rate.) In pancreatic juice, there is reciprocal relationship between the Cl^- and HCO_3^- concentrations, which is maintained by the Cl^--HCO_3 exchanger in the apical membrane of ductal cells. At the highest pancreatic flow

rates (more than 30 μL/min • g), the HCO3− concentration of pancreatic juice is highest (and much higher than plasma HCO3 −) and the Cl− concentration is lowest. At the lowest flow rates, HCO3 − is lowest and Cl− is highest. The relationship between flow rate and the relative concentrations of Cl− and HCO3 − is explained as follows: At low (basal) rates of pancreatic secretion, the pancreatic cells secrete an isotonic solution composed mainly of Na+, *Cl−*, and H2O. However, when stimulated (e.g., by secretin), the centroacinar and ductal cells secrete even greater amounts of an isotonic solution with a different composition, mainly Na+, *HCO3−*, and H2O.

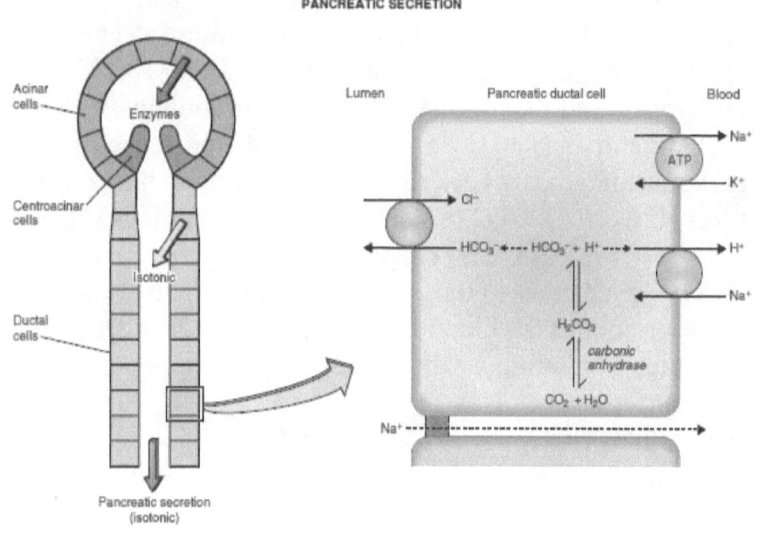

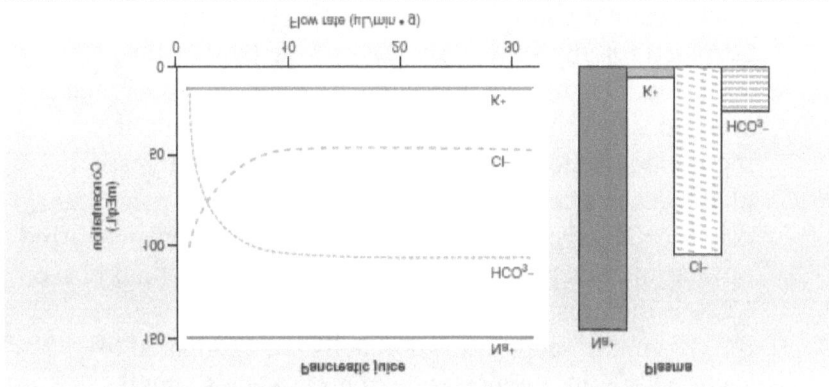

Regulation of Pancreatic Secretion

Pancreatic secretion has two functions: (1) to secrete the enzymes necessary for digestion of carbohydrates, proteins, and lipids; the enzymatic portion of pancreatic secretion performs these digestive functions; and (2) to neutralize H+ in the chyme delivered to the duodenum from the stomach. The aqueous portion of pancreatic secretion contains HCO3−, which performs the neutralizing function. Therefore, it is logical that the enzymatic and aqueous portions are regulated separately:

The aqueous secretion is stimulated by the arrival of H+ in the duodenum, and the enzymatic secretion is stimulated by products of digestion (small peptides, amino acids, and fatty acids).

Like gastric secretion, pancreatic secretion is divided into cephalic, gastric, and intestinal phases. In the pancreas, the cephalic and gastric phases are less important than the intestinal phase. Briefly, the cephalic
phase is initiated by smell, taste, and conditioning and is mediated by the vagus nerve. The cephalic phase produces mainly an enzymatic secretion. The gastric phase is initiated by distention of the stomach and is also mediated by the vagus nerve. The gastric phase produces mainly an enzymatic secretion.

The intestinal phase is the most important phase and accounts for approximately 80% of the pancreatic secretion. During this phase, *both* enzymatic and aqueous secretions are stimulated. The hormonal and neural regulation of the acinar and ductal cells in the intestinal phase. Acinar cells (enzymatic secretion). The pancreatic acinar cells have receptors for CCK (CCKA receptors) and muscarinic receptors for ACh. During the intestinal phase, CCK is the most important stimulant for the enzymatic secretion. The I cells are stimulated to secrete CCK by the presence of amino acids, small peptides, and fatty acids in the intestinal lumen. Of the amino acids stimulating CCK secretion, phenylalanine, methionine, and tryptophan are most potent. In addition, ACh stimulates enzyme secretion and potentiates the action of CCK by vagovagal reflexes. Ductal cells (aqueous secretion of Na^+, HCO_3^-, and H_2O). The pancreatic ductal cells have receptors for CCK, ACh, and secretin. Secretin, which is secreted by the S cells of the duodenum, is the major stimulant of the aqueous HCO_3^--rich secretion. Secretin is secreted in response to H^+ in the lumen of the intestine, which signals the arrival of acidic chyme from the stomach. To ensure that pancreatic lipases will be active (because they are inactivated at low pH), the acidic chyme requires rapid neutralization by the HCO_3^--containing pancreatic juice. The effects of secretin are potentiated by both CCK and ACh.

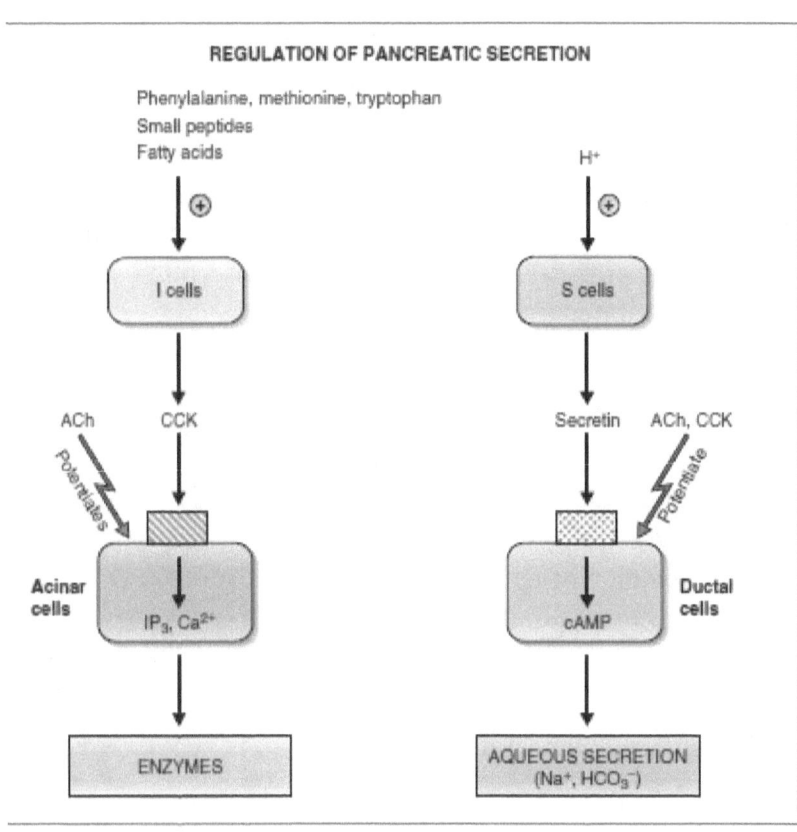

Malabsorption can affect macronutrients (eg, proteins, carbohydrates, fats), micronutrients (eg, vitamins, minerals), or both, causing excessive fecal excretion, nutritional deficiencies, and GI symptoms. Malabsorption may be global, with impaired absorption of almost all nutrients, or partial (isolated), with malabsorption of only specific nutrients.

Pathophysiology:

Digestion and absorption occur in three phases:

- Intraluminal hydrolysis of fats, proteins, and carbohydrates by enzymes—bile salts enhance the solubilization of fat in this phase

- Digestion by brush border enzymes and uptake of end-products

- Lymphatic transport of nutrients

The term malabsorption is commonly used when any of these phases is impaired, but, strictly speaking, impairment of phase 1 is maldigestion rather than malabsorption.

Pancreatic enzymes (lipase and colipase) split long-chain triglycerides into fatty acids and monoglycerides, which combine with bile acids and phospholipids to form micelles that pass through jejunal enterocytes. Absorbed fatty acids are resynthesized and combined with protein, cholesterol, and phospholipid to form chylomicrons, which are transported by the lymphatic system. Medium-chain triglycerides are absorbed directly. Unabsorbed fats trap fat-soluble vitamins (A, D, E, K) and possibly some minerals, causing deficiency. Bacterial overgrowth results in deconjugation and dehydroxylation of bile salts, limiting the absorption of fats. Unabsorbed bile salts stimulate water secretion in the colon, causing diarrhea. Carbohydrates The pancreatic enzyme amylase and brush border enzymes on microvilli lyse carbohydrates and disaccharides into constituent monosaccharides. Colonic bacteria ferment unabsorbed carbohydrates into CO_2, methane, H_2, and short-chain fatty acids (butyrate, propionate, acetate, and lactate). These fatty acids cause diarrhea. The gases cause abdominal distention and bloating. Proteins Gastric pepsin initiates digestion of proteins in the stomach (and also stimulates release of cholecystokinin that is critical to the secretion of pancreatic enzymes). Enterokinase, a brush border enzyme, activates trypsinogen into trypsin, which converts many pancreatic proteases into their active forms. Active pancreatic enzymes hydrolyze proteins into oligopeptides, which are absorbed directly or hydrolyzed into amino acids.

Symptoms and Signs:

The effects of unabsorbed substances, especially in global malabsorption, include diarrhea, steatorrhea, abdominal bloating, and gas. Other symptoms result from nutritional deficiencies. Patients often lose weight despite adequate food intake. Chronic diarrhea is the most common symptom and is what usually prompts evaluation of the patient. Steatorrhea—fatty stool, the hallmark of malabsorption—occurs when 7 g/day of fat are excreted. Steatorrhea causes foul-smelling, pale, bulky, and greasy stools. Severe vitamin and mineral deficiencies occur in advanced malabsorption; symptoms are related to the specific nutrient deficiency (see Symptoms of Malabsorption). Vitamin B_{12} deficiency may occur in blind loop syndrome or after extensive resection of the distal ileum or stomach. Iron deficiency may be the only symptom in a patient with mild malabsorption.

Symptoms of Malabsorption

Symptom	Malabsorbed Nutrient
1. Anemia (hypochromic, microcytic)	
2. Anemia (macrocytic)	Vitamin B 12, folate
3. Bleeding, bruising, petechiae	Vitamins K and C
4. Carpopedal spasm	Ca, Mg
5. Edema	Protein
6. Glossitis	Vitamins B 2 and B 12, folate, niacin, iron
7. Night blindness	Vitamin A
8. Pain in limbs, bones, pathologic fractures	K, Mg, Ca, vitamin D
9. Peripheral neuropathy	Vitamins B 1, B 6, B 12

Confirming malabsorption

Tests to confirm malabsorption are appropriate when symptoms are vague and the etiology is not apparent. Most tests for malabsorption assess fat malabsorption because it is relatively easy to measure. Confirmation of carbohydrate malabsorption is not helpful once steatorrhea is documented. Tests for protein malabsorption are rarely used because fecal nitrogen is difficult to measure.

Direct measurement of fecal fat from a 72-h stool collection is the gold standard test for establishing steatorrhea but unnecessary with gross steatorrhea of obvious cause. However, this test is available routinely in only a few centers. Stool is collected for a 3-day period during which the patient consumes 100 g fat/day. Total fat in the stool is measured. Fecal fat 7 g/day is abnormal. Although severe fat malabsorption (fecal fat 40 g/day) suggests pancreatic insufficiency or small-bowel mucosal disease, this test cannot determine the specific cause of malabsorption. Because the test is messy, unpleasant, and time consuming, it is unacceptable to most patients and difficult to do.

Sudan III staining of a stool smear is a simple and direct, but nonquantitative, screening test for fecal fat. Acid steatocrit is a gravimetric assay done on a single stool sample; it has a reported high sensitivity and specificity (using 72-h collection as the standard). Near-infrared reflectance analysis (NIRA) simultaneously tests stool for fat, nitrogen, and carbohydrates and may become the preferred test in the future; this test is currently available in only a few centers.

Measurement of elastase and chymotrypsin in the stool can also help differentiate pancreatic and intestinal causes of malabsorption; both are decreased in pancreatic exocrine insufficiency, whereas both are normal in intestinal causes. The -xylose absorption test can be done if the etiology is not obvious; however, it is currently rarely used because of the advent of advanced endoscopic and imaging tests. Although it can noninvasively assess intestinal mucosal integrity and help differentiate mucosal from pancreatic disease, an abnormal -xylose test result requires an endoscopic examination with biopsies of the small-bowel mucosa. As a result, small-bowel biopsy has replaced this test to establish intestinal mucosal disease. -Xylose is absorbed by passive diffusion and does not require pancreatic enzymes for digestion. A normal -xylose test result in the presence of moderate to severe steatorrhea indicates pancreatic exocrine insufficiency rather than small-bowel mucosal disease. Bacterial overgrowth syndrome can cause abnormal results because the enteric bacteria metabolize pentose, thus decreasing the -xylose available for absorption. After fasting, the patient is given 25 g of -xylose in 200 to 300 mL of water po. Urine is collected over 5 h, and a venous sample is obtained after 1 h. Serum -xylose 20 mg/dL or 4 g in the urine sample indicates abnormal absorption. Falsely low levels can also occur in renal diseases, portal hypertension, ascites, or delayed gastric emptying time.

Carbohydrates

Carbohydrates constitute about 50% of the typical American diet. Ingested carbohydrates are polysaccharides, disaccharides (sucrose, lactose, maltose, and trehalose), and small amounts of monosaccharides (glucose and fructose).

Digestion of Carbohydrates

Only monosaccharides are absorbed by the intestinal epithelial cells. Therefore, to be absorbed, all ingested carbohydrates must be digested to monosaccharides: glucose, galactose, or fructose. The pathways for carbohydrate digestion. Starch is first digested to disaccharides, and then disaccharides are digested to monosaccharides. Digestion of **starch** begins with **α-amylase.** Salivary amylase starts the process of starch digestion in the mouth; it plays little role overall, however, because it is inactivated by the low pH of the gastric contents. Pancreatic amylase digests interior 1,4-glycosidic bonds in starch, yielding three disaccharides, α-limit dextrins, maltose, and maltotriose. These disaccharides are further digested to monosaccharides by the intestinal brush-border enzymes, **α-dextrinase, maltase,** and **sucrase.** The product of each of these final digestive steps is glucose. Glucose, a monosaccharide, can be absorbed by the epithelial cells. The three **disaccharides** in food are trehalose, lactose, and sucrose. They do not require the amylase digestive step because they already are in the disaccharide form. Each molecule of disaccharide is digested to two molecules of monosaccharide by the enzymes **trehalase, lactase,** and **sucrase.** Thus, trehalose is digested by trehalase to two molecules of glucose; lactose is digested by lactase to glucose and galactose; and sucrose is digested by sucrase to glucose and fructose. To summarize, there are three end products of carbohydrate digestion: glucose, galactose, and fructose; each is absorbable by intestinal epithelial cells.

Absorption of Carbohydrates

The mechanism of monosaccharide absorption by intestinal epithelial cells .Glucose and galactose are absorbed by mechanisms involving Na^+-dependent cotransport. Fructose is absorbed by facilitated diffusion. **Glucose and galactose** are absorbed across the apical membrane by secondary active transport mechanisms similar to those found in the early proximal convoluted tubule. Both glucose and galactose move from the intestinal lumen into the cell on the **Na^+-glucose cotransporter (SGLT 1),** against an electrochemical gradient. The energy for this step does not come directly from adenosine triphosphate (ATP) but from the Na^+ gradient across the apical membrane; the Na^+ gradient is, of course, created and maintained by the Na^+-K^+ ATPase on the basolateral membrane. Glucose and galactose are extruded from the cell into the blood, across the basolateral membrane, by facilitated diffusion (**GLUT 2**). **Fructose** is handled differently from glucose and galactose. Its absorption does not involve an energy requiring step or a cotransporter in the apical membrane. Rather, fructose is transported across both the apical and basolateral membranes by facilitated diffusion; in the apical membrane, the fructose-specific transporter is called GLUT 5, and in the basolateral membrane, fructose is transported by GLUT 2. Because only facilitated diffusion is involved, fructose cannot be absorbed against an electrochemical gradient (in contrast to glucose and galactose).

Disorders of Carbohydrate Digestion and Absorption

Most disorders of carbohydrate absorption are the result of a failure to break down ingested carbohydrates to an absorbable form (i.e., to monosaccharides). If nonabsorbable carbohydrates (e.g., disaccharides) remain in the gastrointestinal lumen, they "hold" an equivalent amount of water to keep the intestinal contents isosmotic. Retention of this solute and water in the intestine causes osmotic diarrhea.

Lactose intolerance, which is caused by **lactase deficiency,** is a common example of failure to digest a carbohydrate to an absorbable form. In this disorder, the brush-border lactase is deficient or lacking and lactose is not digested to glucose and galactose. If lactose is ingested in milk or milk products, the lactose remains undigested in the lumen of the intestine. Lactose, a disaccharide, is nonabsorbable, holds water in the lumen, and causes **osmotic diarrhea.** Persons with lactose intolerance either may avoid ingesting milk products or may ingest milk products supplemented with lactase

Proteins

Dietary proteins are digested to absorbable forms (i.e., amino acids, dipeptides, and tripeptides) by proteases in the stomach and small intestine and then absorbed into the blood. The proteins contained in gastrointestinal secretions (e.g., pancreatic enzymes) are similarly digested and absorbed.

Digestion of Proteins

The digestion of protein begins in the stomach with the action of pepsin and is completed in the small intestine with pancreatic and brush-border proteases . The two classes of proteases are endopeptidases and exopeptidases.

Endopeptidases hydrolyze the interior peptide bonds of proteins. The endopeptidases of the gastrointestinal tract

are pepsin, trypsin, chymotrypsin, and elastase.
Exopeptidases hydrolyze one amino acid at a time from the C-terminal ends of proteins and peptides. The exopeptidases of the gastrointestinal tract are carboxypeptidases A and B. As noted, protein digestion begins with the action of **pepsin** in the **stomach.** The gastric chief cells secrete the inactive precursor of pepsin, pepsinogen.

At low gastric pH, pepsinogen is activated to pepsin. There are three isozymes of pepsin, each of which has a pH optimum ranging between pH 1 and 3; above pH 5, pepsin is denatured and inactivated. Therefore, pepsin is active at the low pH of the stomach, and its actions are terminated in the duodenum, where pancreatic HCO_3- secretions neutralize gastric $H+$ and increase the pH. Interestingly, pepsin is not essential for normal protein digestion. In persons whose stomach has been removed or persons who do not secrete gastric $H+$ (and cannot activate pepsinogen to pepsin), protein digestion and absorption are normal. These examples demonstrate that pancreatic and brush-border proteases alone can adequately digest ingested protein. Protein digestion continues in the **small intestine** with the combined actions of pancreatic and brushborder proteases. Five major pancreatic proteases are secreted as inactive precursors: trypsinogen, chymotrypsinogen, proelastase, procarboxypeptidase A, and procarboxypeptidase B.

The first step in intestinal protein digestion is the activation of trypsinogen to its active form, **trypsin,** by the brush-border enzyme **enterokinase.** Initially, a small amount of trypsin is produced, which then catalyzes the conversion of all of the other inactive precursors to their active enzymes. Even the remaining
trypsinogen is autocatalyzed by trypsin to form more trypsin. The activation steps yield five active enzymes for protein digestion: trypsin, chymotrypsin, elastase, carboxypeptidase A, and carboxypeptidase B. These

pancreatic proteases then hydrolyze dietary protein to amino acids, dipeptides, tripeptides, and larger peptides called oligopeptides. Only the amino acids, dipeptides, and tripeptides are absorbable. The oligopeptides are further hydrolyzed by brush-border proteases, yielding the smaller absorbable molecules. Finally, the pancreatic proteases digest themselves and each other!

Absorption of Proteins

As previously described, the products of protein digestion are amino acids, dipeptides, and tripeptides. Each form can be absorbed by intestinal epithelial cells. Especially note the contrast between proteins and carbohydrates: Carbohydrates are absorbable in the monosaccharide form only, whereas proteins are absorbable in larger units. The **L-amino acids** are absorbed by mechanisms analogous to those for monosaccharide absorption. The amino acids are transported from the lumen into the cell by Na^+-amino acid cotransporters in the apical membrane, energized by the Na^+ gradient. There are four separate cotransporters: one each for neutral, acidic, basic, and imino amino acids. The amino acids then are transported across the basolateral membrane into the blood by facilitated diffusion, again by separate mechanisms for neutral, acidic, basic, and imino amino acids. Most ingested protein is absorbed by intestinal epithelial cells in the **dipeptide** and **tripeptide** forms rather than as free amino acids. Separate H^+-dependent cotransporters in the apical membrane transport dipeptides and tripeptides from the intestinal lumen into the cell, utilizing an H^+ ion gradient created by an Na^+-H^+ exchanger in the apical membrane . Once inside the cell, most of the dipeptides and tripeptides are hydrolyzed to amino acids by cytosolic peptidases, producing amino acids that exit the cell by facilitated diffusion; the remaining dipeptides and tripeptides are absorbed unchanged.

Disorders of Protein Digestion and Absorption

Disorders of protein digestion or absorption occur when there is a deficiency of pancreatic enzymes or when there is a defect in the transporters of the intestinal epithelial cells. In disorders of the exocrine pancreas such as **chronic pancreatitis** and **cystic fibrosis,** there is a deficiency of all pancreatic enzymes including the proteases. Dietary protein cannot be absorbed if it is not digested by proteases to amino acids, dipeptides, and tripeptides. The absence of trypsin alone makes it appear as if all of the pancreatic enzymes are missing because trypsin is necessary for the activation of all precursor enzymes (including trypsin itself) to their active forms. Several diseases are caused by a defect in or absence of an Na+-amino acid cotransporter. **Cystinuria** is a genetic disorder in which the transporter for the dibasic amino acids cystine, lysine, arginine, and ornithine is absent in both the small intestine and the kidney. As a result of this deficiency, none of these amino acids is absorbed by the intestine or reabsorbed by the kidney.

The intestinal defect results in failure to absorb the amino acids, which are excreted in feces. The renal defect results in increased excretion of these specific amino acids and gives the disease its name, cystinuria or excess cystine excretion.

Lipids

The dietary lipids include triglycerides, cholesterol, and phospholipids. A factor that greatly complicates lipid digestion and absorption is their insolubility in water (their hydrophobicity). Because the gastrointestinal tract is filled with an aqueous fluid, the lipids must somehow be solubilized to be digested and absorbed. Thus, the mechanisms for processing lipids are more complicated than those for carbohydrates and proteins, which are water soluble.

GI HORMONES:

These are released from endocrine cells in the GI mucosa into the portal circulation enter the general circulation, and have physiologic actions on the target cells.

OFFICIAL HORMONES:

Substances must be secreted in response to a physiologic stimulus and carried in blood stream to a distant site where it produces physiologic actions. Its function must be independent of any neural activity. It must have been isolated, purified, chemically identified and synthesized.

Four substances meet the requirements to be considered "official GI hormones"; others are considered as: candidate hormones".

The four official GI hormones are:

1. Gastrin
2. CCK
3. Secretin
4. Glucose-dependent insilinotropic peptide(GIP)

GASTRIN:

ACTION: Hydrogen ion secretion by gastric parietal cells.

GASTRIN: It is 17 amino acid straight chain peptide secreted by G (gastrin) cells in the antrum of the stomach. It is also known as little gastrin which is secreted in response to a meal. Big gastrin (34 amino acid peptides) is secreted during the interdigestive period (between meals).

Minimum fragment necessary for biologic activity of gastrin is the C-terminal tetra peptide.

STIMULUS FOR SECRETION:

1. Products of protein digestion (e.g. small peptides and amino acids)-phenylalanine and tryptophan.
2. Distension of stomach by food.
3. Vagal stimulation.

INHIBITED BY:

1. Low pH of gastric contents.
2. Somatostatin.

ACTIONS OF GASTRIN:

1. It stimulates Hydrogen secretion by gastric parietal cells.
2. It stimulates the growth of gastric mucosa.

ZOLLINGER ELLISON SYNDROME:

GASTRIN SECRETING TUMOR:

1. Hydrogen ion secretion is increased.
2. Gastric mucosa is hypertrophied.
3. Elevated gastrin levels in blood.
4. Duodenal ulcers.
5. Steatorrhea.

CHOLECYSTOKININ:

It promotes fat digestion and absorption. It is CCK-33 amino acid peptide. The minimum fragment necessary for its biologic activity is the C-terminal hepta peptide. CCK is secreted by the I cells of the duodenal and jejunal mucosa of small intestine.

STIMULUS FOR SECRETION:

1. Fatty acids and monoglycerides but not triglycerides.
2. Small peptides and amino acids.

ACTIONS OF CCK:

1. CONTRACTION OF GALLBLADDER: with relaxation of sphincter of oddi ejects bile from the gallbladder into the lumen of small intestine, which is needed for emulsification and solubilization of dietary lipids.
2. SECRETION OF PANCREATIC ENZYMES:
   PANCREATIC LIPASES: converts lipids to fatty acids, monoglycerides and cholesterol.
   PANCREATIC AMYLASES: digests carbohydrates.
   PANCREATIC PROTEASES: digest proteins.
3. SECRETION OF HCO_3 FROM THE PANCREAS:
4. GROWTH OF EXOCRINE PANCREAS AND GALLBLADDER.
5. INHIBITION OF GASTRIC EMPTYING. Crucial for processes of fat digestion and absorption and slows the delivery of chyme from stomach to small intestine.

SECRETIN:

It is 27 amino acid peptide. It is secreted by S cells of the duodenum in response to Hydrogen ions and fatty acids in the lumen of small intestine.

ACTIONS OF SECRETIN:

It promotes secretion of pancreatic and biliary HCO3, which neutralizes hydrogen ions in the lumen of the small intestine. It also inhibits the effects of gastrin on the parietal cells.

GIP:

GIP is 42-amino acid peptide. It is secreted by K cells of the duodenal and jejunal cells. Only GI hormone secreted in response to all three types of nutrients: glucose, amino acids and fatty acids.

ACTIONS OF GIP:

Stimulation of Insulin secretion by the pancreatic beta cells: also called as INCRETIN (A GI hormone that promotes the secretion of insulin). It causes inhibition of gastric hydrogen ion secretion and inhibition of gastric emptying.

CANDIDATE HORMONES: They fail to meet one or more criteria necessary to be classified as "Official "GI hormones.

1. Motilin
2. Pancreatic polypeptide
3. Enteroglucagon
4. Glucagon like peptide-1 (GLP-1)

MOTILIN:

It is 22 amino acid peptide. It is secreted by upper duodenum during fasting state. It increases GI motility. It initiates interdigestive myoelectric complexes that occur at 90 minute intervals.

PANCREATIC POLYPEPTIDE:

It is 36 amino acid peptide. It is secreted in response to ingestion of carbohydrates, proteins and lipids. It inhibits pancreatic secretion of HCO3 and enzymes.

ENTEROGLUCAGON:

It is released from the intestinal cells in response to a decrease in blood glucose. It directs the liver to increase glycogenolysis and gluconeogenesis.

GLP -1:

It is secreted by L cells of small intestine. It is also called INCRETIN. It stimulates insulin secretion and inhibits glucagon secretion and decreases gastric emptying. It inhibits appetite.

GIT HAS FOUR TYPES OF MOTILITY PATTERNS:

1. Tonic contractions.
2. Segmental contractions.
3. Propagated contractions (Peristalsis).
4. Inhibited contractions.

ESOPHAGUS:

1. PRIMARY ESOPHAGEAL PERISTALSIS: It is initiated by swallowing i-e part of swallowing and is thus co-ordinated by vagal fibers emerging from swallowing center. As soon as food bolus enters the esophagus from pharynx, the UES contracts to prevent regurgitation of food onto mouth and primary esophageal peristalsis begins which propel food downwards. The LES relaxes as the peristaltic wave approaches the sphincter and allows the bolus of food to enter the stomach without causing any resistance.
2. SECONDARY ESOPHAGEAL PERISTALSIS: When the primary esophageal peristalsis is not able to push a bolus of solid food all the way down the esophagus, the food remaining in the esophagus stretches mechanical receptors and initiates another peristaltic wave called secondary esophageal peristalsis. Secondary esophageal peristalsis is co-ordinated by intrinsic nervous system of the esophagus.

STOMACH:

1. MOTILITY OF EMPTY STOMACH:
   a. Migrating motor complex.
   b. Hunger contractions.

2. **GASTRIC MOTILITY RELATED TO MEAL:**
    a. Receptive relaxation.
    b. Mixing peristaltic waves.
    c. Gastric emptying.

MMC:

Peristaltic waves that begin in the esophagus, and travels through the entire GIT during inter digestive period. It removes any food remaining in the stomach and intestine during interdigestive period in preparation for next meal. The hormone MOTILIN, released from the endocrine cells in the epithelium of small intestine, increase the strength of MMC> MMC are abolished immediately after the entry of food in the stomach.

HUNGER CONTRACTIONS:

Occur in the empty stomach, which over a period of hours increase in intensity and are called Hunger contractions. MMC are responsible for hunger contractions when they become extremely strong they fuse to cause tetanic contraction lasting for 2-3 minute, which can be felt and may be painful. They are associated with sensation of hunger.

RECEPTIVE RELAXATION:

The passage of each bolus of food stimulates the stretch receptors of oral region and produces relaxation. By the end of the meal, about 1-2 liters of food can be accompanied. It is vagovagal reflex initiated by distension of stomach and is synchronized with primary peristalsis in esophagus.

MIXING PERISTALTIC WAVES:

The presence of food in the distal body and antral part of stomach increases the contractile activity of this part of stomach. The combination of peristaltic waves and retropulsion is called mixing peristaltic waves. Chyme is formed after mixing of food with stomach acid and enzymes.

GASTRIC EMPTYING:

The process by which, the chyme is pushed from stomach into duodenum.

SMALL INTESTINE:

MOTILITY OF SMALL INTESTINE:

MOTILITY OF SMALL INTESTINE DURING INTERDIGESTIVE PERIOD:

- A. MOTOR MIGRATING COMPLEX:
  This is a peristaltic wave that begins in the esophagus and travels through the entire gastrointestinal tract during interdigestive period. The MMC's sweep out the chyme, remaining in the small intestine. MMC's occur every 60-90 minutes and last for about 10 minutes.

MOTILITY OF SMALL INTESTINE DURING DIGESTIVE PERIOD:

- A. MIXING MOVEMENTS: (SEGMENTATION CONTRACTION)
  These contractions mix the intestinal contents. A section of small intestine contracts, that sends the intestinal contents (chyme) in both orad and caudad directions. That section of small intestine then relaxes, and the contents move back into the segment.

This back and forth movement produced by segmentation contractions causing mixing without net forward movement of chyme.

B. **PROPULSIVE MOVEMENT: (PERISTALTIC CONTRACTIONS)**

It is the law of intestine which co-ordinated within enteric nervous system. Stretch afferents stimulate interneurons.

PROXIMAL TO THE SITE OF DISTENSION (BOLUS): Excitatory motor neurons stimulated that releases acetylcholine and substance P that causes smooth muscle contraction.

DISTAL TO THE SITE OF BOLUS: Inhibitory interneurons are stimulated that release NO, VIP and ATP that result in smooth muscle relaxation.

CONTROL OF PERISTALTIC CONTRACTIONS:

NEURAL CONTROL:

A. **PARASYMPATHETIC:**
   Through vagus nerve, it increases intestinal motility. (Strong emotions)

B. **SYMPATHETIC:**
   Through thoracolumbar outflow, it decreases intestinal motility (Anger and pain)

HORMONAL CONTROL:

A. **INCREASED BY:**
   Gastrin, CCK, 5HT, Thyroxine, Insulin.

B. **DECREASED BY:**
   Secretin and glucagon

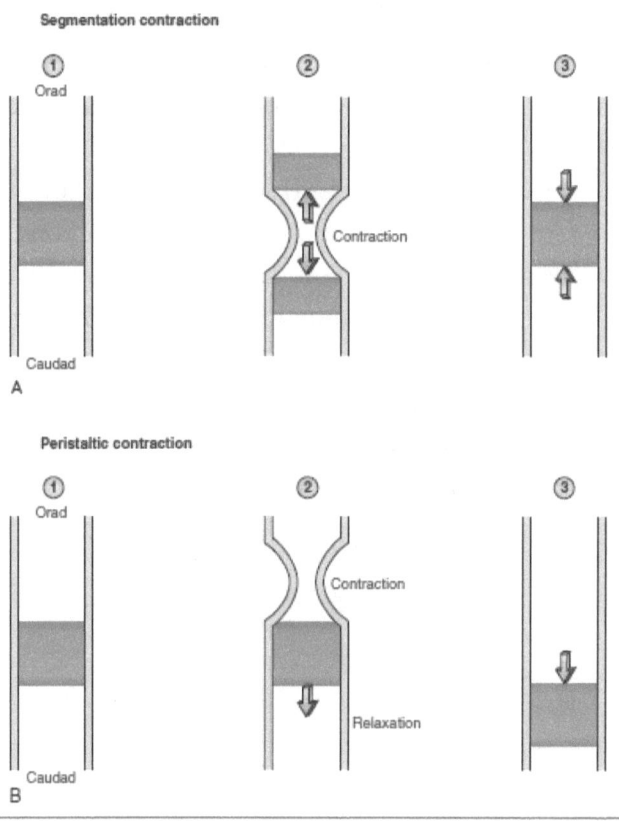

MOTILITY OF LARGE INTESTINE:

- A. HAUSTRAL CONTRACTIONS: Similar to segmentation contractions of small intestine and vigorously mix the contents of colon and by exposing more the contents to mucosa.(Facilitate absorption)
- B. PERISTALSIS: Progressive contractile wave preceded by a wave of relaxation. Small pressure

waves of prolonged duration which propels the contents towards the rectum very slowly (5cm/hr). It can take 48 hours for the chyme to traverse the colon.

C. MASS MOVEMENTS: Observed in colon and are special types of peristaltic contractions. These occurs every 3-4 times a day generally after meals and each contraction lasts for about 3 minutes. The mass movements force the fecal material rapidly en mass down the colon. They also move material into the rectum and rectal distension initiates the defecation reflex.

GI REFLEXES:

LOCAL REFLEXES:

Reflexes that are integrated entirely within the gut wall enteric nervous system. These include reflexes that control:

1. GI secretions
2. GI peristalsis
3. Mixing contractions
4. Local inhibitory effects.

SHORT REFLEXES:

Reflexes from the gut to preverteberal sympathetic ganglion and then back to GIT. These reflexes transmit signals long distances to other areas of GIT.

1. Gastrocolic
2. Enterogastric
3. Coloileal
4. Ileogastric.

LONG REFLEXES:

Reflexes from gut to spinal cord or brain stem and then back to GIT.

1. Vagovagal reflexes.
2. Pain reflexes
3. Defecation reflex
4. Vomiting reflex.

SHORT REFLEXES:

1. **GASTROCOLIC (GASTROILEAL REFLEX):**
   Stomach activity leads to ileocecal relaxation and increased mass movements in the colon. These reflexes are mediated through both long and short nervous pathways (extrinsic and intrinsic) and hormones (CCK and gastrin). It is most evident after first meal of the day, often followed by urge to defecate. Newborn children routinely defecate after meals.

2. **ENTEROGASTRIC REFLEX:**
   When fat or protein chyme reaches the duodenum, receptors detect and send impulses to enteric nerves of stomach that causes inhibition of stomach motility and secretion. It delays gastric emptying.

3. **INTESTINO-INTESTINAL REFLEX:**
   Distension of one portion of intestine leads to decreased contractions caudad of the bolus. It depends on extrinsic neural connections.

4. **GASTROILEAL REFLEX:**
   Signals from the stomach causes increased motility of ileum and increased movements of chyme through ileocecal valve. It is mediated by extrinsic ANS and possibly by gastrin.

5. **ILEOGASTRIC REFLEX:**
   Distension of ileum inhibits gastric motility.

6. **COLOILEAL RELFEX:**
   Reflexes from the colon inhibit emptying of ileal contents/ Filled colon inhibits movements of ileum.

7. RECTOSPHHINCTERIC REFLEX:
   As the rectum fills with fecal material, it contracts and the internal anal sphincter relaxes (rectosphincteric reflex).

   LONG RELFEXES:
   1. VAGOVAGAL RELFEX:
      Reflexes from stomach and duodenum to brainstem and back to stomach by way of vagus to control gastric motor and secretory activity.
   2. PAIN RELFEXES:
      It causes general inhibition of entire GIT.

   3. DEFECATION RELFEX:
      A. As the rectum fills with fecal material, it contracts and the internal anal sphincter relaxes (rectosphincteric reflex).
      B. Distension of rectum causes stimulation of stretch receptors that leads to stimulation of myenteric plexus in sigmoid colon that result in increased peristalsis.
      C. Distension of rectum causes stimulation of stretch receptors that leads to stimulation of parasympathetic neurons in sacral spinal cord. There is increased peristalsis throughout large intestine.
      D. Once rectum is filled to about 25% of its capacity, there is an urge to defecate. However defecation is prevented because the external anal sphincter is tonically contracted.

E. Distension of rectum causes stimulation of stretch receptors that leads to stimulation of parasympathetic neurons in sacral spinal cord. It causes the stimulation of somatic motor neurons that causes involuntary contraction of external anal sphincter.
F. Voluntary relaxation of the external anal sphincter can override the contraction directed by somatic motor neurons.

4. VOMITING RELFEX:
    a. A wave of reverse peristalsis begins in the small intestine, moving the GI contents in the orad direction. The gastric contents are pushed into the esophagus.
    b. If the upper esophageal sphincter is closed then retching occurs, if the pressure in the esophagus is high enough to open the upper esophageal sphincter, vomiting occurs.
    c. The Vomiting center in the medulla is stimulated by tickling the back of the throat, gastric distension and vestibular distension (motion sickness)
    d. The Chemoreceptor trigger zone in the fourth ventricle is activated by emetics, radiation and vestibular stimulation.

TEMPERATURE REGULATION:

Humans maintain a normal body temperature at a set point of 37*C (98.6*F). Because environmental temperatures vary greatly, the body has mechanisms, coordinated in the anterior hypothalamus, for both heat generation and heat loss to keep body temperature constant. When the environmental temperature decreases, the body generates and conserves heat. When the environmental temperature increases, the body temperature increases, the body reduces heat production and dissipates heat.

MECHANISMS FOR GENERATING HEAT:

When environmental temperature is less than body temperature, mechanisms are activated that increase heat production and reduce heat loss. These mechanisms include:

1. Stimulation of thyroid hormone production
2. Activation of Sympathetic nervous system
3. Shivering

THYROID HORMONES:

These hormones are thermogenic. Their actions on target tissues result in heat production. Major actions are:

a. Stimulation of Na K ATPase
b. Increased oxygen consumption
c. Increased metabolic rate
d. Increased heat production

As thyroid hormones are thermogenic, it follows that an excess or deficit of thyroid hormones would cause disturbances in the regulation of body temperature. In hyperthyroidism, the metabolic rate increases, oxygen consumption increases and heat production increases. In hypothyroidism, metabolic rate decreases, decreased oxygen consumption and decreased heat production and extreme sensitivity to cold occur.

SYMPATHETIC NERVOUS SYSTEM:

Cold environmental temperature activates the sympathetic nervous system.

    a. Stimulation of the beta receptors in brown fat, which increases metabolic rate and heat production .This action, is synergistic with the actions of thyroid hormones.

    b. Stimulation of alpha 1 receptors in vascular smooth muscle of skin blood vessels, produces vasoconstriction .Vasoconstriction reduces blood flow to the surface of the skin and consequently reduces heat loss.

SHIVERING:

It involves rhythmic contraction of skeletal muscle, and is the most potent mechanism for increasing heat production in the body. Cold environmental temperature activates centers in the posterior hypothalamus, which then activate the alpha and gamma motor neurons innervating the skeletal muscle. The skeletal muscles contract rhythmically, generating heat and raising body temperature.

MECHANISMS FOR DISSIPATING HEAT:

When the environmental temperature increases, mechanisms are activated that result in heat loss from the body by radiation and convection. Since heat is a normal byproduct of metabolism, the body must dissipate this heat just to maintain body temperature at a set point. When the environmental temperature is increased, more heat than usual must be dissipated.

Mechanisms for dissipating heat are co-ordinated in the anterior hypothalamus. Increased body temperature decreases sympathetic activity in skin blood vessels. This decrease in sympathetic tone results in increased blood flow through skin arterioles and greater arteriovenous shunting of blood to venous plexuses near the surface of the skin. In effect, warm blood from the body core is shunted to the body surface and heat is then lost by radiation and convection. Shunting of blood to the surface is evidenced by redness and warmth of the skin. There also is increased activity of the sympathetic cholinergic fibers innervating thermoregulatory sweat glands to produce increased sweating (cooling). The behavioral components to dissipate heat include increasing the exposure of skin to the air (e.g. removing clothing and fanning).

REGULATION OF BODY TEMPERATURE:

The temperature regulating center is located in anterior hypothalamus. This center receives information about the environmental temperature from thermoreceptors in the skin and about the core temperature from thermoreceptors in the anterior hypothalamus itself. The anterior hypothalamus then orchestrates the appropriate responses, which may involve heat generating or heat dissipating mechanisms.

If core temperature is below the set point temperature, then heat –generating and heat retaining mechanisms are activated. These mechanisms include increased metabolic rate (thyroid hormones, sympathetic nervous system), shivering and vasoconstriction of blood vessels of the skin (increased sympathetic tone).

If the core temperature is above the set point temperature, then heat dissipating mechanisms are activated. These mechanisms include vasodilation of the blood vessels of the skin (decreased sympathetic tone) and increased activity of sympathetic cholinergic fibers to sweat glands.

FEVER:

Fever is an abnormal elevation of body temperature. Pyrogens produce fever by increasing the hypothalamic set point temperature. The result of such a change in set point is that a normal core temperature is "seen" by the hypothalamic center as too low relative to the new set point. The anterior hypothalamus then activates heat generating mechanisms (e.g. shivering) to raise body temperature to the new set point.

At the cellular level, the mechanism of pyrogen action is increased production of interleukin 1(IL-1) in phagocytic cells. IL-1 then acts on the anterior hypothalamus to increase local production of prostaglandins which increases the set point temperature.

Fever can be reduced by aspirin, which inhibits the cyclooxygenase enzyme, necessary for the synthesis of prostaglandins. By inhibiting the production of prostaglandins aspirin interrupts the pathway that pyrogens utilize to raise the set point temperature. When fever is treated with aspirin, the temperature sensors in the anterior hypothalamus now "see " body temperature as too high relative to the set point temperature and set in motion the mechanisms for dissipating heat including vasodilation and sweating.

DISTURBANCES OF TEMPERATURE REGULATION:

HEAT EXHAUSTION: It can occur as a consequence of body's responses to elevated environmental temperature. Normally, the responses to increased temperature includes

HEAT STROKE:

MALIGNANT HYPERTHERMIA:

It is characterized by a massive increase in metabolic rate, increased oxygen consumption and increased heat production in skeletal muscle. The heat dissipating mechanisms are unable to keep pace with the excessive heat production and if hyperthermia is not treated, body temperature may increase to dangerously high or even fatal levels. In susceptible individuals, malignant hyperthermia can be caused by inhalation anesthetics.

Heat exchange with the environment occurs by three processes:

CONDUCTION: The transfer of heat energy from a warmer object to a cooler object in the form of electromagnetic waves (heat waves) which travel through space. It occurs to or from molecules in contact with the skin (or GIT) or pulmonary epithelia.

RADIATION: The transfer of energy from a warmer to a cooler object that is in direct contact with the warmer one.

It occurs by infra red rays to or from bodies at different temperatures from that of the skin.

EVAPORATION: The conversion of a liquid such as sweat into a gaseous vapor, a process that requires heat (the heat of vaporization) which is absorbed from the skin. It occurs through sweat or respiratory secretions from the body.

CONVECTION: The transfer of heat energy by air currents. Cool air warmed by the body through conduction rises and is replaced by more cool air.

Radiation and conduction can increase or decrease total body heat content. Both conduction and evaporation heat loss are increased by convection of air around the body.

The body regulates heat content by regulating skin, temperature, sweat production and heat production. Skin temperature depends on the insulating properties of subcutaneous fat, which is not subject to rapid regulation and cutaneous blood flow. Through changes in the diameter of the arteries and precapillary sphincters, blood flow into cutaneous circulation can be regulated dramatically, from slightly more than 0% up to 30% of cardiac output. Local heating dilates the precapillary sphincters, increasing cutaneous blood flow locally. Cutaneous heating or irritation also triggers spinal reflexes that dilate arterioles across the wider area. Thermoreceptors are present in skin and preoptic anterior hypothalamus, where the thermoreceptors are much more sensitive to small changes in temperature than the peripheral receptors are. An increase in core temperature warms the hypothalamus and evokes a reduction in tonic activity in sympathetic fibers innervating arterioles, permitting the arterioles to dilate all over the body surface. The increased blood flow to the skin shifts part of the heat content of the body to the surface where it can be lost by conduction, convection, evaporation and radiation.

Cooling has the opposite effects. Local cooling of the skin causes precapillary sphincters to constrict, whereas a drop in the core temperature increases sympathetic outflow to cutaneous arterioles, with the resulting constriction reducing cutaneous blood flow and thus heat loss to the environment. Increased sympathetic activity also causes Piloerection (goose flesh).

The control of sweat production is critical for survival under conditions in which conduction, convection and radiation of heat from the skin cannot offset heat absorption and heat production (e.g. when the environment is hotter than the body or during intense exercise). Eccrine sweat glands are activated by sympathetic fibers, which release acetylcholine rather than norepinephrine (NE), and can secrete up to approx. 1.5 l/hr in normal adults. After chronic adaptation to a hot climate, this rate can increase to 4l/hr. This is accompanied by increases in plasma aldosterone levels to reduce the loss of sodium and water. Heat production in a normal adult during maximal exercise can be 20 times the level at rest. During extreme heat, behavioral changes (lethargy) that lead to decrease physical activity reduce heat production. During cold exposure behavioral changes such as stomping the feet and clapping the hands increase heat production. In addition, shivering occurs by involuntary asynchronous contraction of skeletal muscles. This is produced, at least in part by facilitation of stretch reflex and can increase heat production 5 fold to 6 fold.

Release of epinephrine and norepinephrine from the adrenal medulla also occurs during cold exposure and this increases metabolic heat production (chemical thermogenesis) esp. in brown adipose tissue (in humans this is abundant only in infants).Chronic cols exposure also causes a persistent increase in thyroxin production, which uncouples oxidative phosphorylation and increases the metabolic rate in many tissues (as catecholamines do in adipose tissue).

If body temperature falls below 33*C, mental confusion occurs as CNS function begins to be impaired. Below 30*C thermoregulatory control by the CNS is lost, shivering stops, consciousness is lost, slow atrial fibrillation and finally ventricular fibrillation occur.

Body temperature is regulated by a center in hypothalamus. The temperature set point varies slightly (by 0.6*C) each day in a circadian rhythm, with the lowest temperature occurring just before waking in the morning. In women, a small monthly elevation (0.2*C-0.6*C) is associated with ovulation. Fever can be triggered by infection, dehydration or thyrotoxicosis, involves an elevation of temperature set point in the hypothalamus. During infection, exogenous pyrogens associated with invading microorganisms trigger the release of endogenous pyrogens such as interleukin 1 beta (IL-1beta), IL-6 and tumor necrosis factor (TNF) from the leukocytes; this causes the production of PGE2 and thromboxane which elevate the set point temperature. Heat conservation responses (cutaneous vasoconstriction, inhibition of sweating), increased heat production (shivering) and behavioral responses (e.g. pulling the covers) continue until the new set point temperature is attained.

Heat exhaustion is where you become very hot and start to lose water or salt from your body which leads to symptoms of; tiredness, dizziness, headache, muscle cramps, heavy sweating and intense thirst.110*F (43.3*C) is considered the upper limit compatible with life. Temperatures above result in denaturing of enzymes and blocking of metabolic pathways. Temperature below than that slows down metabolism and affects brain. Heat stroke is where the body is no longer able to cool itself and a person's body temperature becomes dangerously high. The symptoms are confusion, disorientation (seizures) and a loss of consciousness.

CORE BODY TEMPERATURE:

It is the temperature of the internal environment of the body. This includes organs such as heart, liver and the blood.

Normal (36.5-37.5*C) (97.7-99.5*F)

Fever >37.5 or 38.3(99.5 or 100.9*F)

Body temperature is a measure of the body's ability to generate and get rid of heat.

SITES FOR MONITORING BODY TEMPERATURE:

The oral and axillary temperature are comparable whereas rectal temperature averages about 1*F higher.

BODY FLUIDS:

Total body water (TBW) is approximately 60% of body weight.

The percentage of TBW is highest in newborns and adult males and lowest in adult females and in adults with a large amount of adipose tissue.

DISTRIBUTION OF WATER:

1. **INTRACELLULAR FLUID (ICF):** It is two thirds of TBW. The major cations of ICF are K+ and Mg+. The major anions of ICF are proteins and organic phosphates (ATP, ADP and AMP)
2. **EXTRACELLULAR FLUID (ECF):** It is one third of TBW. It is composed of interstitial fluid and plasma. The major cation of ECF is Na^+. The major anions of ECF are Cl and HCO_3.
   a. Plasma is one fourth of the ECF. Thus it is one – twelfth of TBW (1/4 x 1/3)
      The major plasma proteins are albumin and globulin
   b. Interstitial fluid is three fourths of the ECF. Thus, it is one fourth of TBW (3/4 x 1/3). The composition of interstitial fluid is the same as that of plasma except that it has little protein. Thus, interstitial fluid is an ultra-filtrate of plasma.
3. 60-40-20 rule
   TBW is 60% of body weight.
   ICF is 40% of body weight.
   ECF is 20% of body weight.

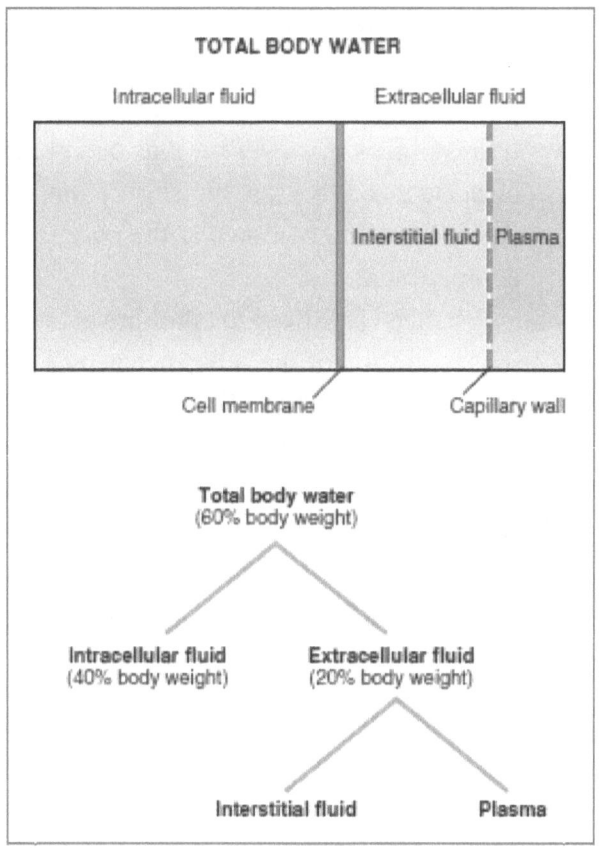

B. Measuring the volumes of the fluid compartments:

DILUTION METHOD:

    A. A known amount of a substance is given whose volume of distribution is the body fluid compartment of interest.
    For example:
        1. Tritiated water is a marker of TBW that distributes wherever water is found.

2. Mannitol is a marker for ECF because it is a large molecule that cannot cross cell membranes and is therefore excluded from the ICF.
3. Evans blue is a marker for plasma volume because it is a dye that binds to serum albumin and is therefore confined to the plasma compartment.

B. The substance is allowed to equilibrate.
C. The concentration of the substance is measured in plasma , and the volume of distribution is calculated as follows: Volume =Amount /Concentration
Where Volume = volume of distribution or volume of the body fluid compartment (L)
Amount= amount of substance (mg)
Concentration = concentration of plasma (mg/L)

BODY WATER AND BODY FLUID COMPARTMENTS:

BODY FLUID COMPARTMENT	MARKERS USED TO MEASURE VOLUME	MAJOR CATIONS	MAJOR ANIONS
TBW	TRITIATED WATER D_2O ANTIPYRENE	-	-
ECF	SULFATE	Na	Cl and HCO_3

	INULIN MANNITOL		
PLASMA	RISA EVANS BLUE	Na	Cl, HCO3 and Plasma protein
INTERSTITIAL	ECF-PLASMA VOLUME (INDIRECT)	Na	Cl and HCO3
ICF	TBW-ECF (INDIRECT)	K	ORGANIC PHOSPHATES AND PROTEIN

SHIFTS OF WATER BETWEEN COMPARTMENTS:
1. BASIC PRINCIPLES:
   A. OSMOLARITY: it is the concentration of solute particles.
   B. PLASMA OSMOLARITY: it is estimated as 2xNa + Glucose /18 + BUN /2.8
   C. At steady state, ECF osmolarity and ICF osmolarity are equal.
   D. To achieve this equality, water shifts between ECF and ICF compartments.
   E. It is assumed that solutes such as NaCl and mannitol do not cross cell membranes and are confined to ECF.
2. EXAMPLES OF SHIFTS OF WATER BETWEEN COMPARTMENTS:

A. **INFUSION OF ISOTONIC NaCl- ADDITION OF ISOTONIC FLUID**
   It is also called isosmotic volume expansion.
   (i) ECF volume increases, but no change occurs in the osmolarity of ECF or ICF. Because osmolarity is unchanged, water does not shift between the ECF and ICF compartments.
   (ii) Plasma protein concentration and hematocrit decrease because the addition of fluid to the ECF dilutes the protein and red blood cells (RBCs). Because ECF osmolarity is unchanged, the RBCs will not shrink or swell.
   (iii) Arterial blood pressure increases because ECF volume increases.

B. **DIARRHEA: LOSS OF ISOTONIC FLUID:**
   It is also called isosmotic volume contraction
   (i) ECF volume decreases, but no change in the osmolarity of ECF or ICF. Because osmolarity is unchanged, water does not shift between the ECF and ICF compartments.
   (ii) Plasma protein concentration and hematocrit increase because the loss of ECF concentrates the protein and RBCs. Because ECF osmolarity is

unchanged, the RBCs will not shrink or swell.
- (iii) Arterial blood pressure decreases because ECF volume decreases.

C. **EXCESSIVE NaCl INTAKE-ADDITION OF NaCl**

It is called hyperosmotic volume expansion.
- (i) The osmolarity of ECF increases because osmoles (NaCl) have been added to the ECF.
- (ii) Water shifts from ICF to ECF. As a result of this shift, ICF osmolarity increases until it equals that of ECF.
- (iii) As a result of the shift of water out of the cells, ECF volume increases (volume expansion) and ICF volume decreases.
- (iv) Plasma protein concentration and hematocrit decrease because of the increase in the ECF volume.

D. **SWEATING IN A DESERT:LOSS OF WATER:**

It is also called hyperosmotic volume contraction.
- (i) The osmolarity of the ECF increases because sweat is hyoosmotic (relatively more water than salt is lost)
- (ii) ECF volume decreases because of the loss of volume in the sweat. Water shifts out of ICF: as a result of the shift, ICF osmolarity increases

until it is equal to ECF osmolarity and ICF volume decreases.
(iii) Plasma protein concentration increases because of the decrease in ECF volume. Although hematocrit might also be expected to increase, it remain unchanged because water shifts out of the RBC's, decreasing their volume and offsetting the concentrating effect of the decreased ECF volume.

E. <u>SYNDROME OF INAPPROPRIATE ANTIDIURETIC HORMONE(SIADH)- GAIN OF WATER:</u>
It is called hypoosmotic volume expansion.
(i) The osmolarity of ECF decreases because excess water is retained.
(ii) ECF volume increases because of the water retention. Water shifts into the cells; as a result of this shift, ICF osmolarity decreases until it equal ECF osmolarity, and ICF volume increases.
(iii) Plasma protein concentration decreases because of the increase in ECF volume. Although hematocrit might also be expected to decrease, it remains unchanged because water shifts into the RBC's, increasing their volume and offsetting the diluting effect of the gain of ECF volume.

F. <u>ADRENOCORTICAL INSUFFICIENCY-LOSS OF NaCl:</u>

It is called hypoosmotic volume contraction

(i) The osmolarity of ECF volume decreases. As a result of the lack of aldosterone in adrenocortical insufficiency, there is decreased NaCl reabsorption, and the kidneys excrete more NaCl than water.

(ii) ECF volume decreases. Water shifts into the cells; as a result of this shift, ICF osmolarity decreases until it equals ECF osmolarity and ICF volume increases.

(iii) Plasma protein concentration increases because of the decrease in ECF volume. Hematocrit increases because of the decreased ECF volume and because the RBC's swell as a result of water entry.

(iv) Arterial blood pressure decreases because of the decrease in ECF volume.

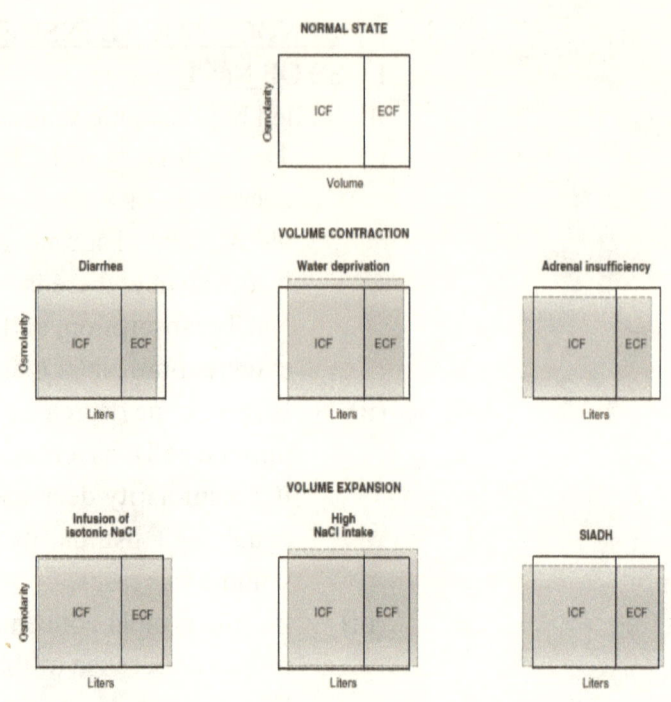

SHIFTS OF WATER BETWEEN BODY FLUID COMPARTMENTS

FUNCTIONS OF DIFFERENT SEGMENTS OF NEPHRON:

EARLY PROXIMAL TUBULE:

It contains brush border, reabsorbs all the glucose, amino acids and most of the HCO_3, Na, Cl, phosphate and water. Isotonic reabsorption occurs here. It generates and secretes ammonia which acts as a buffer for secreted H^+. The hormone PTH inhibits Na/ phosphate cotransport resulting in phosphate excretion. Angiotensin II stimulates Na^+/H^+ exchange resulting in increased sodium, water and HCO3 reabsorption. Hence 65-80% Na is reabsorbed here.

THIN DESCENDING LOOP OF HENLE:

It is passively permeable to water via medullary hyper tonicity and impermeable to sodium. It is called the concentrating segment. It makes urine hypertonic.

THICK ASCENDING LOOP OF HENLE:

It actively reabsorbs sodium, potassium and chloride. Indirectly induces paracellular reabsorption of Mg^+ and Ca^+ through positive lumen potential generated by K^+ back leak. It is impermeable to water. It makes urine less concentrated as it ascends. 10-20% Na^+ is reabsorbed.

EARLY DISTAL CONVOLUTED TUBULE:

It actively reabsorbs Na+ and Cl .It makes urine hypotonic .Under the influence of PTH, there is increased calcium /sodium exchange leading to increased Ca reabsorption. 5-10% of Na^+ is reabsorbed.

COLLECTING TUBULE:

It reabsorbs Na+ in exchange for secreting K^+ and H^+ (regulated by aldosterone). Aldosterone acts as a mineralocorticoid leading to insertion of Na^+ channel on luminal side. ADH acts on the V_2 receptor leading to insertion of aquaporin H_2O channels on the luminal side. 3-5 % Na is reabsorbed.

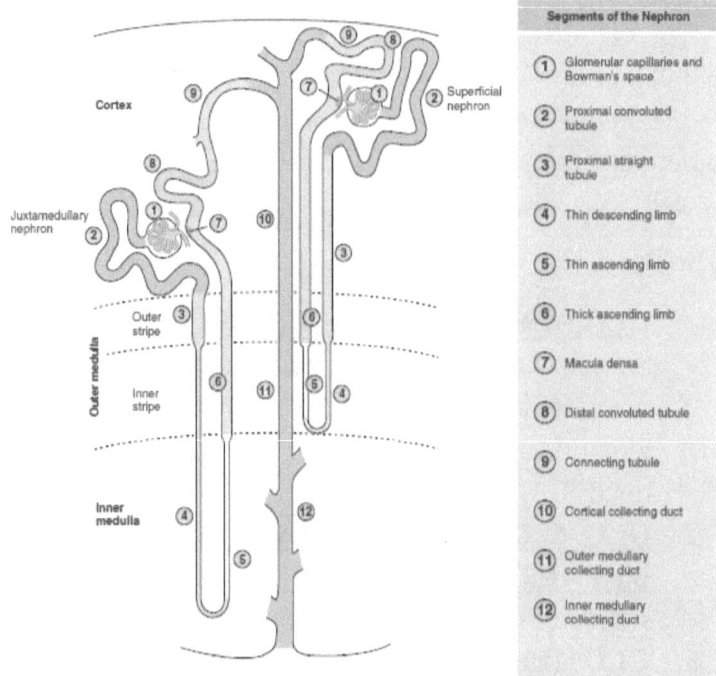

SEGMENTS OF NEPHRON

GENERAL PRINCIPLES OF RENAL TUBULAR TRANSPORT:

TUBULAR REABSORPTION:

It is the Active transport of solutes and passive movement of water from the tubular lumen into peritubular capillaries. Reabsorption is the removal of substances of nutritive value such as glucose, amino acids, and electrolytes from the glomerular filtrate. Small proteins and peptides are reabsorbed in the proximal tubules by endocytosis.

TUBULAR SECRETION:

It is the transport of solutes from the peritubular capillaries into the tubular lumen i-e- addition of a substance to the glomerular filtrate.

DIFFERENT PATTERNS OF RENAL HANDLING OF A SUBSTANCE:

1. **GLOMERULAR FILTRATION ONLY**: Substances are freely filtered but neither reabsorbed nor secreted (e.g. inulin). Such substances are called glomerular markers and have renal clearance equal to GFR.
2. **GLOMERULAR FILTERATION FOLLOWED BY PARTIAL REABSORPTION:** Such substances have renal clearance less than GFR.
3. **GLOMERULAR FILTERATION FOLLOWED BY COMPLETE TUBULAR REABSORTION**: Such substances have lowest renal clearance e.g. Na^+, amino acids, HCO_3 and Cl. The substances that are not filtered at all e.g. protein, also have lowest clearance.
4. **GLOMERULAR FILTRATION FOLLOWED BY TUBULAR SECRETION:** Such substances that are both filtered across glomerular capillaries and secreted from the peritubular capillaries into urine have the highest renal clearance e.g. PAH.
5. **GLOMERULAR FILTRATION FOLLOWED BY PARTIAL REABSORPTION AND SECRETION**: In this circumstance, depending on which two processes are dominant, there may be net reabsorption or net secretion of the substance. Net absorption is said to occur if the amount of

substance excreted in urine is less than GFR in the same time. Similarly, net secretion is said to occur when the amount is more than GFR, in the same time.

6. **<u>NO GLOMERULAR FILTRATION, NO ABSORPTION ONLY SECRETION:</u>** Many organic compounds are bound to plasma proteins and therefore unavailable for ultrafiltration. Secretion is thus major route of excretion in urine.

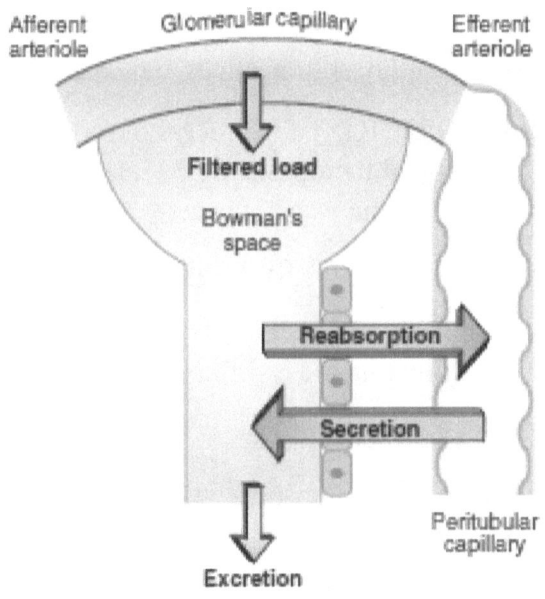

PROCESSESS OF FILTRATION REABSORPTION AND SECRETION IN A NEPHRON

TRANSPORT OF SODIUM ACROSS DIFFERENTSEGMENTS OF RENAL TUBULE:

TRANSPORT ACROSS PROXIMAL TUBULE:

The proximal tubule reabsorbs approx. 67%of filtered water, Na^+, Cl^-,K^+ and other solutes almost all the glucose and amino acids filtered by the glomerulus. It does not reabsorb inulin, creatinine, sucrose and mannitol. It secretes H^+, PAH, urate, penicillin, sulfonamides and creatinine.

SODIUM REABSORPTION: The process of sodium reabsorption in proximal tubule is ISOOSMOTIC i-e reabsorption of sodium and water is exactly proportional.

MECHANISMS OF SODIUM REABSORPTION:

Mechanism of sodium reabsorption in the early proximal tubule and late proximal tubule is different:

IN EARLY PROXIMAL TUBULE:

Sodium is reabsorbed by cotransport with hydrogen or organic solutes (glucose, amino acids, phosphate and lactate). The sodium reabsorption is a two step process:

ACROSS THE BASOLATERAL MEMBRANE:

Sodium moves against an electrochemical gradient via Na K ATPase pump, which pumps Na into the paracellular spaces and lowers the intracellular Na concentration.

ACROSS THE APICAL MEMBRANE:

The sodium moves down an electrochemical gradient as above. The entry of Na is mediated by specific antiporter and symporter proteins:

These include;

a. Na-H antiporter is the main determinant of Na and H2O reabsorption in the proximal tubule. Na-H exchange is linked directly to the reabsorption of HCO3.
b. Na –glucose (and other organic solutes) symporter mechanisms are also involved in the entry of Na in the proximal cells. The glucose, amino acids, phosphate and lactate are almost completely absorbed along with Na by the symporter (carrier) proteins which are different for different molecules.

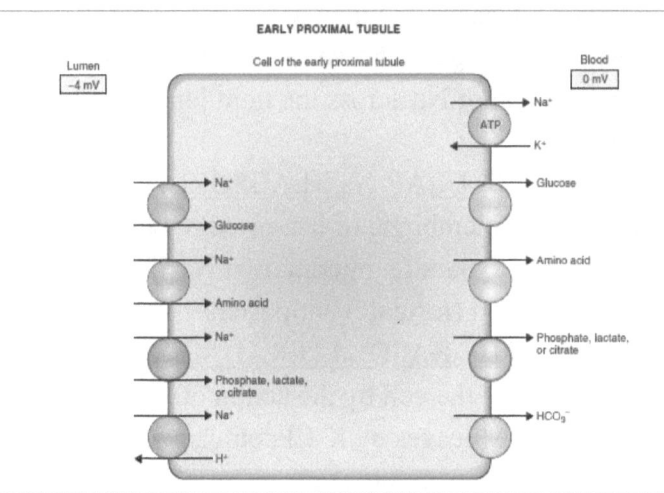

IN THE LATE PROXIMAL TUBULE:

The Na is reabsorbed primarily by chloride driven transport mechanism across both the transcellular and paracellular pathways.

a. <u>REABSORPTION VIA PARACELLULAR PATHWAY:</u> The filtered glucose, amino acids and HCO3 have already been almost completely removed from the tubular fluid by reabsorption in the early proximal tubule. So the fluid entering the late proximal tubule contains very little of these substances but contains a higher concentration of chloride (140 mE/l) compared with that of early proximal tubule (105mE/L). This high concentration of Cl in the lumen of late proximal tubule and comparatively low concentration (105 mE/L) in the interstitium creates a concentration gradient which favors the diffusion of Cl from the tubular lumen across the tight junctions into lateral inter cellular space. Movement of negatively charged Cl causes the tubular fluid to become positively charged relative to the blood. This causes the diffusion of Na across the tight junctions into the blood.
b. <u>TRANSCELLULAR Na REABSORPTION:</u> across the luminal membrane of late proximal tubule cells occurs due to parallel operation of Na-H and one or more Cl anion (formate) antiporters.
c. <u>ACROSS THE BASOLATERAL MEMBRANE:</u> the Na leaves the cell by the action of Na K-ATPase pump, and Cl leaves by K-Cl cotransporter.

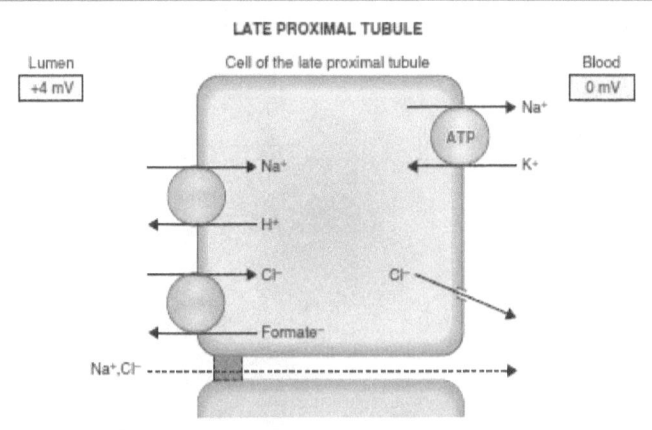

THICK ASCENDING LIMB OF THE LOOP OF HENLE:

It reabsorbs 25% of the filtered Na+. It contains a Na+–K+–2Cl– cotransporter in the luminal membrane.

It is the site of action of the loop diuretics (furosemide, ethacrynic acid, bumetanide), which inhibit the Na+–K+–2Cl– cotransporter.

It is impermeable to water. Thus, NaCl is reabsorbed without water. As a result, tubular fluid [Na+] and tubular fluid osmolarity decrease to less than their concentrations in plasma (i.e., TF/PNa+ and TF/Posm < 1.0). This segment, therefore, is called the diluting segment.

It has a lumen-positive potential difference. Although the Na+–K+–2Cl– cotransporter appears to be electroneutral, some K+ diffuses back into the lumen, making the lumen electrically positive.

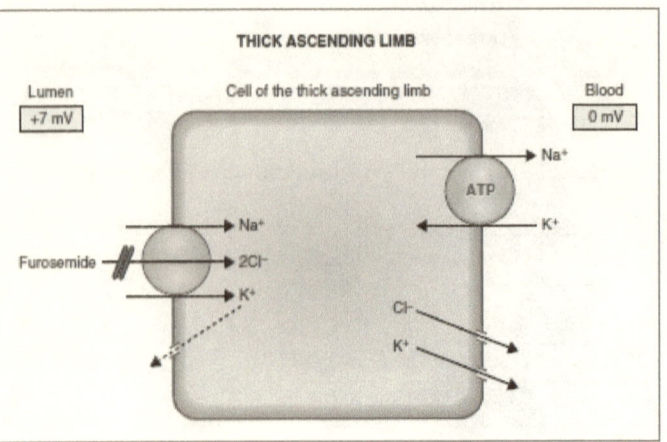

SODIUM REABSORPTION IN THICK ASCENDING LIMB OF HENLE

DISTAL TUBULE AND COLLECTING DUCT

It together reabsorbs 8% of the filtered Na+.

a. EARLY DISTAL TUBULE—SPECIAL FEATURES

It reabsorbs NaCl by a Na+-Cl- cotransporter. It is the site of action of thiazide diuretics. It is impermeable to water, as is the thick ascending limb. Thus, reabsorption of NaCl occurs without water, which further dilutes the tubular fluid. It is called the cortical diluting segment.

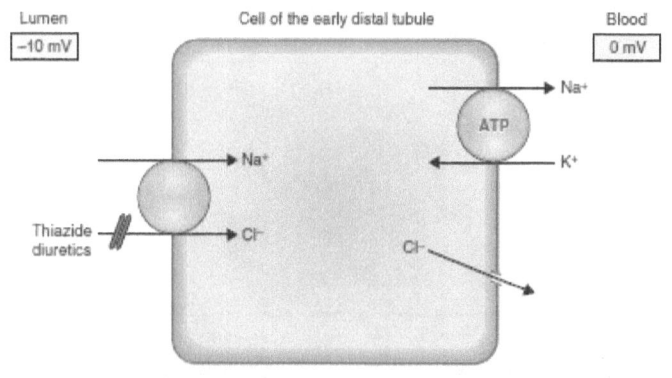

SODIUM REABSORPTION IN EARLY DISTAL TUBULE

b. Late distal tubule and collecting duct—special features
They have two cell types.
(1) *Principal cells*
It reabsorbs Na+ and H2O. It secretes K+. Aldosterone increases Na+ reabsorption and increases K+ secretion. Like other steroid hormones, the action of aldosterone takes several hours to develop because new protein synthesis of Na+ channels (ENaC) is required. About 2% of overall Na+ reabsorption is affected by aldosterone. Antidiuretic hormone (ADH) increases H2O permeability by directing the insertion of H2O channels in the luminal membrane. In the absence of ADH, the principal
cells are virtually impermeable to water.
 K+-sparing diuretics (spironolactone, triamterene, amiloride) decrease K+ secretion.
(2) *α-Intercalated cells*
It secretes H+ by an H+-adenosine triphosphatase (ATPase), which is stimulated by aldosterone.
    a. It reabsorb K+ by an H+,K+-ATPase.

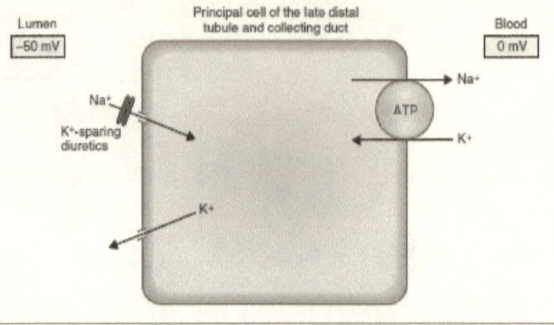

SODIUM REABSORPTION IN LATE DISTAL TUBULE

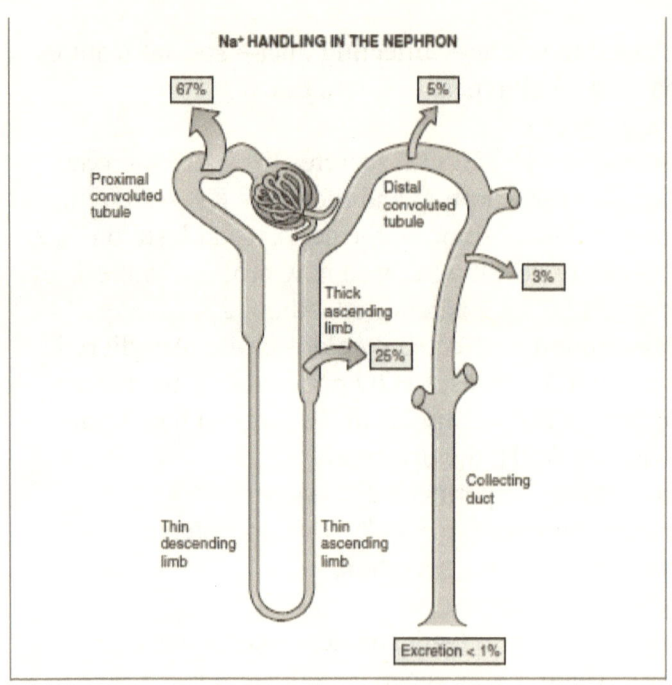

SODIUM HANDLING IN THE NEPHRON

TRANSPORT OF POTASSIUM ACROSS MAJOR NEPHRON:

GLOMERULAR FILTRATION: Filtration occurs freely across the glomerular capillaries, potassium is not bound to plasma proteins.

TUBULAR REBSORPTION AND SECRETION:

67% of filtered K^+ is reabsorbed in the proximal tubule. 20% in loop of Henle, and 10 % is delivered to early distal tubule. In contrast to PCT and loop of Henle, which are capable of only reabsorbing K^+, distal tubule (DT) and collecting duct, are able to either reabsorb or secrete K^+. The role of reabsorption or secretion by DT and CD depends on a variable hormones and factors.

REABSORPTION OF K^+ BY PROXIMAL TUBULE:

In proximal tubule, approx. 7% of filtered K^+ is reabsorbed passively in proportion to H2O reabsorption (solvent drag) and about 60% of filtered K+ is reabsorbed actively by paracellular transport mechanism. **REABSORPTION OF K^+ BY LOOP OF HENLE:**

20% of the filtered K+ is reabsorbed in the thick ascending limb (TAL) of loop of Henle along with Na^+ reabsorption.

REABSORPTION AND SECRETION OF K^+ BY DISTAL TUBULE AND COLLECTING DUCT:

Reabsorption of K+ occurs only when the dietary intake is very low (i-e during K+ depletion).Under these circumstances K+ excretion can be as low as 1% of filtered load because the kidneys conserve as much K+ as possible. Secretion of K+ is variable and accounts for wide range of urinary K+ excretion, depending upon the dietary K+

intake, aldosterone levels, acid base status and urine flow rate.

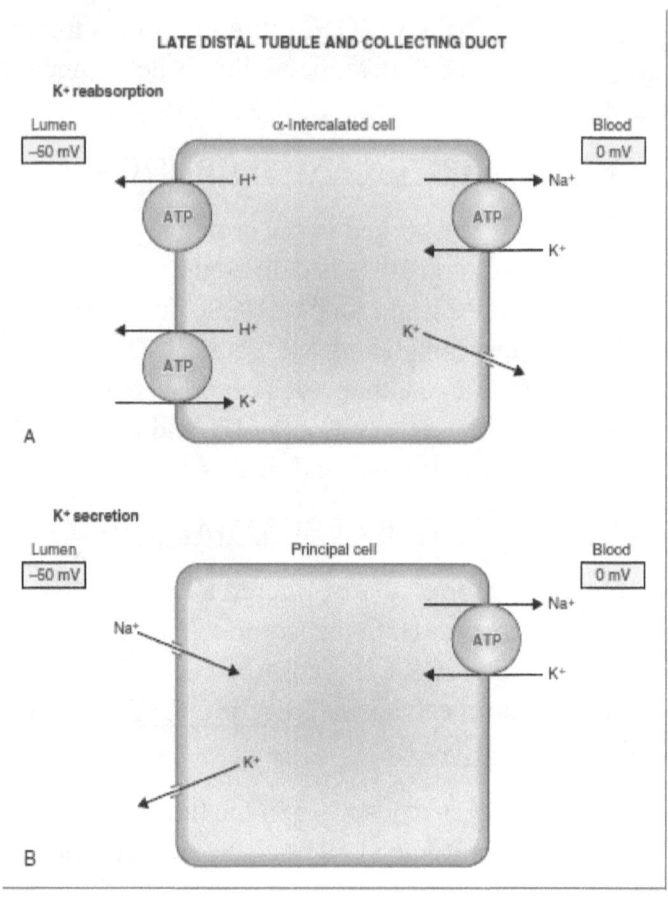

HORMONES AND FACTORS THAT REGULATE URINARY K+ EXCRETION:

1. Plasma K+ level
2. Aldosterone
3. Glucocorticoids
4. ADH
5. Acid base balance

6. Flow of tubular fluid
7. Luminal anions.

PLASMA K^+ LEVELS:

Dietary intake of K^+; Hyperkalemia resulting from high K^+ diet or rhabdomyolysis stimulates secretion within minutes. Hypokalemia from a low K^+ diet or other factors (e.g. diarrhea) decreases K^+ secretion.

ALDOSTERONE:

Aldosterone secretion is increased by hyperkalemia and angiotensin II (after activation of renin-angiotensin system). Aldosterone secretion is decreased by hypokalemia and atrial natriuretic peptide. Chronic rise in aldosterone level increases K+ secretion by principal cells by the following mechanisms;

a. BY INCREASING Na^+K^+ ATPase ACTIVITIY: Aldosterone increases amount of Na^+K^+ ATPase in principal cells. This leads to increased pumping of Na^+ out of the cell at basolateral membrane and increased Na^+ entry into the cells across the luminal membrane.
b. BY MAKING THE TRANSEPITHELIAL POTENTIAL DIFFERENCE MORE LUMEN NEGATIVE. By increasing Na+ reabsorption from lumen, the aldosterone makes the TEPD more lumen negative which turns favors K^+ secretion.
c. BY INCREASING THE PERMEABILITY OF APICAL MEMBRANE TO K^+: Aldosterone increases K+ secretion.

3. **GLUCO-CORTICOIDS:** It indirectly increases K^+ excretion by increasing GFR, which increases tubular flow. Increased tubular flow increases K^+ secretion.

4. **ANTIDIURETIC HORMONE:** ADH increases Na^+ and water reabsorption and decreases the tubular flow which in turn decreases K^+ secretion.

5. **FLOW OF TUBULAR FLUID:** Increase in tubular fluid increases K+ secretion rapidly while decrease in tubular fluid flow decreases the secretion of K^+ by distal tubule and collecting ducts.

6. **ACID BASE STATUS:** Acute acidosis reduces K^+ secretion by 2 mechanisms.

a. By decreasing Na^+K^+ ATPase activity across basolateral membrane it reduces the intracellular K^+ concentration and thus reduces the electrochemical driving force for K^+ exit across apical membrane.

b. By reducing the permeability of apical membrane K^+, it decreases K^+ secretion and also tends to increase the intracellular K^+ concentration.

Acute alkalosis: has exactly the opposite effects to acute acidosis and thus as a net result increase K+ secretion by the principal cells.

8. **LUMINAL ANIONS:**
Excess anions (e.g.HCO_3) in the lumen cause an increase in K+ secretion by increasing the negativity of the lumen and increasing the driving force for K+ secretion.

CHANGES IN DISTAL K+ SECRETION:

CAUSES OF INCRESED DISTAL K+SECRETION	CAUSES OF DECREASED DISTAL K+SECRETION
HIGH K+ DIET	LOW K+ DIET
HYPERALDOSTERONISM	HYPOALDOSTERONISM
ALKALOSIS	ACIDOSIS
THIAZIDE DIURETICS	K+SPARING DIURETICS.
LOOP DIURETICS	
LUMINAL ANIONS	

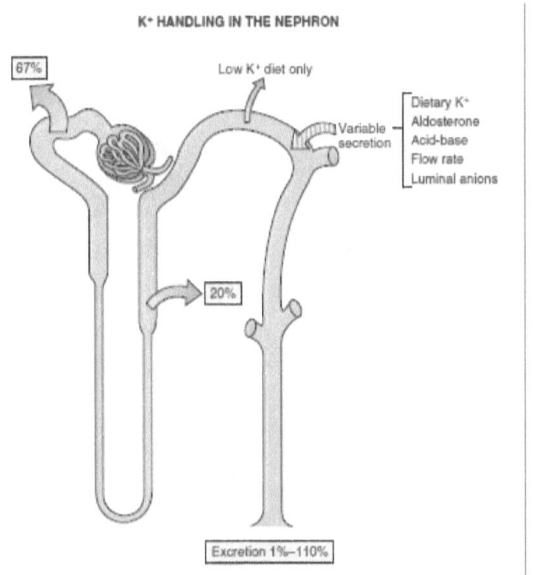

UREA:

Urea is reabsorbed and secreted in the nephron by diffusion, either simple or facilitated depending on the segment of the nephron. Fifty percent of the filtered urea is reabsorbed in the proximal tubule by simple diffusion. Urea is secreted into the thin descending limb of Henle by simple diffusion (from the high concentration of urea in the medullary interstitial fluid). The distal tubule, cortical collecting ducts and outer medullary collecting ducts are impermeable to urea; thus no urea is reabsorbed by these segments. ADH stimulates a facilitated diffusion transporter for urea (UTI) in the inner medullary collecting ducts. Urea reabsorption from the inner medullary collecting ducts contributes to urea recycling in the inner medulla and to the addition of urea to the corticopapillary osmotic gradient.

Urea excretion varies with urine flow rate. At high levels of water reabsorption (low urine flow rate), there is greater urea reabsorption and decreased urea excretion. At low levels of water reabsorption (high urine flow rate), there is less urea reabsorption and increased urea excretion.

PHOSPHATE:

85% of the filtered phosphate is reabsorbed in the proximal tubule by Na phosphate cotransport. Because distal segments of the nephron do not reabsorb phosphate, 15% of the filtered load is excreted in urine. Parathyroid (PTH) inhibits phosphate reabsorption in the proximal tubule by activating adenylate cyclase, generating cyclic AMP (cAMP), and inhibiting Na phosphate cotransport. Therefore, PTH causes phosphaturia and increased urinary cAMP.

Phosphate is a urinary buffer for H^+; excretion of H_2PO_4 is called titrable acid.

PHOSPHATE HANDLING IN THE NEPHRON

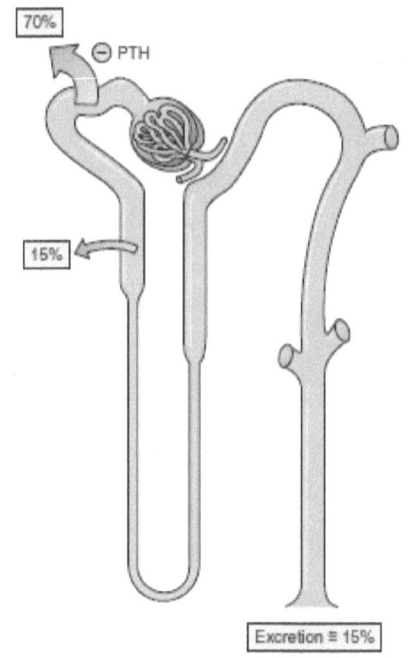

CALCIUM (Ca^+):

Sixty percent of the plasma calcium is filtered across the glomerular capillaries. Together, the proximal tubule and thick ascending limb reabsorb more than 90% of the filtered Ca+ by passive processes that are coupled to Na^+ reabsorption. Loop diuretics (e.g. furosemide) cause increased urinary calcium excretion. Because Ca^+

233

reabsorption is linked to Na^+ reabsorption in the loop of Henle, inhibiting Na^+ reabsorption with a loop diuretic also inhibits calcium reabsorption. If volume is replaced, loop diuretics can be used in the treatment of hypercalcemia.

Together, the distal tubule and collecting duct reabsorb 8% of the filtered Ca^+ by an active process.

1. PTH increases Ca^+ reabsorption by activating adenylate cyclase in the distal tubule.
2. Thiazide diuretics increase Ca^+ reabsorption in the early distal tubule and therefore decrease Ca^+ excretion. For this reason thiazide diuretics are used in the treatment of idiopathic hypercalciuria.

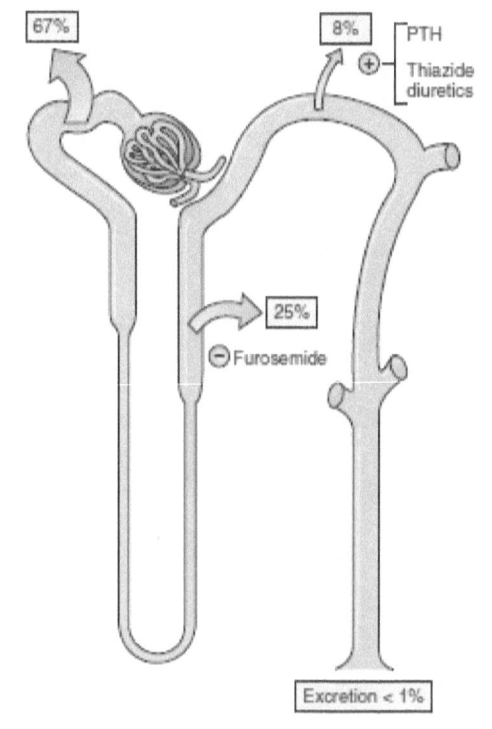

MAGNESIUM:

It is reabsorbed in the proximal tubule, thick ascending limb of the loop of henle, and distal tubule. In the thick ascending limb Mg^+ and Ca^+ compete for reabsorption; therefore hypercalcemia causes an increase in Mg^+ excretion.by inhibiting Mg^+ reabsorption). Likewise hypermagnesemia causes an increase in Ca^+ excretion by inhibiting Ca^+ reabsorption.

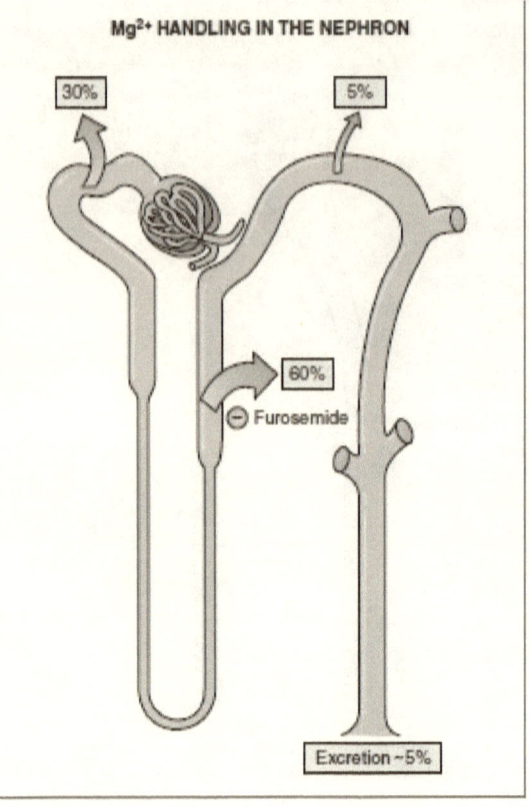

ACID BASE BALANCE:

It is concerned with maintaining a normal hydrogen ion concentration in the body fluids. This balance is achieved by:

a. Utilization of buffers in extracellular fluid and intracellular fluid.
b. Respiratory mechanisms that excrete CO_2
c. Renal mechanisms that reabsorb HCO_3^- and secrete H+ ions

The normal range of arterial pH is 7.37 to 7.42.
Acidemia =<7.37
Alkalemia=>7.42

The mechanisms for buffering and respiratory compensation occur rapidly within minutes to hours. The mechanisms for renal compensation are slower requiring hours to days.

ACID PRODUCTION IN THE BODY:

Arterial pH is slightly alkaline despite acid production in the body. There are two forms of acids.
a. Volatile acid (CO_2)
b. Nonvolatile of fixed acid.

CO_2:

13,000- 20,000 millimoles daily is the rate of generation. When it reacts with H_2O it forms H_2CO_3 by the action of enzyme carbonic anhydrase. CO_2 is produced by the cells is added to venous blood, converted to H+ and HCO_3^- within the red blood cells, and carried to the lungs. In the lungs the reaction occurs in reverse and CO_2 is generated and expired. (CO_2 is therefore called volatile acid). Thus buffering of H+ by venous blood is only a temporary problem.

FIXED ACID:

Catabolism of proteins and phospholipids result in approx. 50 meq/day of fixed acid production. Proteins containing sulfur containing amino acids generate H_2SO_4 and phospholipids generate phosphoric acid. As these are not volatile they need to be buffered in body fluids until they can be excreted by the kidneys. In addition to above acids β hydroxybutyrate and acetoacetic acid are also generated in diabetic ketoacidosis and lactic acid is generated during strenuous exercise or when tissues are hypoxic. Salicylic acid is produced in salicylate poisoning, formic acid in methanol poisoning and glycolic and oxalic acid in ethylene glycol poisoning. Over production of fixed acids result in METABOLIC ACIDOSIS.

RENAL MECHANISMS IN ACID BASE BALANCE:
    A. Reabsorption of HCO_3^-
    B. Excretion of H+
        i.   Excreted as titrable acid
        ii.   Excretion of H+ as NH4+

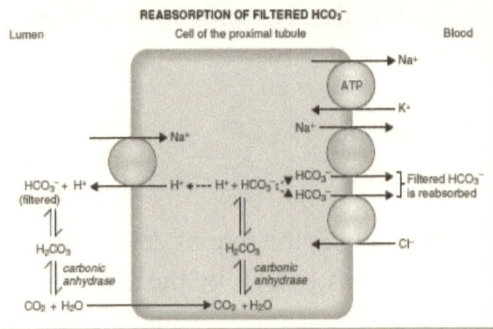

REABSORPTION OF FILTERED HCO_3^-:

About 99.9% of filtered HCO_3^- is reabsorbed. If GFR is 180l/day and plasma HCO_3^- concentration is 24 meq/l then filtered load is (180x24) =4320 meq/day. The measured excretion rate is merely 2 meq/l therefore 4318 meq/day (99.9% of filtered load is reabsorbed. Most filtered HCO_3^- is reabsorbed in PCT, only small quantities are reabsorbed in loop of Henle, distal tubule and collecting duct.

STEPS IN REABSORPTION OF HCO_3^- IN PROXIMAL TUBULE:
1. Luminal membrane has Na^+ H^+ exchanger, Na^+ moves in and H^+ moves out in the lumen.
2. In the lumen H^+ combines with HCO_3^- to form H_2CO_3 under the influence of carbonic anhydrase, H_2CO_3 dissociates into H_2O and CO_2.
3. CO_2 diffuses inside the tubular epithelial cells, where it combines with H_2O to form again H_2CO_3 which dissociates into H^+ and HCO_3^-
4. H^+ transported again into lumen by Na^+ H^+ exchanger
5. HCO_3^- is reabsorbed by Cl^- HCO_3^- exchanger and $Na\ HCO_3$ cotransporter.

EXCRETION OF H^+ AS TITRABLE ACID:

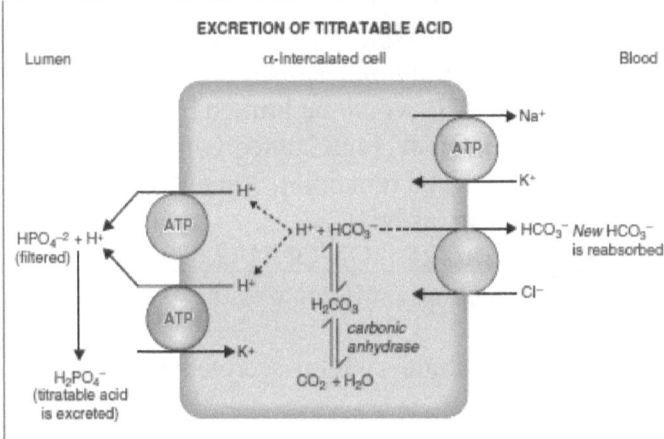

By definition titrable acid is H^+ excreted with urinary buffers. Inorganic phosphate is the most important buffer because of its relatively high concentration in urine and its ideal pk. 85% of filtered phosphate is reabsorbed, only 15% of filtered phosphate is left to be excreted as titrable acid.

MECHANISM OF EXCRETION OF TITRABLE ACID:
Titrable acid is excreted throughout the nephron, but primarily in α intercalated cell of the late distal tubule and collecting duct.

There are 2 mechanisms for secretion of H^+ in α intercalated cell of DCT and CD.
  a. H^+ ATPase (under the influence of Aldosterone)
  b. H^+K^+ ATPase.

In the lumen, H^+ secreted combines with the A^- form of phosphate buffer HPO_4^{-2} to produce the HA form of the buffer, H_2PO_4 which is a titrable acid and is excreted in urine.

The H^+ secreted by the H^+ATPase is produced in the renal cells from CO_2 and H_2O, which combine to form H_2CO_3 in the presence of intercellular carbonic anhydrase. H_2CO_3 dissociates into H^+, which is secreted and HCO_3 which is reabsorbed into blood via Cl^- HCO_3^- exchanger.

EXCRETION OF H^+ AS NH_4:
If titrable acid were the only mechanism for excreting H^+, then excretion of fixed H^+ would be limited by the amount of phosphate in urine. On average 20meq/l of fixed H^+ is excreted as titrable H^+. The remaining 30meq/l is excreted by a second mechanism, as NH_4.

MECHANISM OF EXCRETION OF H^+ AS NH_4:
Three segments of nephron participate in the excretion of H^+ as NH_4.
  1. The proximal tubule. (NH_4 is secreted by Na^+ H^+ exchanger

2. Thick ascending loop of Henle. (The NH_4 that was previously secreted in proximal tubule is reabsorbed and added to corticopapillary gradient.
3. α intercalated cells of collecting ducts.(NH3 and H+ are secreted and combine to form NH_4 and is excreted.

PROXIMAL TUBULE: In the cells of proximal tubule, the enzyme glutaminase metabolizes glutamine to glutamate and NH_4. The glutamate is metabolized to αketoglutarate, which is metabolized to CO_2 and H_2O and then HCO_3. The HCO_3 is reabsorbed across the basolateral membrane into blood via Na^+HCO_3 cotransport.

In the proximal tubule cell, NH_4 is in equilibrium with NH_3 and H^+ being lipid soluble diffuses down its concentration gradient from cell to lumen and H^+ is secreted into the lumen on the Na^+H^+ exchanger. Once in the lumen NH_3 and H^+ recombines with NH_4.

1. Part of it is excreted in the urine.
2. Part of it is reabsorbed in Thick Ascending limb to be resecreted in CD for excretion in urine.

THICK ASCENDING LIMB OF LOOP OF HENLE:

NH_4 is reabsorbed by $Na^+K^+2Cl^-$ cotransporter in place of K^+ and participates in counter current multiplication.

COLLECTING DUCT :(α intercalated cells)
There as 2 mechanisms for secretion of H^+:
1. H^+ ATPase
2. H^+K^+ATPase.

As H^+ is secreted into tubular fluid ,NH_3 diffuses from its high concentration in the medullary interstitium into the lumen of the collecting ducts, where it combines with secreted H+ to form NH4. (Diffusion of NH3 occurs as it is lipid soluble and not that of NH4 which is not lipid soluble)NH4 trapped in tubular fluid is excreted.

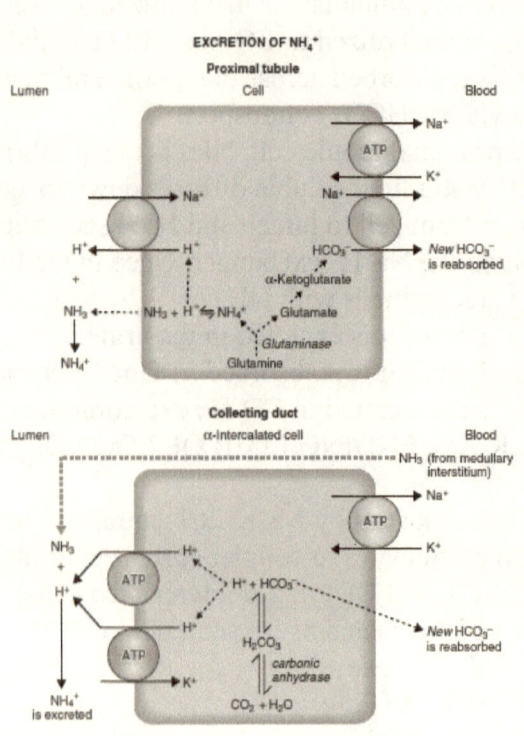

GLOMERULAR FILTRATION RATE:

The amount of filtrate formed in all the renal corpuscles of both kidneys each minute is the glomerular filtration rate (GFR). In adults the GFR averages 125ml/min. Homeostasis of body fluids require that the kidneys maintain a relatively constant GFR. If the GFR is too high, needed substance may pass so quickly through renal tubules that some are not reabsorbed and are lost in the urine. If the GFR is too low, nearly all the filtrate may be reabsorbed and certain waste products may not be excreted.

COMPOSITION OF GLOMERULAR FILTRATE:

Composition of glomerular filtrate is that of plasma except for absence of proteins (colloids) and cells.

DYNAMICS OF GLOMERULAR FILTRATION:

According to starling hypothesis, the GFR can be expressed as:

$GFR = K_f\{(P_{Gc} - P_{Bs})\_(\pi_{GC} - \pi_{BS})\}$

GFR is the filtration across the glomerular membrane.

The filtration co-efficient (K_f) normally equals $12.5 m^2/min/mmHg$

P_{Gc}=Glomerular capillary hydrostatic pressure=45mmHg

P_{Bs}=Bowman's space hydrostatic pressure=10mmHg.

π_{GC}=Glomerular capillary oncotic pressure=25mmHg

π_{BS}=Bowman's space oncotic pressure=0mmHg because glomerular filtrate contains no proteins.

Effective filtration pressure (EFP) is the net outward force calculated as the difference between outward (PGc and π_{BS}) and inward (PBs and π_{GC}) directed forces. Thus under normal circumstances:

GFR=12.5{(45-10)-(25-0)} =125ml/min

NORMAL GFR:

125ml/min (90-140ml/min)

180l/day of plasma is filtered at the glomerulus .99%of it is reabsorbed and only 1%is excreted as urine. After age 30 GFR declines with age.

FACTORS AFFECTING GFR:

1. FILTRATION CO-EFFICIENT (Kf):
   Increased Kf raises GFR while decreased Kf reduces GFR. Kf is the product of permeability and filtration area of the glomerular capillary membrane.
   a. Permeability of the glomerular capillaries is increased in abnormal conditions like hypoxia and presence of toxic agents. In such conditions, GFR is increased because plasma proteins are also filtered to a variable degree.
   b. Alterations in GFR filtration area of glomerular capillaries can alter the Kf .Thus Contraction of mesangial cells causes decreased Kf and relaxation of mesangial cells result in increased Kf.
2. HYDROSTATIC PRESSURE INBOWMAN'S SPACE FLUID (P_{BS}):
   Force opposing filtration (10mmHg) because of fluid in the lumen of the nephron.s

It opposes filtration and therefore GFR is inversely related to it. It decreases in acute obstruction of urinary tract (e.g. ureteric obstruction by stone).

3. **GLOMERULAR CAPILLARY HYDROSTATIC PRESSURE(P_{GC}):**
   Force favoring filtration (45mmHg). It remains constant along the entire length of glomerular capillary.
   GFR is directly related to P_{GC} which is mainly dependent on arterial pressure, renal blood flow, afferent arteriolar resistance and efferent arteriolar resistance. In ARF, GFR declines because of fall in P_{GC}.

4. **GLOMERULAR CAPILLARY ONCOTIC PRESSURE(π_{GC}):**
   Force opposing filtration (25mm Hg) It is determined by protein concentration of glomerular capillary blood. It does not remain constant along the capillary length rather it increases as fluid is filtered out of the capillary.
   GFR is inversely proportional to π_{GC}. In hyperproteinemia, in hemoconcentration the π_{GC} is raised leading to decreased GFR. Conversely in hypoproteinemia and hemodilution the πGC is reduced leading to increased GFR.
   GFR= Kfxnet ultrafiltration pressure
   Net ultrafiltration pressure is the sum of starling pressures
   For glomerular capillaries, net ultrafiltration pressure always favor filtration, so the direction of fluid movement is always OUT of the capillaries. The greater the net pressure, the higher rate of glomerular filtration.

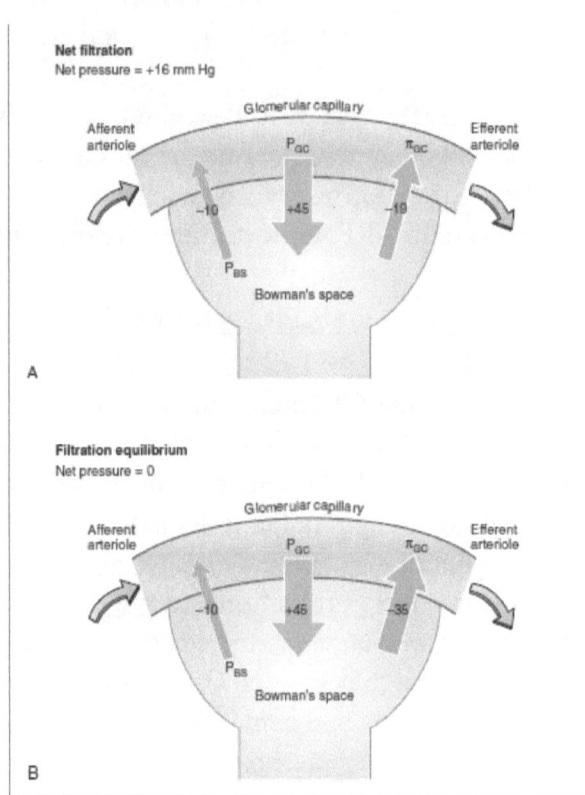

STARLING FORCES ACROSS GLOMERULAR MEMBRANE

RENAL CLEARANCE:

Clearance is a general concept that describes the rate at which substances are removed from plasma. Thus whole body clearance means the total rate of removal of a substance by all organs, hepatic clearance means the rate of removal by the liver, and renal clearance means the rate of removal by the kidneys.

Renal Clearance: It is the volume of plasma completely cleared of a substance by the kidneys per unit time. The higher the renal clearance, the more plasma is cleared of the substance. Substances with highest renal clearances may be completely removed on a single pass of blood through the kidneys. Substances with the lowest renal clearance are not removed at all.

The equation for renal clearance is as follows:

$C = UV/P$

Where: C=Clearance (ml/min)

U=Urine concentration of substance X (mg/ml)

V= Urine flow rate per minute (ml/min)

P=Plasma concentration of substance X (mg/ml)

Thus renal clearance is the ratio of urinary excretion UxV to Plasma concentrations.

CLEARANCE OF VARIOUS SUBSTANCES:

Renal clearance can be calculated for any substance. Renal clearance can vary from zero to greater than 600 ml/min.

1. Renal clearance of albumin is zero =not filtered across glomerular basement membrane.
2. Renal clearance of glucose is zero= filtered but completely reabsorbed.
3. Renal clearance of Na, Urea, Phosphate Cl=higher than zero=filtered and partially reabsorbed.
4. Renal clearance of inulin=125ml/min=Exactly as GFR= freely filtered neither reabsorbed nor secreted
5. Renal clearance of PAH=Highest clearance=Filtered and secreted

Both BUN and creatinine can be used be used to estimate GFR because both urea and creatinine are filtered across the glomerular capillaries. Inulin is the perfect glomerular marker; the closest substance is creatinine which is freely filtered across the glomerular capillaries but also secreted to a small extent. Thus the clearance of creatinine slightly overestimates the GFR. Creatinine is an endogenous substance and needs not be infused in order to measure GFR. Inulin is required to be infused.

RENAL THRESHOLD:

Plasma concentration at which a substance first appears in the urine. For glucose it is 180mg/dl

TRANSPORT MAXIMUM:

The Maximal amount of solute that can be actively transported (reabsorbed or secreted) per minute by the renal tubules. The point at which the carriers are saturated is the Tm. It is important to note that Tm pertains to solutes that are actively transported only and the substances that are passively transports (e.g. urea) do not exhibit Tm.

Substances that have Tm are Phosphate, sulfate, glucose, many amino acids, uric acid, albumin, and acetoacetate and beta hydroxybutyrate.

Substances that do not have Tm include reabsorption of Na along the nephron and HCO3.

CLEARANCE RATIO:

Clearance of a substance X can be compared to clearance of inulin and is expressed as the clearance ratio. Thus clearance ratio = C_x/C_{inulin}

When $C_x/C_{inulin}=1$ clearance of X is equal to inulin.

When $C_x/C_{inulin}=<1$ clearance of X is lower than clearance of inulin either substance is not filtered or is filtered but reabsorbed e.g. glucose, Na and PO4

When $C_x/C_{inulin} =>1$ the clearance of X is higher than the clearance of inulin. The substance is filtered and secreted e.g. organic acids and bases.

Inulin has unique property that it is the only substance whose clearance is exactly equal to GFR. It is freely filtered but neither reabsorbed nor secreted. Thus the amount of inulin filtered will be exactly equal to the amount of inulin excreted. For these reasons, inulin is a reference substance called a glomerular marker.

FILTRATION FRACTION:

It is the ratio of GFR to renal plasma flow (RPF). At normal values of GFR, 125ml/min and RPF is 650ml/min, filtration fraction is approximately 0.2 %(125/650). Thus 20 % of renal plasma flow is actually filtered per minute.

JG APPARATUS:

The JG apparatus is a specialized region of a nephron where the afferent arteriole and the distal convoluted tubule (DCT) come into direct contact with each other. The JG apparatus as a whole works to regulate filtrate formation and systemic blood pressure. The specialized cells of arteriole at this region are called JG cells. The JG cells contain an enzyme renin and function as mechanoreceptors to sense blood pressure. The specialized cells of DCT at the point of contact with afferent arteriole are the MACULA DENSA CELLS. These cells function as chemoreceptor to sense changes in the solute concentration and flow rate of the filtrate. When systemic blood pressure, decreases there is decreased amount of Na and Cl reaching the DCT and there is decreased stretch of JG cells which leads to release of renin. Renin release causes activation of renin angiotensin mechanism which ultimately leads to increased blood pressure.

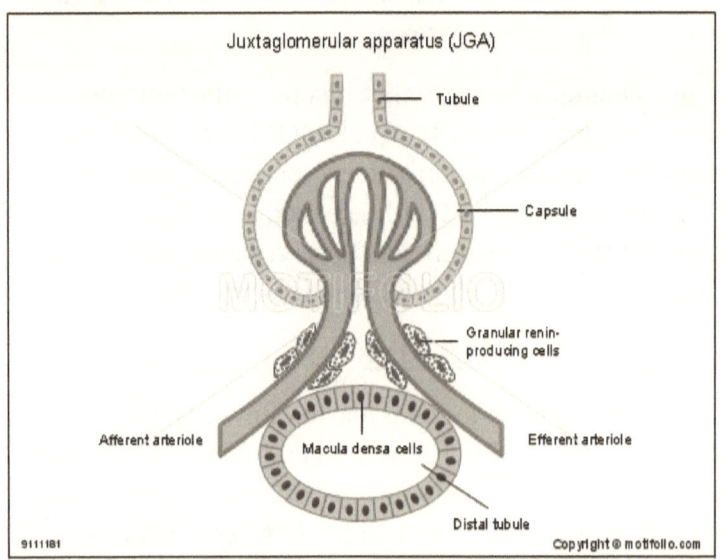

FILTRATION MEMBRANE:

It consists of:

1. Capillary endothelium
2. Glomerular basement membrane
3. Bowman's visceral epithelium(podocytes)

CHARACTERISTIC FEATURES OF FILTRATION MEMBRANE:

HIGH PERMEMEABILITY: Highly permeable to water and 100% dissolved substances because of its porous nature.

PERMEABILITY SELECTIVITY: depends on pore size and electrical charge in the filtration membrane.

PORE SIZE: Capillary endothelial cells have pores 70-90 nm in diameter, GBM has no pores but permeability corresponds to pore size of 8nm.

<4nm is freely filtered

>8nm has zero permeability

4-8nm (filtration is inversely proportional to diameter)

ELECTRICAL CHARGE:

The pores in the filtration membrane are negatively charged due to presence of glycoproteins rich in sialic acid. Thus albumin with a diameter of 7nm is not filtered because of negative charge. Neutral and cationic particles pass easily.

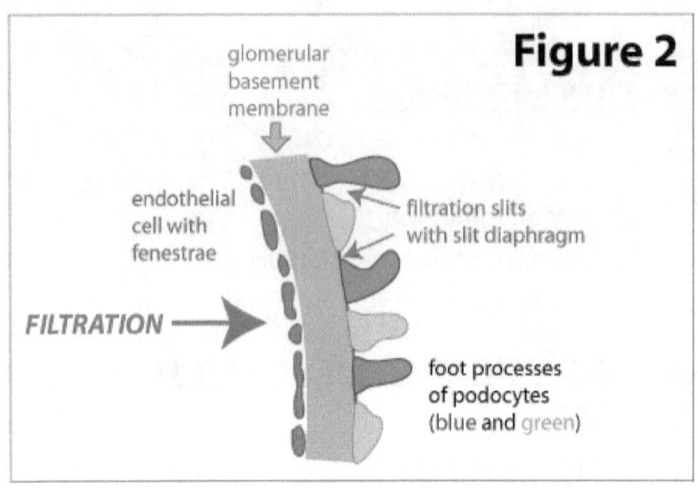

Figure 2

AUTOREGULATION: The maintenance of normal blood flow to an organ during periods of altered arterial pressure.

AUTOREGULATION OF RENAL BLOOD FLOW:

RBF is auto regulated over a wide range of mean arterial pressure. Renal arterial pressure can vary from 80-200 mmHg, yet RBF will be kept constant .Only when arterial pressure decreases to less than 80 mm of HG does RBF also decrease. The way to maintain this constancy of blood flow in face of changing arterial pressure is by varying the resistance of the arterioles.

RBF is 25% of cardiac output, which is 5l/min so RBF is 1.25l/min

For renal auto regulation, the resistance is controlled primarily at the level of afferent arteriole rather than efferent arteriole .Mechanism of auto regulation is not completely understood; clearly autonomic nervous system is not involved as denervated kidney auto regulates as well as an intact kidney.

MYOGENIC HYPOTHEIS:

Increased arterial pressure stretches the blood vessels, which causes reflex contraction of smooth muscle in the blood vessel walls and consequently increased resistance to blood flow. The increase in resistance then balances the increase in arterial pressure and RBF is kept constant.

TUBULOGLOMERULAR FEEDBACK:

The process by which alterations in renal tubular flow are sensed by specialized cells in the macula densa and signal the afferent arteriole to constrict or dilate to bring about alterations in GFR, thereby negating the alterations in tubular flow.

When renal arterial pressure increases, both RBF and GFR increase. The increase in GFR results in increased delivery of solutes and water to the macula densa region of the early distal tubule, which senses some component of increased delivery load. The macula densa responds to the increased delivery load by secreting a vasoactive substance that constricts afferent arterioles via a paracrine mechanism. Local vasoconstriction of afferent arteriole then reduces RBF and GFR back to normal.

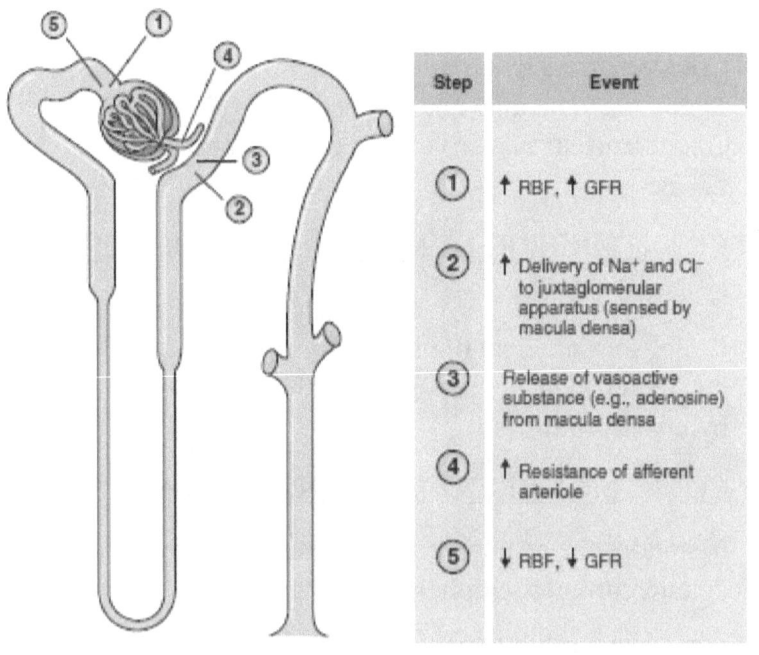

MECHANISM OF TUBULOGLOMERULAR FEEDBACK

COUNTERCURRENT MECHANISM:

Countercurrent exists when fluids flow in opposite directions in parallel and adjacent tubes. There are two countercurrent systems and an osmotic equilibrating device.

COUNTERCURRENT MULTIPLIER: (LOOP OF HENLE)

Establishes gradient of osmolarity from cortex (300 mosmoles/liter) to the papilla (1200 mosmoles/liter) aided by urea cycling.

COUNTERCURRENT EXCHANGER :(VASA RECTA)

Maintains the osmotic gradient established by countercurrent multiplier.

OSMOTIC EQUILIBRATING DEVICE: (COLLECTING DUCT)

Depending on the plasma level of ADH, collecting duct urine is allowed to equilibrate with the hyperosmotic medullary gradient resulting from counter current system.

COUNTERCURRENT MULTIPLICATION:

1. Descending limb of loop of Henle doesn't reabsorb solute but does absorb water (concentrates urine).
2. Ascending limb of loop of Henle doesn't reabsorb water but does absorb solute actively (dilutes urine and the urine leaving ascending limb of loop of Henle is hyposmotic-100 mosmoles/liter)

STEPS:

1. As NaCl is reabsorbed from thick ascending limb by NaK2Cl cotransport, it creates a gradient in the interstitium (max 200 mosmoles/liter) at a time because paracellular diffusion of ions back into eventually counterbalances transport of ions out of lumen when 200 mosmoles/liter gradient is achieved.
2. Urine in the descending limb now equilibrates osmotically with the interstitium and water leaves.
3. Flow of fluid now moves hyperosmotic urine into the ascending limb and NaCl transport creates another gradient
4. .The loop configuration creates a counter current multiplier for the effect of Na+pump to create the cortico- medullary gradient (300-1200mosmoles/liter).

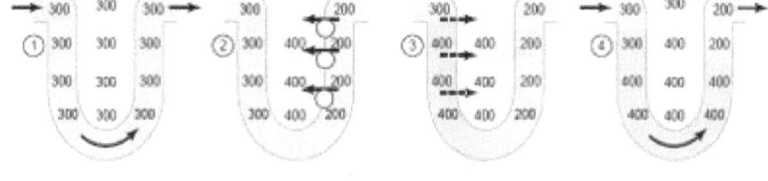

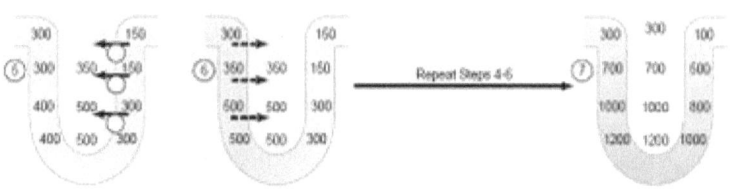

Countercurrent multiplier system in the loop of Henle for producing a hyperosmotic renal medulla. (Numerical values are in milliosmoles per liter.)

COUNTERCURRENT EXCHANGER:

1. Vasa recta are freely permeable to both solutes and water throughout the length, water diffuses along

the osmotic gradient and NaCl diffuses along its concentration gradient.

2. Blood entering the descending limb of vasa recta is 300 mosmoles/liter and blood leaving the ascending limb of vasa recta is 325 mosmoles/liter. Only slight increase in the solute content of the blood going out of the medulla shows that the medullary concentration gradient is maintained as most of the solute is left in the interstitium.

3. Urine osmolarity is inversely related to medullary (vasa recta) blood flow. Faster the blood flows; there is less time for equilibration and increased solute leave blood leading to decreased medullary concentration gradient.

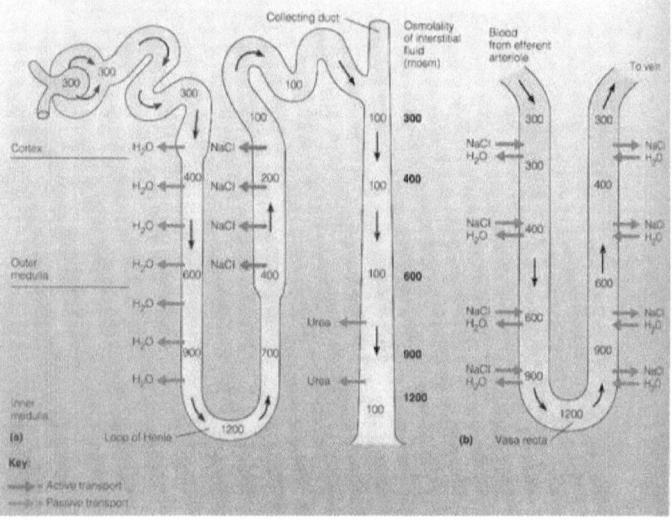

As the blood descends through the descending limb of vasa recta, water diffuses out and NaCl diffuses into equilibrate with the increasing osmolarity of medullary interstitial fluid from top to bottom established by countercurrent multiplier. As the blood ascends through the ascending limb of vasa recta, water diffuses in and NaCl diffuses out to equilibrate with the decreasing osmolarity of medullary interstitium from bottom to top. The process continues and the equilibrium is never reached.

ROLE OF UREA RECYCLING IN MEDULLARY CONCENTRATION GRADIENT:

Absorption of urea in the collecting tubules, under the influence of ADH and secretion in the loop of Henle contributes 50% of medullary concentration gradient.

OSMOTIC EQUILIBRATING DEVICE:

1. **WHEN ADH PLASMA LEVELS ARE INCREASED DURING NEGATIVE WATER BALANCE:**
   The collecting ducts become highly permeable to water and water moves out of the collecting duct into hyperosmotic medullary interstitium down its chemical gradient until the collecting duct lumen and corresponding medullary interstitium have equal water concentrations. So much water leaves by the end of the collecting duct that urine volume is low (perhaps 500 ml/day) and the urine osmolarity is high (1200 mosmoles/liter. The kidneys have saved volume.

2. **WHEN ADH PLASMA LEVELS ARE REDUCED DURING POSITIVE WATER BALANCE:**
   Water is trapped in the collecting ducts and some solute removal still occurs in the collecting ducts and therefore a very large volume of dilute urine (upto 100 mosmoles/liter) is formed.

ENDOCRINE FUNCTIONS OF KIDNEY:

1. **ERYTHROPOEITIN:** released by the interstitial cells in the peritubular bed in response to hypoxia.
2. **1, 25(OH)$_2$ VIT D:** Proximal tubule cells convert 25(OH) vitamin to 1, 25(OH)$_2$ vitamin D (Active form) by the enzyme 1αhydroxylase which is stimulated by PTH.
3. **RENIN:** secreted by JG cells in response to decreased renal arterial pressure and increased renal sympathetic discharge(β1 effect)
4. **PROSTAGLANDINS:** several prostaglandins (PGE2 and PGI2) are produces locally in the kidneys and cause vasodilation of both afferent and efferent arterioles. Vasodilatory effects of prostaglandins are protective for RBF. Thus prostaglandins modulate the vasoconstriction produced by the sympathetic nervous system and angiotensin II. Unopposed this vasoconstriction can cause a profound reduction in RBF, resulting in renal failure. NSAIDS inhibit synthesis of prostaglandins and therefore, interfere with the protective effects of prostaglandins on renal function following a hemorrhage.

HORMONES ACTING ON THE KIDNEY:

1. **ATRIAL NATRIURETIC PEPTIDE:** ANP and BNP both cause dilation of afferent arteriole and constriction of efferent arteriole: there is an overall decrease in renal vascular resistance and resulting increase in RBF. Dilation of afferent arteriole and

constriction of efferent arteriole both lead to increased GFR. It is secreted in response to increased atrial pressure causes increased GFR and increased sodium filtration with no compensatory sodium reabsorption in distal nephron. Net effect: Na loss and volume loss.

2. **PARATHYROID HORMONE:** secreted in response to decreased plasma Ca, increased plasma PO4 or decreased plasma 1, 25 (OH) $_2$.
It causes increased Ca reabsorption (DCT), decreased PO_4 reabsorption (PCT) and increased 1, 25(OH) $_2$ vitamin D production. Additional effect is increased Ca and PO_4 absorption from gut.

3. **RENIN:** In response to decreased blood volume angiotensinogen is converted to angiotensin 1 which is converted by Angiotensin converting enzyme in the lungs to angiotensin 2. This is synthesized in response to decreased B.P. The net effect is efferent arteriolar constriction leading to increased GFR and increased FF.

4. **ANGIOTENSIN II:** Following hemorrhage there is activation of renin angiotensinogen system leading to production of Angiotensin II which is a potent vasoconstrictor of both afferent and efferent arterioles that increases resistance and decrease blood flow and GFR.
LOW LEVELS OF ANGIOTENSIN II: Increase in GFR by constricting arteriole.
HIGH LEVELS OF ANGIOTENSIN II:
Decrease in GFR by constricting afferent and efferent arteriole.

5. **ALDOSTERONE:** secreted in response to decreased blood volume (via ATII) and increased

plasma K^+: causes increased sodium reabsorption, increased K+ secretion and increased H^+ secretion.

6. **<u>ADH (VASOPRESSIN):</u>** secreted in response to increased plasma osmolarity and decreased blood volume. It binds to receptors on principal cells causing increased number of water channels and increased H_2O reabsorption.

PHYSIOLOGY OF MICTURITION:

Micturition is the process by which urinary bladder empties when filled. The main physiological events of micturition are:

1. Filling of urinary bladder.
2. Emptying of urinary bladder.

FILLING OF URINARY BLADDER:

TRANSPORT OF URINE THROUGH URETERS:

As urine collects in the renal pelvis, the pressure in the pelvis increases and initiates a peristaltic contraction beginning in the pelvis and spreading along the ureter to force urine towards the bladder.

CAPACITY OF THE BLADDER:

Physiological capacity of the bladder varies with age, being:

20-50ml at birth, about 200 ml at one year and 600 ml in young adult males. In all cases the physiological capacity is about twice at which the first desire to void is felt.

VOLUME AND PRESSURE CHANGES IN BLADDER DURING FILLING:

The normal bladder is completely empty at the end of micturition and the intravesical pressure is equal to the intrabdominal pressure. As the bladder is filled up, it adjusts its tone and a fairly large volume of urine can be accommodated with minimal alterations in the intravesical pressure.

CYSTOMETRY:

Refers to a process of studying the relationship between the intravesical volume and pressure, the cystometrogram refers to graphical record of this relationship.

NORMAL CYSTOGRAM: shows three phases of filling:

PHASE IA: It is the initial phase of filling in which pressure rises from 0-10 cm of H2O, when about 50 ml of fluid is collected in the bladder.

PHASE IB: It is the phase of plateau which lasts till the bladder volume is 400ml. During this phase the pressure in the bladder does not change much and remains approximately at 10 cm H2O. This is because of adaptation of urinary bladder by relaxation.

PHASE II: This phase starts beyond 400ml volume when pressure begins to rise markedly, triggering the micturition reflex. Normally the voiding contractions raises the intravesical pressure by about 20-40 cm 0f H2O. If voiding is avoided, the pressure rises from 10cm of H2O onward. Beyond 600 ml the urge to void urine becomes almost unbearable.

EMPTYING OF THE BLADDER:

Emptying of the bladder is basically a reflex called the micturition reflex, which is controlled by supraspinal centers and is assisted by contraction of perineal and abdominal muscles. Therefore, emptying the urinary bladder focuses on:

1. Micturition reflex.
2. Voluntary control of micturition

3. Role of perineal and abdominal muscles in micturition.

MICTURITION REFLEX:

<u>INITIATION</u>: Micturition reflex is initiated by stimulation of the stretch receptors located in wall of urinary bladder.

<u>STIMULUS</u>: Filling of the bladder by 300 to 400 ml of urine in adults constitutes the adequate stimulus for the micturition reflex to occur.

<u>AFFERENTS:</u> The afferents from the stretch receptors in the detrusor muscle and urethra travel along the pelvic splanchnic nerves and enter the spinal cord through dorsal roots to S2, S3 and S4 segments to reach the sacral micturition center.

<u>SACRAL MICTURITION CENTER:</u> Is formed by the sacral detrusor nucleus and sacral pudendal nucleus.

<u>EFFERENTS</u>: Efferents arising from the sacral detrusor nucleus are the preganglionic parasympathetic fibers which relay in the ganglia near or within the bladder and urethra. The postganglionic parasympathetic fibers are excitatory to the detrusor muscle and inhibitory to internal sphincter.

<u>RESPONSE:</u> Once micturition reflex is initiated, it is self-regenerative, i-e initial contraction of bladder wall. Further activates the receptors to increase sensory impulses (afferents) from the bladder and urethra which cause further increase in reflex contraction of detrusor muscle of the bladder. The cycle thus keeps on repeating itself again and again until the bladder has reached a strong degree of contraction.

Once the micturition reflex becomes powerful enough this cause another reflex which passes through pudendal nerves to external sphincter to cause its inhibition. If this inhibition is more potent than the voluntary constrictor signals from brain, then urination will not occur. If not so, urination will not occur unless the bladder fills still more and micturition reflex becomes more powerful.

VOLUNTARY CONTROL OF MICTURITION:

The micturition reflex is a spinal reflex facilitated and inhibited by higher brain centers (supraspinal centers). In infants and young children, micturition is purely a reflex action.

Voluntary control is gradually acquired as a learned ability of the toilet training. Once voluntary control is acquired, the supraspinal control exerts final control of micturition by following means:

The higher centers keep the micturition reflex partially inhibited all the time except when it is desired to micturate. When the convenient time to urinate present, the higher centers facilitate the sacral micturition center (SMC) to initiate a micturition reflex and inhibit the external urinary sphincter so that urination can occur.

Supraspinal control centers: which control the micturition reflex (a completely automatic cord reflex) include pontine micturition center (PMC) and supraspinal centers.

ROLE OF PERINEAL AND ABDOMINAL MUSCLES IN MICTURITION:

1. At the onset of micturition, the levator ani and perineal muscles are relaxed, thereby shortening post-urethra and decreasing urethral resistance.
2. The diaphragm descends.

3. The abdominal muscles contract, accelerating the filling of urine by raising the intrabdominal pressure which in turn secondarily increases the intravesical pressure thereby increasing the flow of urine.

4.

ACID BASE DISORDERS:

Disturbance of blood pH can be caused by a primary disturbance of HCO_3 concentration or a primary disturbance of PCO_2.

METABOLIC: acid base disorders are primary disorders involving HCO_3

METABOLIC ACIDOSIS: Decrease in HCO_3, caused by gain of fixed acid H^+ or loss of HCO_3

METABOLIC ALKALOSIS: Increase in HCO_3, caused by loss of fixed acid H^+ or gain of HCO_3

RESPIRATORY: acid base disturbances are primary disorders of PCO_2.

RESPIRATORY ACIDOSIS: Increase PCO_2 caused by hypoventilation.

RESPIRATORY ALKALOSIS: Decrease PCO_2 caused by hyperventilation.

RULE OF THUMB:
1. If primary disturbance is metabolic, respiratory compensation will occur.
2. If primary disturbance is respiratory, renal compensation will occur.
3. The compensatory response is in the same direction as the original disturbance.

DISORDER	PCO2	H+	HCO3	RESPIRATORY COMPENSATION	RENAL COMPENSATION/
METABOLIC ACIDOSIS	DECREASED	INCREASED	DECREASED	HYPERVENTILATION	INCREASED HCO_3 REABSORPTION
METABOLIC ALKALOSIS	INCREASED	DECREASED	INCREASED	HYPOVENTILATION	DECREASED HCO_3 REABSORPTION
RESPIRATORY ACIDOSIS	INCREASED	INCREASED	INCREASED	NONE	INCREASED HCO_3 REABSORPTION
RESPIRATORY ALKALOSIS	DECREASED	DECREASED	DECREASED	NONE	DECREASED HCO_3 REABSORPTION

ANION GAP OF PLASMA:

The major cation if Na and major anion is HCO_3 and Cl. When the Na concentration is compared with the sum of HCO3 and Cl, there is an anion gap that is Na concentration is greater than the sum of HCO3 and Cl concentration. The unmeasured anions that make up the "gap" are plasma proteins, phosphate, citrate and sulphate.

Anion gap= Na-(HCO3 +Cl)

= (140)-(24+105)

= 11meq/l (8-16meq/l)

Anion gap is used to differentiate the cause of metabolic acidosis.

1. NORMAL ANION GAP; if HCO3 is replaced by Cl anion gap is normal ,e.g. Diarrhea and renal tubular acidosis
2. INCREASED ANION GAP; if HCO3 is replaced by unmeasured anions , the anion gap is increased ,e.g. DKA, Lactic acidosis, salicylate poisoning ,methanol poisoning , ethylene glycol poisoning and chronic renal failure.

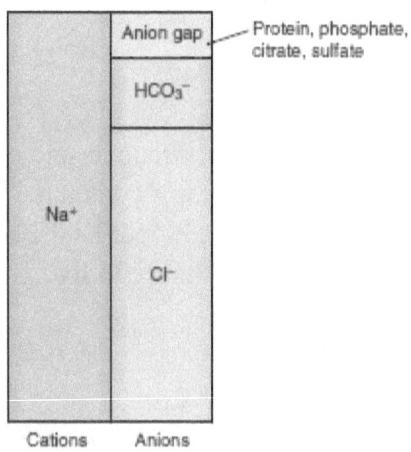

DIALYSIS AND TRANSPLANTATION:

DIALYSIS:

The process of removing waste products and excess fluid form the body. Dialysis is necessary when the kidneys are not able to adequately filter the blood. Dialysis allows the patients with kidney failure a chance to live productive lives.

TYPES:

HEMODIALYSIS AND PERITONEAL DIALYSIS:

Hemodialysis uses a special type of filter to remove excess waste products and water from the blood. Peritoneal dialysis uses a fluid that is placed into the patient's abdominal cavity through a special plastic tube to remove excess waste products and fluid from the body.

Peritoneal dialysis uses the peritoneum as a natural permeable membrane through which water and solutes can equilibrate. It is less physiologically stressful than hemodialysis, does not require vascular access, can be performed at home and allows patients much greater flexibility.

PRINCIPLES OF DIALYSIS:

Dialysis works on the principles of diffusion of solutes and ultrafiltration of fluid across a semi-permeable membrane. Blood flows by one side of a semipermeable membrane and a dialysate flows by opposite direction. A semi-permeable membrane is a thin layer of material that contains various sized holes or pores. Smaller solutes and fluid pass through the membrane, but the membrane blocks the passage of larger particles.

Patient's blood is pumped into a dialyzer containing two fluid compartments configured as bundles of hollow fiber capillary tubes. Blood in the first compartment is pumped along one side of semi-permeable membrane while a crystalloid solution is pumped along other side, in a separate compartment in opposite direction. Concentration gradients of solute between blood and dialysate lead desired changes in patient's serum solutes such as reduction in BUN and creatinine, an increase in HCO_3 and equilibration of Na, Cl, K and Mg. The dialysate compartment is under negative pressure relative to blood compartment to prevent filtration of dialysate with blood stream and to remove the excess fluid from the patient. The dialyzed blood is returned to the patient.

INDICATIONS OF URGENT DIALYSIS:

1. Severe acidosis
2. Pulmonary edema
3. Hyperkalemia
4. Uremic pericarditis
5. Severe uremic symptoms
    a. Encephalopathy
    b. Vomiting.

CONTRAINDICATIONS OF DIALYSIS:
A. Unco-operative patient
B. Hemodynamically unstable patient

TRANSPLANTATION:
INDICATIONS:
1. Organ failure

CONTRAINDICATIONS OF LIVING DONOR:
1. Mental disease.
2. Diseased organ
3. Mortality and morbidity risk

4. ABO incompatibility
5. Cross matching incompatibility.
6. Transmissible disease.

DIFFERENT TYPES OF REJECTION:
1. **HYPERACUTE:** it occurs within minutes and hours, observed typically with xenografts. It is caused by pre-formed antibodies directed to components of the grafts typically endothelial cells. Such antibodies activate complement system and endothelial injury leads to platelet adhesion and thrombosis. The graft thus never becomes vascularized.
2. **ACUTE:** this occurs over a period of 7-10 days (primary response) or 2-3 days (in secondary response). It involves both cell-mediated and antibody mediated immunity. The cell mediated reaction leads to necrosis of parenchyma and is associated with lymphocyte and macrophages infiltrates. Cell lysis mediated by cytotoxic lymphocyte constitutes the dominant component of allograft rejection. The antibody mediated reaction leads to necrosis of individual endothelial cells and to vasculitis rather than thrombosis.
3. **CHRONIC:** this occurs after weeks or months and is characterized by fibrosis and arteriosclerosis. Arteriosclerosis is common in kidney and heart transplant and is major cause of late graft failure. It is due to extensive intimal proliferation of smooth muscle.

INTRODUCTION TO ENDOCRINOLOGY:

The endocrine system in concert with the nervous system is responsible for homeostasis. Growth, development, reproduction, blood pressure, concentration of ions and other substances in blood, and even behavior are regulated by the endocrine system. Endocrine physiology involves the secretion of hormones and their subsequent actions on the target tissues.

A hormone is a chemical substance that is classified as a peptide, steroid or amine. Hormones are secreted in the circulation in small amounts and delivered to target tissues, where they produce physiologic responses. Hormones are synthesized and secreted by endocrine cells usually found in the endocrine glands.

The classical endocrine glands are the hypothalamus, anterior and posterior lobes of the pituitary, thyroid, parathyroid, adrenal cortex, adrenal medulla, gonads, placenta and pancreas. The kidney is also considered to be an endocrine gland, and endocrine cells are found throughout the gastrointestinal gland.

CLASSIFICATION OF HORMONES:

DEPENDING UPON THE CHEMICAL NATURE:

1. **AMINES OR AMINO ACID DERIVATIVES:**
    a. Catecholamines (epinephrine and norepinephrine)
    b. Throxine (T4) and Triiodothyronine(T3)
2. **PROTEINS AND POLYPEPTIDES:**
    a. Posterior pituitary hormones(ADH and oxytocin)

      b. Insulin
      c. Glucagon
      d. Parathormone
      e. Other anterior pituitary hormones.
3. <u>STEROID HORMONES:</u>
      a. Glucocorticoids
      b. Mineralocorticoid
      c. Sex steroids
      d. Vitamin D

<u>DEPENDING UPON THE MECHANISM OF ACTION:</u>

1. <u>GROUP 1 HORMONES:</u> These act by binding to intracellular receptor and mediate their actions via formation of a hormone receptor complex. These include steroid, retinoid and thyroid hormones.
2. <u>GROUP 2 HORMONES:</u> These involve second messenger to mediate their effect. Depending upon the chemical nature of the second messengers, group II hormones are further divided into 4 subgroups, A, B, C and D.

GROUP	SECOND MESSENGER	HORMONES
GROUP II A	Cyclic AMP	ACTH ADH Angiotensin II Calcitonin CRH Catecholamine (beta 2 adrenergic) FSH Glucagon LH PTH

		Somatostatin TSH
GROUP II B	Cyclic GMP	ANP NO
GROUP II C	Calcitonin phosphatidyl inositol/or both	Ach Catecholamines (alpha 1 adrenergic) Gastrin Oxytocin TRH GnRH PDGF
GROUP II D	Kinase or phosphatase cascade	HCS Erythropoietin GH Insulin IGF NGF Prolactin

MECHANISM OF ACTION:

The main mechanisms of action of hormones are:

a. Action through change in membrane permeability.
b. Action through effect on gene expression by binding of hormones to intracellular receptors.
c. Action through secondary messengers which activate intracellular enzymes when hormones combine with membrane receptors.
d. Action through tyrosine kinase activation.

ACTION THROUGH CHANGE IN MEMBRANE PERMEABILITY:

Certain hormone bind with receptors present in the cell membrane(external receptors) and cause conformational change in the proteins of the receptors, this results in either opening or closing of the ion channels (such as Na channels ,K channels and Ca channels)The movement of the ions causes the subsequent effect, e.g adrenaline, noradrenaline act by this mechanism.

ACTION THROUGH EFFECT ON GENE EXPRESSION BY BINDING OF HORMONES WITH INTRACELLULAR RECEPTORS:

Group 1 hormones act by their effect on the gene expression include steroid hormones, retinoids and thyroid hormones. These hormones are lipophilic in nature and can easily pass through the cell membrane. They act through intracellular receptors located in the cytosol or in the nucleus.

a. <u>TRANSPORT</u>: After secretion the hormone is carried to the target tissue on serum binding protein.
b. <u>INTERNALIZATION:</u> Being lipophilic the hormone easily diffuses through the plasma membrane.
c. <u>RECEPTOR HORMONE COMPLEX</u>: It is formed by binding of hormone to the specific receptor inside the cell.
d. <u>CONFORMATIONAL CHANGE</u>: Occurs in receptor proteins leading to activation of receptors.
e. The activated receptor hormone complex then diffuses into the nucleus and binds on the specific region on the DNA known as Hormone responsive elements (HRE), which initiates gene expression.

f. Binding of the receptor hormone complex to DNA alters the rate of transcription of messenger RNA (mRNA).
g. The mRNA diffuses in the cytoplasm, where it promotes the translation process at the ribosomes. In this way new proteins are formed which result in specific responses. Some of the new proteins synthesized are enzymes.

ACTION THROUGH SECOND MESSENGERS:

The peptides and biogenic amines are two principal classes of hormones which act through second messengers and are classified as group II hormones. Such hormones are also called first messengers. The release of the second messengers is mediated by GTP binding protein also called G proteins.

COUPLING BY G PROTEINS:

Group II hormones are water soluble and bind to the plasma membrane of the target cell via cell surface receptors. The hormone bearing receptor then interacts with a G protein and activates it by binding GTP.

There are two classes of G proteins: stimulatory G protein (Gs) and inhibitory G protein (Gi). In its activated ("on") state, the G protein interacts with one or more of the effector protein (most of which are enzymes or ion channels such as adenylyl cyclase; Ca or K channels or phospholipase C, A2 or D) to activate or inhibit them.

The changed effector molecules, in turn, generate second messenger that mediates the hormone intracellular action.

SECOND MESSENGER SYSTEMS:

The second messenger systems that are activated through coupling of hormone receptor complexes by G protein include:

a. Adenylyl cyclase –cAMP system
b. Guanyl cyclase- cGMP system
c. Membrane phospholipase- phospholipid system
d. Calcium calmodulin system.

MECHANISM OF ACTION OF HORMONES VIA TYROSINE KINASE ACTIVATION:

Certain hormones act by activating tyrosine kinase system and have been classified as group –II D hormones. This mechanism of signal generation from plasma membrane receptors does not require G protein intermediaries. These receptors have an extracellular hormone binding portion, a single trans membrane portion and an intra cytoplasmic C terminal portion.

The activation of tyrosine kinase occurs by two mechanisms:

1. Hormone receptors possessing intrinsic tyrosine activity, e.g those for insulin and epidermal growth factor(EGF) involving following steps:
   a. Binding of hormone to the receptor changes its conformation and exposes sites on its intracellular portion that are capable of receptor autophosphorylation at specific tyrosine sites.
   b. As a result, the receptor itself becomes tyrosine kinase that phosphorylates tyrosine residue on intracellular substrates.

c. This latter activity sets into motion a cascade of events leading to enzyme activation and gene transcription.
2. Hormone receptors that do not possess intrinsic tyrosine kinase activity, e.g, those for growth hormones, cytokines etc acts as follows:
   a. Hormone binding to the extracellular portion of the receptor changes it intracytoplasmic tail.
   b. The changes produced in intracytoplasmic tail of receptor exposes sites which attract and dock the intracytoplasmic tyrosine kinases (such as JAK kinases and STAT kinases) and then activate them.
   c. The activated intracytoplasmic tyrosine kinases phosphorylate cytoplasmic substrates such as transcription factor proteins and ultimately modulate gene expression.

HORMONE SYNTHESIS:

Hormones are categorized in one of the three classes: peptides and proteins, steroids, or amines. Each class differs in its biosynthetic pathway: Peptides and protein hormones are synthesized from amino acids; steroid hormones are derived from cholesterol; and amine hormones are derivatives of tyrosine.

PEPTIDE AND PROTEIN HORMONE SYNTHESIS:

Most hormones are peptides and proteins in nature. The biosynthetic pathways are familiar from biochemistry. The primary amino acid sequence of the peptide is dictated by specific messenger ribonucleotide (mRNA), which has been transcribed from the gene for that hormone.

1. In the nucleus, the gene is transcribed into an **mRNA.** Generally, a single gene is responsible for directing the primary structure of each peptide hormone. (Because the genes for almost all peptide hormones have been cloned, recombinant DNA technology makes it possible to synthesize human peptide hormones.)
2. The mRNA is transferred to the cytoplasm and translated on the **ribosomes** to the first protein product, a **preprohormone.** Translation of the mRNA begins with a signal peptide at the N terminus. Translation ceases, and the signal peptide attaches to receptors on the endoplasmic reticulum via "docking proteins." Translation then continues on the endoplasmic reticulum until the entire peptide sequence is produced (i.e., the preprohormone).

3. The signal peptide is removed in the **endoplasmic reticulum,** converting the preprohormone to a **prohormone.** The prohormone contains thecomplete hormone sequence plus other peptide sequences, which will be removed in a final step. Some of the "other" peptide sequences in the prohormone are necessary for proper folding of the hormone (e.g., formation of intramolecular linkages).
4. The prohormone is transferred to the **Golgi apparatus,** where it is packaged in secretory vesicles. In the secretory vesicles, proteolytic enzymes cleave peptide sequences from the prohormone to produce the final **hormone.** Other functions of the Golgi apparatus include glycosylation and phosphorylation of the hormone.
5. The final hormone is stored in **secretory vesicles** until the endocrine cell is stimulated. For example, parathyroid hormone (PTH) is synthesized and stored in vesicles in the chief cells of the parathyroid gland. The stimulus for secretion of PTH is low extracellular calcium (Ca^{2+}) concentration. When sensors on the parathyroid gland detect a low extracellular Ca^{2+} concentration, the secretory vesicles are translocated to the cell membrane, where they extrude PTH into the blood by exocytosis. The other constituents of the secretory vesicles, including copeptides and cleavage enzymes, are extruded with PTH.

PEPTIDE HORMONE SYNTHESIS

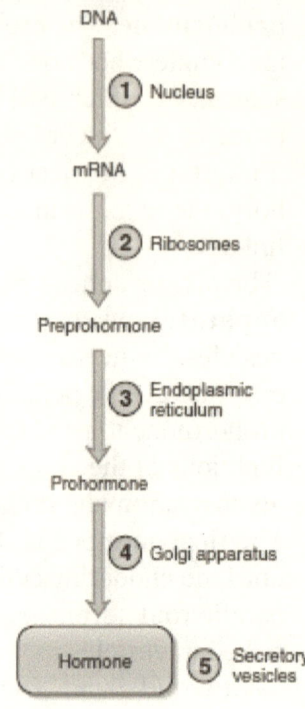

STEROID HORMONE SYNTHESIS:

Steroid hormones are synthesized and secreted by the adrenal cortex, gonads, corpus luteum, and placenta. The steroid hormones are cortisol, aldosterone, estradiol and estriol, progesterone, testosterone, and 1,25-dihydroxycholecalciferol. All steroid hormones are derivatives of **cholesterol,** which is modified by removal or addition of side chains, hydroxylation, or aromatization of the steroid nucleus.

AMINE HORMONE SYNTHESIS:

The amine hormones are catecholamines (epinephrine, norepinephrine, and dopamine) and thyroid hormones. The amine hormones are derivatives of the amino acid **tyrosine.**

REGUALTION OF HORMONE SYTHESIS:

To maintain homeostasis, the secretion of hormones must be turned on and off as needed. Adjustments in secretory rates may be accomplished by neural mechanisms or by feedback mechanisms.

Neural mechanisms are illustrated by the secretion of catecholamines, where preganglionic sympathetic nerves synapse on the adrenal medulla and, when stimulated, cause secretion of catecholamines into the circulation.

Feedback mechanisms are more common than neural mechanisms. The term "feedback" means that some element of the physiologic response to a hormone "feeds back," either directly or indirectly, on the endocrine gland that secreted the hormone, changing its secretion rate. Feedback can be negative or positive. Negative feedback is the most important and common mechanism for regulating hormone secretion; positive feedback is rare.

Negative Feedback

The principles of negative feedback underlie the homeostatic regulation of virtually all organ systems. For example, A decrease in arterial blood pressure is detected by baroreceptors, which activate coordinated mechanisms that increase blood pressure. As blood pressure returns to normal, a disturbance is no longer sensed by the baroreceptors and those mechanisms previously activated will be turned off. The more sensitive the feedback mechanism, the smaller the "excursions" of blood pressure above or below normal. In endocrine systems, negative feedback means that *some feature of hormone action, directly or indirectly, inhibits further secretion of the hormone.* Negative feedback loops are illustrated in Figure 1 For illustrative purposes, the hypothalamus is shown in relation to the anterior pituitary, which is shown in relation to a peripheral endocrine gland. In the figure, the hypothalamus secretes a releasing hormone, which stimulates secretion of an anterior pituitary hormone. The anterior pituitary hormone then acts on a peripheral endocrine gland (e.g., the testis) to cause secretion of the hormone (e.g., testosterone), which acts on target tissues (e.g.skeletal muscle) to produce physiologic actions. The hormones "feed back" on the anterior pituitary and the hypothalamus to inhibit their hormonal secretions.

Long-loop feedback means that the hormone feeds back *all the way* to the hypothalamic-pituitary axis. **Short-loop feedback** means that the anterior pituitary hormone feeds back on the hypothalamus to inhibit secretion of hypothalamic-releasing hormone. Not shown in the figure is a third possibility called **ultrashort-loop feedback,** in which the hypothalamic hormone inhibits its own secretion (e.g., growth hormone–releasing hormone [GHRH] inhibits GHRH secretion). The net result of any version of negative feedback is that when hormone levels are judged (by their physiologic actions) to be adequate or high, further secretion of the hormone is inhibited. When hormone levels are judged to be inadequate or low, secretion of the hormone is stimulated. There are other examples of negative feedback that do not utilize the hypothalamic-pituitary axis. For example, **insulin** regulates blood glucose concentration. In turn, insulin secretion is turned on or off by changes in the blood glucose concentration. Thus, when blood glucose concentration is high, insulin secretion from the pancreas is turned on; insulin then acts on its target tissues (liver, muscle, and adipose) to decrease the blood glucose concentration back toward normal. low enough, insulin is no longer needed and its secretion is turned off.

Positive Feedback

Positive feedback is uncommon. With positive feedback, some feature of hormone action causes *more* secretion of the hormone (see Fig. 1) When compared with negative feedback, which is self-limiting, positive feedback is self-augmenting. Although rare in biologic systems, when positive feedback does occur, it leads to an explosive event. A nonhormonal example of positive feedback is the opening of nerve sodium (Na^+) channels during the **upstroke of the action potential.** Depolarization opens voltage-sensitive Na+ channels and causes Na+ entry into the cell, which leads to more depolarization and more Na+ entry. This self-reinforcing process produces the rapid, explosive upstroke.

In hormonal systems, the primary example of positive feedback is the effect of **estrogen** on the secretion of follicle-stimulating hormone (**FSH**) and luteinizing hormone (**LH**) by the anterior pituitary at the midpoint of the menstrual cycle. During the follicular phase of the menstrual cycle, the ovaries secrete estrogen, which acts on the anterior pituitary to produce a rapid burst of FSH and LH secretion. FSH and LH have two effects on the ovaries: ovulation *and* stimulation of estrogen secretion. Thus, estrogen secreted from the ovaries acts on the anterior pituitary to cause secretion of FSH and LH, and these anterior pituitary hormones cause *more* estrogen secretion. In this example, the explosive event is the burst of FSH and LH that precedes ovulation.

A second example of hormonal positive feedback is **oxytocin**. Dilation of the cervix causes the posterior pituitary to secrete oxytocin. In turn, oxytocin stimulates uterine contraction, which causes further dilation of the cervix. In this example, the explosive event is parturition, the delivery of the fetus.

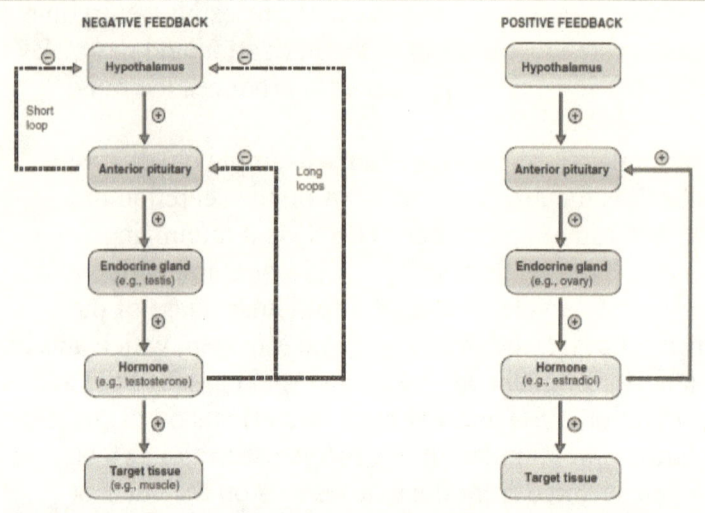

The responsiveness of a target tissue to a hormone is expressed in the dose-response relationship in which the magnitude of response is correlated with hormone concentration. As the hormone concentration increases, the response usually increases and then levels off. Sensitivity is defined as the hormone concentration that produces 50% of the maximal response. If more hormones is required to produce 50% of the maximal response, then there has been a decrease in sensitivity of the target tissue. If fewer hormones is required, there has been an increase in sensitivity of the target tissue. The responsiveness or sensitivity of a target tissue can be changed in one of two ways: by changing the number of receptors or by changing the affinity of the receptors for the hormone. The greater the number of receptors for a hormone, the greater the maximal response. The higher the affinity of the receptor for the hormone, the greater the likelihood of a response. A change in the number or affinity of receptors is called down-regulation or up-regulation. Downregulation means that the number of receptors or the affinity of the receptors for the hormone has decreased. Up-regulation means that the number or the affinity of the receptors has increased. Hormones may downregulate or up-regulate their own receptors in target tissues and even may regulate receptors for other hormones.

Down-Regulation:

Down-regulation is a mechanism in which a hormone decreases the number or affinity of its receptors in a target tissue. Down-regulation may occur by decreasing the synthesis of new receptors, by increasing the degradation of existing receptors, or by inactivating receptors. The purpose of down-regulation is to reduce the sensitivity of the target tissue when hormone levels are high for an extended period of time. As down regulation occurs, the response to hormone declines, although hormone levels remain high. An example of down-regulation is the effect of progesterone on its own receptor in the uterus. Down-regulation can also refer to a hormone's effect on receptors for other related hormones. This type of down-regulation also is illustrated by progesterone. In the uterus, progesterone down-regulates its own receptor and down-regulates the receptors for estrogen. A second example of this type of down-regulation is seen in the thyroid system: Triiodothyronine, or T3, decreases the sensitivity of thyrotropin-releasing hormone (TRH) receptors in the anterior pituitary. The overall effect is that chronically high levels of T3 reduce the overall responsiveness of the hypothalamic-pituitary thyroid axis.

Up-Regulation:

Up-regulation of receptors is a mechanism in which a hormone increases the number or affinity of its receptors. Up-regulation may occur by increasing synthesis of new receptors, decreasing degradation of existing receptors, or activating receptors. For example, prolactin increases the number of its receptors in the breast, growth hormone increases the number of its
receptors in skeletal muscle and liver, and estrogen increases the number of its receptors in the uterus. A hormone also can up-regulate the receptors for other hormones. For example, estrogen not only up-regulates its

own receptor in the uterus, but it also up-regulates the receptors for LH in the ovaries.

ENDOCRINE ROLE OF HYPOTHALAMUS: The hypothalamus is a specialized center in the brain that functions as a master coordinator of hormonal action. It is the part of the brain situated below the thalamus and is very closely connected to the pituitary gland. Thus hypothalamus provides an important link between the endocrine system and the nervous system.

The hypothalamus serves its endocrine function through the neurosecretory cells which are arranged in different nuclei of hypothalamus.

The main functions of hypothalamus are control of:

1. Control of anterior pituitary function
2. Control of posterior pituitary function

CONTROL OF ANTERIOR PITUITARY FUNCTION:

Hypothalamus controls the functioning of anterior pituitary through various hypothalamic-hypophysiotropic hormones i-e various hypothalamic releasing and inhibiting hormones. The hypothalamic releasing and inhibiting hormones are released in response to neural stimuli.

Various hypothalamic releasing and inhibiting hormones include:

   a. Growth hormone releasing hormone(GHRH)
   b. Growth hormone inhibiting hormone (GRIH) also called Somatostatin.
   c. Corticotropin releasing hormone(CRH)
   d. Thyrotropin releasing hormone(TRH)
   e. Gonadotropin releasing hormone(GnRH)

f. Prolactin releasing hormone(PRH)
g. Prolactin inhibiting hormone(PIH)

CONTROL OF POSTERIOR PITUITARY FUNCTION:

The large magnocellular neurosecretory cells forming the supraoptic and paraventricular nuclei of hypothalamus are responsible for synthesis of the two posterior pituitary peptide hormones (oxytocin and ADH) These reach the posterior pituitary through the hypothalamic-hypophyseal tract.

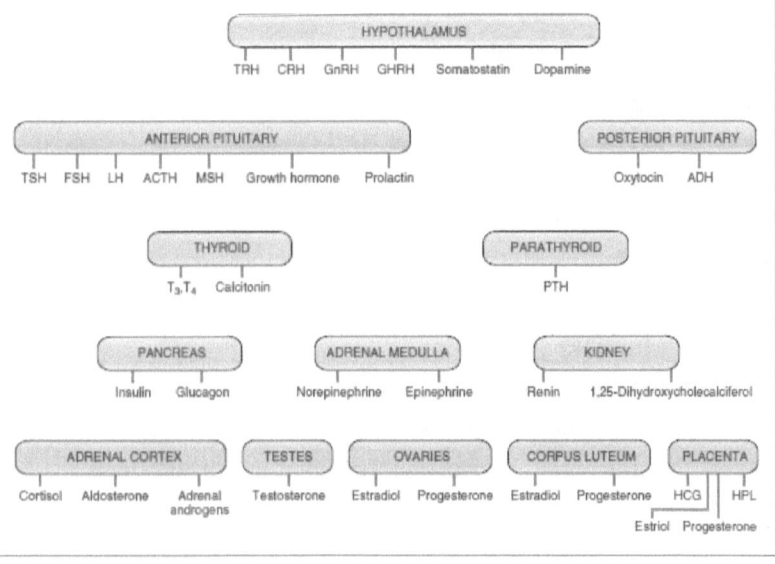

HORMONES OF THE ANTERIOR LOBE OF THE PITUITARY:

These are Growth hormone, prolactin, thyroid stimulating hormone (TSH), LH, Follicle stimulating hormone (FSH), and adrenocorticotropic hormone (ACTH).

1. <u>TSH, LH, and FSH:</u> They all belong to the same glycoprotein family. Each has an alpha subunit and a beta subunit. The alpha subunits are identical. The beta subunits are different and are responsible for the unique biological activity of each hormone.
2. <u>ACTH, MELANOCYTE STIMULATING HORMONE (MSH), BETA –LIPOTROPIN AND BETA ENDORPHIN:</u> These are derived from a single precursor proopiomelanocortin (POMC). Alpha MSH and beta MSH are produced in the intermediary lobe, which is rudimentary in adult humans.
3. <u>GROWTH HORMONE:</u> It is the most important hormone for normal growth to adult size. It is a single –chain polypeptide that is homologous to prolactin and human placental lactogen.
    a. <u>REGULATION OF GROWTH HORMONE SECRETION:</u>
        (I) <u>HYPOTHALAMIC CONTROL-GHRH AND SOMATOSTATIN:</u> GHRH stimulates the synthesis and secretion of growth hormone while Somatostatin inhibits the secretion of growth hormone by blocking the response of the anterior pituitary to GHRH.

- (II) **NEGATIVE FEEDBACK CONTROL BY SOMATOMEDINS:** Somatomedins are produced when growth hormone acts on target tissues and inhibits the secretion of growth hormone by acting directly on the anterior pituitary and by stimulating the secretion of Somatostatin from the hypothalamus.
- (III) **NEGATIVE FEED BACK CONTROL BY GHRH AND GROWTH HORMONE:** GHRH inhibits its own secretion from the hypothalamus. Growth hormone also inhibits its own secretion by stimulating the secretion of Somatostatin from the hypothalamus.
  b. **SECRETION IS INCREASED BY:** Sleep, stress, hormones related to puberty, starvation, exercise and hypoglycemia.
  c. **SECRETION IS DECREASED BY:** Somatostatin, somatomedins, obesity, hyperglycemia and pregnancy.
  d. **ACTIONS OF GROWTH HORMONE:**
     - (i) In the liver, growth hormone generates the production of somatomedins (IGF), which serve as the intermediaries of several physiologic actions.
     - (ii) **DIRECT ACTIONS OF GROWTH HORMONE:**
        1. Decrease uptake of glucose in the cells (diabetogenic)
        2. Increased lipolysis

3. Increased protein synthesis in the muscles and increased lean body mass.
4. Increased production of IGF

(iii) ACTIONS OF GROWTH HORMOONE VIA IGF:
1. Increase protein synthesis in the chondrocytes and increased linear growth (pubertal growth spurt)
2. Increased protein synthesis in the muscles and increased lean body mass
3. Increased protein synthesis in most organs and increased organ size.

e. MECAHNISM OF ACTION OF GH:
(I) The IGF receptor has tyrosine kinase activity similar to insulin receptor
(II) Growth hormone binds to the extracellular domain of the receptor.
(III) The intracellular side of the receptor does not have tyrosine kinase activity but is non –covalently associated with tyrosine kinase (e.g Janus family of receptor associated tyrosine kinase, JAK).
(IV) Binding of growth hormone causes dimerization of the receptor and activation of tyrosine kinase in the associated protein (e.g JAK).
(V) Targets of the JAK include signal transducers and activators of transcription (STAT) which causes

transcription of new mRNAs and new protein synthesis.

(VI) ## PATHOPHYSIOLOGY OF GROWTH HORMONE:

1. ### GROWTH HORMONE DEFECIENCY:
   In children it causes failure to grow, short stature, mild obesity and delayed puberty.
   It can be caused by:
   a. Lack of anterior pituitary growth hormone
   b. Hypothalamic dysfunction(decreased GHRH)
   c. Failure to generate IGF in the liver
   d. Growth hormone receptor deficiency.

2. ### GROWTH HORMONE EXCESS:
   It can be treated with Somatostatin analogue (e.g. octreotide) which inhibits growth hormone secretion.
   Hyper secretion of growth hormone before puberty causes increased linear growth (GIGANTISM)
   Hyper secretion of growth hormone after puberty causes increased periosteal bone growth, increased organ size and glucose intolerance. (ACROMEGALY)

POSTERIOR PITUITARY HORMONES:

The posterior lobe of the pituitary secretes antidiuretic hormone (ADH) and oxytocin. Both ADH and oxytocin. Both ADH and oxytocin are neuropeptides, synthesized in cell bodies of hypothalamic neurons and secreted from nerve terminals in the posterior pituitary.

Synthesis and Secretion of Antidiuretic Hormone and Oxytocin

Synthesis and Processing

ADH and oxytocin are homologous **nonapeptides** (containing nine amino acids) (Figs.) that are synthesized in the supraoptic and paraventricular nuclei of the hypothalamus. The **ADH** neurons have their cell bodies primarily in the **supraoptic nuclei** of the hypothalamus. The **oxytocin** neurons have their cell bodies primarily in **paraventricular nuclei.** While primarily dedicated to producing ADH or oxytocin, each nucleus also produces the "other" hormoneSimilar genes located in close proximity on the chromosome direct synthesis of the preprohormones for ADH and oxytocin. The peptide precursor for ADH is **prepropressophysin,** which comprises a signal peptide, ADH, neurophysin II, and a glycoprotein. The precursor for oxytocin is **prepro-oxyphysin,** which comprises a signal peptide, oxytocin, and neurophysin I. In the Golgi apparatus, the signal peptides are removed from the *prepro*hormones to form the *pro*hormones, *pro*pressophysin and *pro*-oxyphysin, and the prohormones are packaged in secretory vesicles. The secretory vesicles, containing the prohormones, then travel down the axon of the neuron, through the hypothalamic-hypophysial tract, to the posterior pituitary.En route to the posterior pituitary, the neurophysins are cleaved from their respective prohormones within the secretory vesicles.

Secretion

The secretory vesicles that arrive at the posterior pituitary contain either ADH, neurophysin II, and glycoprotein *or* oxytocin and neurophysin I. Secretion is initiated when an action potential is transmitted from the cell body in the hypothalamus, down the axon to the nerve terminal in the posterior pituitary. When the nerve terminal is depolarized by the action potential, Ca2+ enters the terminal, causing exocytosis of the secretory granules containing ADH or oxytocin and their neurophysins. The secreted hormones enter nearby fenestrated capillaries and are carried to the systemic circulation, which delivers the hormones to their target tissues.

1. <u>ADH</u> :

It originates primarily in the **supraoptic nuclei** of the hypothalamus and regulates serum osmolarity by increasing the H2O permeability of the late distal tubules and collecting ducts.

  a. **Regulation of ADH secretion:**

FACTORS INCREASING ADH SECRETION	FACTORS DECREASING ADH SECRETION
INCREASED SERUM OSMOLARITY	DECREASED SERUM OSMOLARITY
VOLUME CONTRACTION	ETHANOL
PAIN	ANP
NAUSEA	ALPHA AGONISTS
HYPOGLYCEMIA	
NICOTINE,OPIATES, ANTINEOPLASTIC DRUGS	

Actions of ADH

(1) ↑ **H2O permeability (aquaporin 2, AQP2)** of the principal cells of the late distal tubule and collecting duct (via a **V2 receptor** and an adenylate cyclase–cAMP mechanism)

(2) **Constriction of vascular smooth muscle** (via a **V1 receptor** and an IP3/Ca2+ mechanism)

c. **Pathophysiology of ADH:**

	SERUM ADH	PLASMA OSMOLARITY	URINE OSMOLARITY	URINE FLOW RATE
PRIMARY POLYDIPSIA	DECREASED	DECREASED	HYPOOSMOTIC	HIGH
CENTRAL DIABETES INSIPIDUS	DECREASED	INCREASED	HYPOOSMOTIC	HIGH
NEOHROGENIC DIABETES INSIPIDUS	INCREASED	INCREASED	HYPOOSMOTIC	HIGH
WATER DEPRIVATION	INCREASED	HIGH NORMAL	HYPEROSMOTIC	LOW
SIADH	INCREASED	DECREASED	HYPEROSMOTIC	LOW

2. **Oxytocin**

It originates primarily in the **paraventricular nuclei** of the hypothalamus. It causes **ejection of milk from the breast** when stimulated by suckling.

a. Regulation of oxytocin secretion

(1) *Suckling*

It is the major stimulus for oxytocin secretion. Afferent fibers carry impulses from the nipple to the spinal cord. Relays in the hypothalamus trigger the release of oxytocin from the posterior pituitary.

The sight or sound of the infant may stimulate the hypothalamic neurons to secrete oxytocin, even in the absence of suckling.

(2) *Dilation of the cervix and orgasm:* It increases the secretion of oxytocin.

b. Actions of oxytocin

(1) *Contraction of myoepithelial cells in the breast*

Milk is forced from the mammary alveoli into the ducts and delivered to the infant.

(2) *Contraction of the uterus*

During pregnancy, oxytocin receptors in the uterus are up-regulated as parturition approaches, although the role of oxytocin in normal labor is uncertain. Oxytocin can be used to induce labor and **reduce postpartum bleeding**

REGULATION OF OXYTOCIN SECRETION:

FACTORS STMULATING OXYTOCIN SECRETION	FACTORS DECREASING OXYTOCIN SECRETION
SUCKLING	OPIODS(ENDORPHINS)
SIGHT,SMELL ,SOUND OF INFANT	
DILATION OF CERVIX	
ORGASM	

GROWTH HORMONE:

This hormone is released in a pulsatile manner.

Secretion is increased by:

1. Sleep.
2. Stress
3. Hormones related to puberty.
4. Starvation.
5. Exercise.
6. Hypoglycemia.

Secretion is decreased by:

1. Somatostatin.
2. Somatomedins.
3. Obesity.
4. Hyperglycemia.
5. Pregnancy.

Regulation of GH secretion:

A. Hypothalamic control.

It is controlled by:

1. GHRH stimulates GH secretion.
2. Somatostatin inhibits GH secretion.

B. Negative feedback control:
   a. Somatomedins inhibit directly Anterior pituitary.
   b. Stimulate secretion of Somatostatin.
   c. Somatomedins inhibit GH secretion.

3. NEGATIVE FEEDBACK CONTROL BY GHRH AND GH:
A. GHRH inhibits own secretion from Hypothalamus.
B. GH also inhibits own secretion by stimulating somatostatin from Hypothalamus.

ACTIONS OF HORMONES:

In Liver, growth hormone generates the production of somatomedins [insulin-like growth factors (IGF)], which serve as the intermediaries of several physiologic actions. The IGF receptor has tyrosine kinase activity, similar to the insulin receptor.
(1) *Direct actions of growth hormone*
(a) ↓ glucose uptake into cells (diabetogenic)
(b) ↑ lipolysis
(c) ↑ protein synthesis in muscle and ↑ lean body mass
(d) ↑ production of IGF
(2) *Actions of growth hormone via IGF*
(a) ↑ protein synthesis in chondrocytes and ↑ linear growth (pubertal growth spurt)
(b) ↑ protein synthesis in muscle and ↑ lean body mass
(c) ↑ protein synthesis in most organs and ↑ organ size

Pathophysiology of growth hormone:
(1) *Growth hormone deficiency:*
In children causes' failure to grow, short stature, mild obesity, and delayed puberty occurs.
It can be caused by:
(a) Lack of anterior pituitary growth hormone
(b) Hypothalamic dysfunction (↓ GHRH)
(c) Failure to generate IGF in the liver
(d) Growth hormone receptor deficiency
(2) *Growth hormone excess:*
It can be treated with somatostatin analogs (e.g., octreotide), which inhibit growth hormone secretion. Hypersecretion of growth hormone causes acromegaly.

(a) Before puberty, excess growth hormone causes increased linear growth (gigantism).
(b) After puberty, excess growth hormone causes increased periosteal bone growth, increased organ size, and glucose intolerance.

PROLACTIN:

It is the major hormone responsible for lactogenesis. It participates with estrogen in breast development. It is structurally homologous to growth hormone.

REGULATION OF PROLACTIN SECRETION:

1. **HYPOTHALAMIC CONTROL BY DOPAMINE AND THYROTROPIN RELEASING HORMONE(TRH):**
   Prolactin secretion is tonically inhibited by dopamine (prolactin inhibiting factor –PIF) secreted by hypothalamus. Thus, interruption of the hypothalamic pituitary tract causes increased secretion of prolactin and sustained lactation. TRH increases prolactin secretion.
2. **NEGATIVE FEEDBACK CONTROL:**
   Prolactin inhibits its own secretion by stimulating the hypothalamic release of dopamine.

FACTORS THAT INCREASE PROLACTIN SECRETION	FACTORS THAT DECREASE PROLACTIN SECRETION
ESTROGEN(PREGNANCY)	DOPAMINE
BREAST FEEDING	BROMOCRIPTINE(DOPAMINE AGONIST)
SLEEP	SOMATOSTATIN
STRESS	PROLACTIN(BY NEGATIVE

	FEEDBACK)
TRH	
DOPAMINE ANTAGONISTS	

ACTIONS OF PROLACTIN:
1. Stimulates milk production in the breast (casein, lactalbumin)
2. Stimulates breast development (in a supportive role with estrogen)
3. Inhibits ovulation by decreasing synthesis and release of gonadotrophin-releasing hormone (GnRH).
4. Inhibits spermatogenesis (by decreasing GnRH)

PATHPHYSIOLOGY OF PROLACTIN:

1. <u>PROLACTIN DEFICIENCY: DESTRUCTION OF ANTERIOR PITUITARY:</u> This results in failure to lactate.
2. <u>PROLACTIN EXCESS:</u> This results from hypothalamic destruction (due to loss of tonic "inhibitory" control by dopamine) or from prolactin secreting tumors (prolactinoma). This causes galactorrhea and decreased libido. It also results in failure to ovulate and amenorrhea because it inhibits GnRH secretion. It can be treated by bromocriptine, which reduces prolactin secretion by acting as a dopamine agonist.

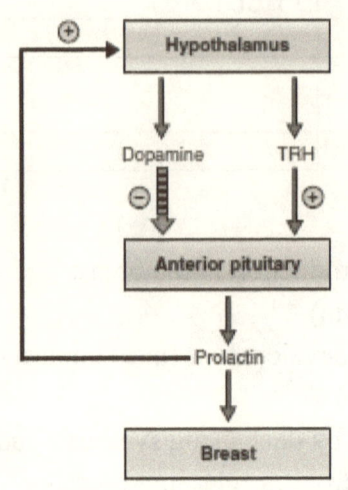

INSULIN:

It contains an A chain and a B chain, joined by two disulfide linkages. It is secreted by beta cells of islets of Langerhan's, which are present on the center of the islet.

Proinsulin is synthesized as a single –chain peptide. Within storage granules, a connecting peptide (C peptide) is removed by proteases to yield insulin. The C peptide is packaged and secreted along with insulin, and its concentration is used to monitor beta cell function in diabetic patients who are receiving exogenous insulin.

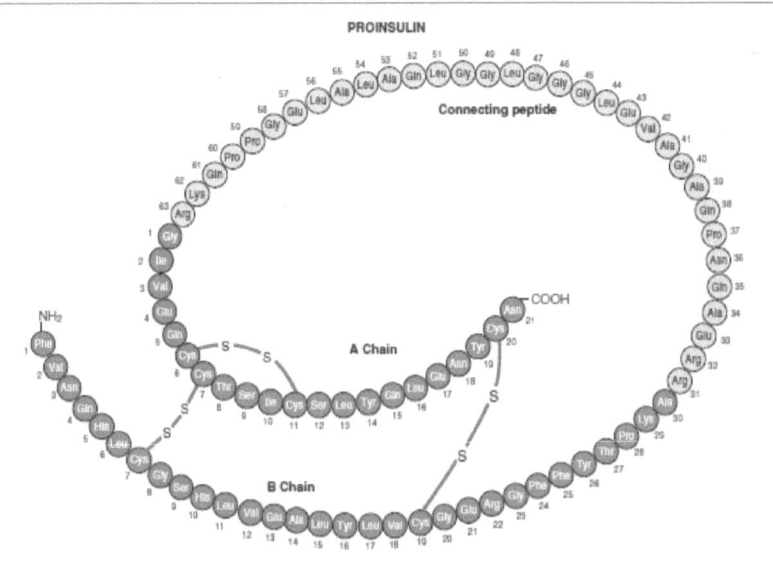

REGULATION OF INSULIN SECRETION:

FACTORS THAT INCREASE INSULIN SECRETION	FACTORS THAT DECREASE INSULIN SECRETION
Increased blood glucose	Decreased blood glucose
Increased amino acids(arginine,lysine,leucine)	Somatostatin
Increased fatty acids	Nor-epinephrine,Epinephrine
Glucagon	
GIP	
Acetylcholine	

BLOOD GLUCOSE CONCENTRATION:

It is the major factor that regulates insulin secretion. Increased blood glucose stimulates insulin secretion. An initial burst of insulin is followed by sustained secretion.

MECHANISM OF INSULIN SECRETION:

Glucose, the stimulant for insulin secretion, binds to the Glut2 receptor on the beta cells of the pancreas. Inside the beta cells, glucose is oxidized to ATP, which closes K channels in the cell membrane and leads to depolarization of the beta cells. Similar to the action of ATP, sulfonylureas drugs (e.g. tolbutamide, glyburide) stimulate insulin secretion by closing these K channels. Depolarization opens Ca channels, which leads to an increase in intracellular Ca and then to secretion of insulin.

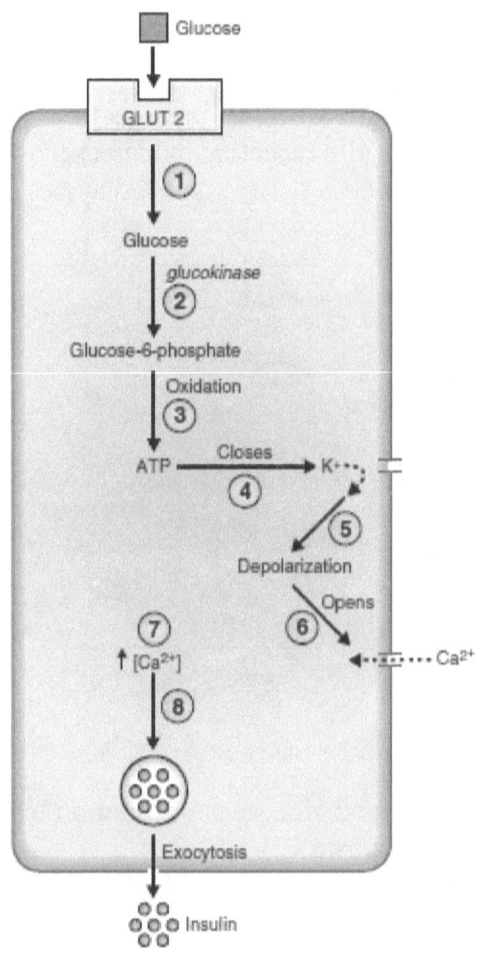

INSULIN SECRETION BY β CELLS

INSULIN RECEPTOR:

It is found on the target tissues for insulin. It is tetramer, with two alpha subunits and two beta subunits. The alpha subunits are located on the extracellular side of the cell membrane. The beta subunits span the cell membrane and have intrinsic tyrosine kinase activity. When insulin binds to the receptor, tyrosine kinase is activated and autophosphorylates the beta subunits. The phosphorylated receptor then phosphorylates intracellular proteins. The insulin –receptor complexes enter the target cells.

Insulin down regulates its own receptors in target tissues. Therefore the number of insulin receptors in increased in starvation and decreased in obesity (e.g. type 2 diabetes mellitus).

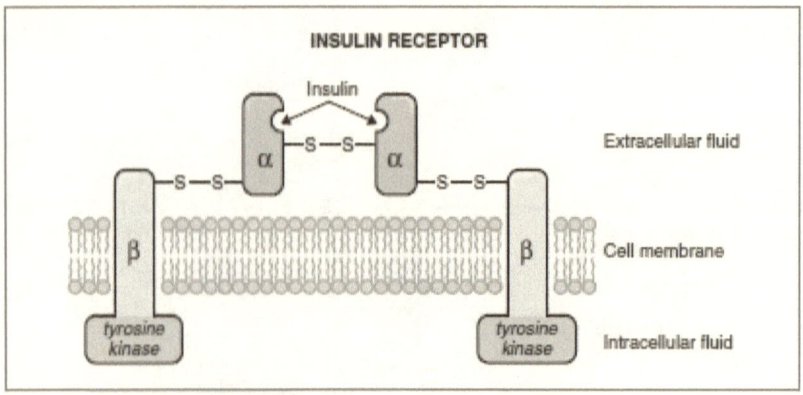

ACTIONS OF INSULIN:

Insulin acts on the liver, adipose tissue and muscle.

    a. Insulin decreases blood glucose concentration by the following mechanisms:
1. It increases uptake of glucose into target cells by directing the insertion of glucose transporters into cell membranes. As glucose enters the cells, the blood glucose concentration decreases.
2. It promotes the formation of glycogen from glucose in muscle and liver, and simultaneously inhibits glycogenolysis.
3. It decreases gluconeogenesis. Insulin increases the production of fructose 2, 6 biphosphate, and increasing phosphofructokinase activity. In effect, substrate is directed away from glucose formation.

b. Insulin decreases blood fatty acid and ketoacid concentrations.
      1. In adipose tissues, insulin stimulates fat deposition and inhibits lipolysis.
      2. Insulin inhibits ketoacid formation in the liver because decreased fatty acid degradation provides less acetyl CoA substrate for ketoacid formation.
   c. Insulin decreases blood amino acid concentration.
      1. Insulin stimulates amino acid uptake into cells, increase protein synthesis, and inhibits protein degradation. Thus, insulin is anabolic.
   d. Insulin decreases blood K concentration
      1. Insulin increases K uptake into cells, thereby decreasing blood K.

INSULIN PATHPHYSIOLOGY-DIABETES MELLITUS:

HYPERGLYCEMIA: It is consistent with insulin deficiency. In the absence of insulin the glucose uptake into the cells is decreased as it is the storage of glucose as glycogen. If tests were performed, the woman's blood would have shown increased levels of both amino acids (because of increased protein catabolism) and fatty acids (because of increased lipolysis).

HYPOTENSION: it is a result of ECF volume contraction. The high blood glucose concentration results in a high filtered load that exceeds the reabsorptive capacity (Tm) of the kidney. The unabsorbed glucose acts as an osmotic diuretic in the urine and causes ECF volume contraction.

METABOLIC ACIDOSIS: It is caused by overproduction of ketoacids (beta hydroxybutyrate and acetoacetate). The increased ventilation rate or Kusmaul respiration is the respiratory compensation for metabolic acidosis.

HYPERKALEMIA: It results from the lack of insulin; normally insulin promotes K uptake into cells.

GLUCAGON:

It is secreted by the alpha cells of the islets of Langerhans of pancreas. Alpha cells are present in the outer rim of the islet.

REGULATION OF GLUCAGON:

FACTORS THAT INCREASE GLUCAGON SECRETION	FACTORS THAT DECREASE GLUCAGON SECRETION
DECREASED BLOOD GLUCOSE	INCREASED BLOOD GLUCOSE
INCREASED AMINO ACIDS ESP ARGININE	INSULIN
CCK (ALERTS ALPHA CELLS TO A PROTEIN MEAL)	SOMATOSTATIN
NOREPINEPHRINE, EPINEPHRINE	FATTY ACIDS
ACETYLCHOLINE	KETO ACIDS

The major factor that regulates glucagon secretion is the blood glucose concentration. Decreased blood glucose stimulates glucagon secretion. Increased blood amino acids stimulate glucagon secretion, which prevents hypoglycemia caused by unopposed insulin in response to a high protein meal.

ACTIONS OF GLUCAGON:

Glucagon acts on the liver and adipose tissue.
The second messenger for glucagon is cAMP.

a. Glucagon increases the blood glucose concentration.
   (1) It increase glycogenolysis and prevents the recycling of glucose into glycogen.
   (2) It increases gluconeogenesis. Glucagon decreases the production of fructose 2,6 bisphosphate, decreasing phosphofructokinase activity; in effect, substrate is directed toward glucose formation rather than toward glucose breakdown.
b. Glucagon increases blood fatty acid and ketoacid concentration.
   (1) Glucagon increases lipolysis. The inhibition of fatty acid synthesis in effect "shunts" substrates towards gluconeogenesis.
   (2) Ketoacids (beta hydroxybutyrate and acetoacetate) are produced from acetyl coenzyme A(CoA), which results from fatty acid degradation.
c. Glucagon increases urea production.
   (1) Amino acids are used for gluconeogenesis(stimulated by glucagon), and the resulting amino acids groups are incorporated into urea.

OVERALL CALCIUM HOMEOSTASIS:

40% of the total calcium is bound to plasma proteins. 60% of the total calcium is not bound to plasma proteins and is ultrafiltrable. Ultrafiltrable calcium includes calcium that is complexes to anions such as phosphate and free ionized calcium. Free ionized calcium is biologically active. Serum calcium is determined by the interplay of intestinal absorption, renal excretion and bone remodeling (bone resorption and formation).Each component is hormonally regulated. To maintain calcium balance net intestinal absorption must be balanced by urinary excretion.

SUMMARY OF HORMONES THAT REGULATE CALCIUM:

	PTH	VITAMIN D	CALCITONIN
STIMULUS FOR SECRETION	DECREASED SERUM Ca	DECREASED SERUM Ca INCREASED PTH DECREASED SERUM PHOSPHATE	INCREASED SERUM Ca
ACTIONS ON:			
BONE	INCREASEED RESORPTION	INCREASED RESORPTION	DECREASED RESORPTION
KIDNEY	DECREASED PHOSPHATE REABSORPTION INCREASED CALCIUM REABSORPTION	INCREASED PHOSPHATE REABSORPTION AND INCREASED CALCIUM REABSORPTION	DECREASED RESORPTION
INTESTINE	INCREASED CALCIUM REABSORPTION BY ACTIVATION OF VIT D	INCREASED CALCIUM REABSORPTION AND INCREASED PHOSPHATE REABSORPTION	DECREASED RESORPTION
OVERALL EFFECT			

ON:			
SERUM Ca	INCREASED	INCREASED	DECREASED
SERUM PHOSPHATE	DECREASED	INCREASED	

POSITIVE CALCIUM BALANCE:

This is seen in growing children. Intestinal absorption exceeds urinary excretion and the excess is deposited in the growing bones.

NEGATIVE CALCIUM BALANCE:

This is seen in women during pregnancy or lactation. Intestinal calcium absorption is less than calcium excretion and the deficit comes from the maternal bones.

1. PARATHYROID HORMONE:

It is the major hormone for regulation of calcium. It is synthesized and secreted by the chief cells of the parathyroid glands.

SECRETION OF PTH:

It is controlled by the serum Ca binding to Ca sensing receptors in the parathyroid cell membrane. Decreased serum Ca increases PTH secretion, whereas increased serum Ca decreases PTH secretion. Decreased serum Ca causes decreased binding to the Ca sensing receptor which stimulates PTH secretion. Mild decreases in serum Mg stimulate PTH secretion. Severe decreases in serum Mg inhibit PTH secretion and produce symptoms of hypoparathyroidism (e.g. hypocalcaemia).The second messenger for PTH secretion by the parathyroid gland is cAMP.

ACTIONS OF PTH:

The actions are co-ordinated to produce an increase in serum Ca and a decrease in serum phosphate. The second messenger for PTH actions on its target tissues is cAMP. PTH increases bone resorption, which brings both Ca and phosphate from bone mineral into ECF alone.

PATHPHYSIOLOGY OF PTH:

a. **PRIMARY HYPERPARATHYROIDISM:**
   It is most commonly caused by parathyroid adenoma. It is characterized by:
   (1) Increased serum calcium(hypercalcemia)
   (2) Decreased phosphate (hypophosphatemia)
   (3) Increased phosphate excretion(phosphaturic effect of PTH)
   (4) Increased urinary calcium excretion (caused by the increased filtered load of calcium)
   (5) Increased urinary cAMP
   (6) Increased bone resorption.

b. **HUMORAL HYPERCALCEMIA OF MALIGNANCY:**
   It is caused by PTH related peptide (PTH-rp) secreted by some malignant tumors (e.g. breast, lung).PTH-rp has all the physiologic actions of PTH, including increased bone resorption, increased renal calcium reabsorption, and decreased renal phosphate reabsorption. It is characterized by:
   (1) Increased serum calcium (hypercalcemia)
   (2) Decreased serum phosphate(hypophosphatemia)
   (3) Increased urinary phosphate excretion (phosphaturic effect of PTH)
   (4) Decreased serum PTH levels due to feedback inhibition from the high serum calcium.

c. **HYPOPARATHYROIDISM:**
   It is most commonly a result of thyroid surgery or it is congenital. It is characterized by:

(1) Decreased serum calcium (hypocalcemia) and tetany.
  (2) Increased serum phosphate (hyperphosphatemia)
  (3) Decreased urinary phosphate excretion.
 d. PSEUDOHYPOPARATHYROIDISM TYPE 1a:
  It is the result of defective Gs protein in the kidney and bone, which causes end organ resistance to PTH. Hypocalcemia and hyperphosphatemia occur (as in hypoparathyroidism), which are not correctible by the administration of exogenous PTH.
  Circulating PTH levels are elevated (stimulated by hypocalcemia)
 e. CHRONIC RENAL FAILURE:
  Decreased glomerular filtration rate (GFR) leads to decreased filtration of phosphate, phosphate retention, and increased serum phosphate.
  Increased serum phosphate complexes calcium and leads to decreased ionized calcium.
  Decreased production of 1,25(OH)2 by the diseased renal tissue also contributes to the decreased ionized calcium(Ca)
  Decreased calcium causes secondary hyperparathyroidism.
  The combination of increased PTH levels and decreased 1, 25 dihydroxycholecalciferol produces renal osteodystrophhy, in which there is increased bone resorption and osteomalacia.
 f. FAMILIAL HYPOCALCEURIC HYPERCALCEMIA(FHH):
  It is an autosomal dominant disorder with decreased urinary calcium excretion and increased serum calcium. It is caused by inactivating mutations of the calcium sensing receptors that regulate PTH secretion.
2. VITAMIN D:

It produces calcium and phosphate to ECF for bone mineralization. In children, vitamin D deficiency causes rickets and in adults, vitamin deficiency causes osteomalacia.

VITAMIN D METABOLISM:

Cholecalciferol, 25-hydroxycholecalciferol and 24,25 dihydroxycholicalceferol are inactive. The active form of vitamin D is 1,25 dihydroxycholecalciferol. The production of 1,25(OH)2 in the kidney is catalyzed by the enzyme 1 α hydroxylase. The activity of this enzyme is increased by the following:

a. Decreased serum calcium
b. Increased PTH levels
c. Decreased serum phosphate.

ACTIONS OF 1, 25(OH) 2:

These are co-ordinated to increase both calcium and phosphate in ECF to mineralize new bone. A. Increased intestinal calcium absorption: Vitamin D dependent Ca binding protein (calbindin D-28K) is induced by 1,25(OH)2 .PTH increases intestinal calcium absorption indirectly by stimulating 1 α hydroxylase and increasing production of the active form of vitamin D.

B. Increased intestinal phosphate absorption.

C. Increased renal absorption of calcium and phosphate, analogous to its action on the intestine.

D. Increase bone resorption, which provides calcium and phosphate from old bone to mineralize new bone.

3. CALCITONIN:

It is synthesized and secreted by the parafollicular cells of the thyroid. Its secretion is stimulated by an increase in serum calcium. It acts primarily to inhibit bone resorption and can be used to treat hypercalcemia.

THYROID HORMONES:

Thyroid hormones are synthesized and secreted by epithelial cells of the thyroid gland. They have effects on virtually every organ system in the body including those involved in normal growth and development. The thyroid gland was the first of the endocrine organs to be described by a deficiency disorder. In 1850, patients without thyroid glands were described as having a form of mental and growth retardation called cretinism. In 1891, such patients were treated by administering crude thyroid extracts (i.e., hormone replacement therapy).

Disorders of thyroid deficiency and excess are among the most common of the endocrinopathies (disorders of the endocrine glands), affecting 4% to 5% of the population in the United States and an even greater percentage of people in regions of the world where there is iodine deficiency.

Synthesis and Transport of Thyroid Hormones:

The two active thyroid hormones are triiodothyronine (T3) and tetraiodothyronine, or thyroxine (T4). The structures of

T3 and T4 differ only by a single atom of Iodine. Although T3 is more active than T4, almost all hormonal output of the thyroid gland is T4. This "problem" of secreting the less active form is solved by the target tissues, which convert T4 to T3. A third compound, reverse T3 has no biologic activity.

Synthesis of Thyroid Hormones:

Thyroid hormones are synthesized by the follicular epithelial cells of the thyroid gland. The follicular epithelial cells are arranged in circular follicles 200 to 300 μm in diameter. The cells have a basal membrane facing the blood and an apical membrane facing the follicular lumen. The material in the lumen of the follicles is colloid, which is composed of newly synthesized thyroid hormones attached to thyroglobulin. When the thyroid gland is stimulated, this colloidal thyroid hormone is absorbed into the follicular cells by endocytosis. The synthesis of thyroid hormones is more complex than that of most hormones. There are three unusual features of the synthetic process:

(1) Thyroid hormones contain large amounts of iodine, which must be adequately supplied in the diet.

(2) Synthesis of thyroid hormones is partially intracellular and partially extracellular, with the completed hormones stored extracellularly in the follicular lumen until the thyroid gland is stimulated to secrete.

(3) As noted, although T4 is the major secretory product of the thyroid gland, it is not the most active form of the hormone.

The circled numbers in the figure correlate with the following steps:

1. Thyroglobulin (TG), a glycoprotein containing large quantities of tyrosine, is synthesized on the rough endoplasmic reticulum and the Golgi apparatus of the thyroid follicular cells. Thyroglobulin is then incorporated into secretory vesicles and extruded across the apical membrane into the follicular lumen. Later, the tyrosine

residues of thyroglobulin will be iodinated to form the precursors of thyroid hormones.

2. Na^+-I^- cotransport, or "I-trap." I^- is actively transported from blood into the follicular epithelial cells against both chemical and electrical gradients. The activity of this pump is regulated by I^- levels in the body. For example, low levels of I^- stimulate the pump. When there is a dietary deficiency of I^-, the Na^+-I^- cotransport increases its activity, attempting to compensate for the deficiency. If the dietary deficiency is severe, however, even the Na^+-I^- cotransport cannot compensate and the synthesis of thyroid hormones will be decreased.

There are several competitive inhibitors of Na^+-I^- cotransport including the anions thiocyanate and perchlorate, which block I^- uptake into follicular cells and interfere with the synthesis of thyroid hormones.

3. Oxidation of I^- to I_2. Once I^- is pumped into the cell, it traverses the cell to the apical membrane, where it is oxidized to I_2 by the enzyme thyroid peroxidase. Thyroid peroxidase catalyzes this oxidation step and the next two steps (i.e., organification of I_2 into thyroglobulin and the coupling reactions). Thyroid peroxidase is inhibited by propylthiouracil(PTU), which blocks the synthesis of thyroid hormones by blocking all of the steps catalyzed by thyroid peroxidase. Thus, administration of PTU is an effective treatment for hyperthyroidism.

4. Organification of I_2. At the apical membrane, just inside the lumen of the follicle, I_2 combines with the tyrosine moieties of thyroglobulin, catalyzed by thyroid peroxidase, to form monoiodotyrosine. (MIT) and diiodotyrosine (DIT). MIT and DIT remain attached to thyroglobulin in the follicularlumen until the thyroid gland is stimulated to secrete its hormones. High levels of I^- inhibit organification and synthesis of thyroid hormones, which is known as the Wolff-Chaikoff effect.

5. Coupling reaction. While still part of thyroglobulin, two separate coupling reactions occur between MIT and DIT,

again catalyzed by thyroid peroxidase. In one reaction, two molecules of DIT combine to form T4. In the other reaction, one molecule of DIT combines with one molecule of MIT to form T3. The first reaction is faster, and as a result, approximately
10 times more T4 is produced than T3. A portion of MIT and DIT does not couple (is "left over") and simply remains attached to thyroglobulin. After the coupling reactions occur, thyroglobulin contains T4, T3, and leftover MIT and DIT. This iodinated thyroglobulin is stored in the follicular lumen as colloid until the thyroid gland is stimulated to secrete its hormones (e.g., by TSH).

6. <u>Endocytosis of thyroglobulin</u>. When the thyroid gland is stimulated, iodinated thyroglobulin (with its attached T4, T3, MIT, and DIT) is endocytosed into the follicular epithelial cells. Pseudopods are pinched off the apical cell membrane, engulf a portion of colloid, and absorb it into the cell. Once inside the cell, thyroglobulin is transported in the direction of the basal membrane by microtubular action.

7. <u>Hydrolysis of T4 and T3 from thyroglobulin by lysosomal enzymes.</u> Thyroglobulin droplets fuse with lysosomal membranes. Lysosomal proteases then hydrolyze peptide bonds to release T4, T3, MIT, and DIT from thyroglobulin. T4 and T3 are transported across the basal membrane into nearby capillaries to be delivered to the systemic circulation. MIT and DIT remain in the follicular cell and are recycled into the synthesis of new thyroglobulin.

8. <u>Deiodination of MIT and DIT</u>. MIT and DIT are deiodinated inside the follicular cell by the enzyme thyroid deiodinase. The I^- generated by this step is recycled into the intracellular pool and added to the I^- transported by the pump. The tyrosine molecules are incorporated into the synthesis of new thyroglobulin to begin another cycle. Thus, both I^- and tyrosine are "salvaged" by the deiodinase enzyme. A deficiency of thyroid deiodinase therefore mimics dietary I^- deficiency.

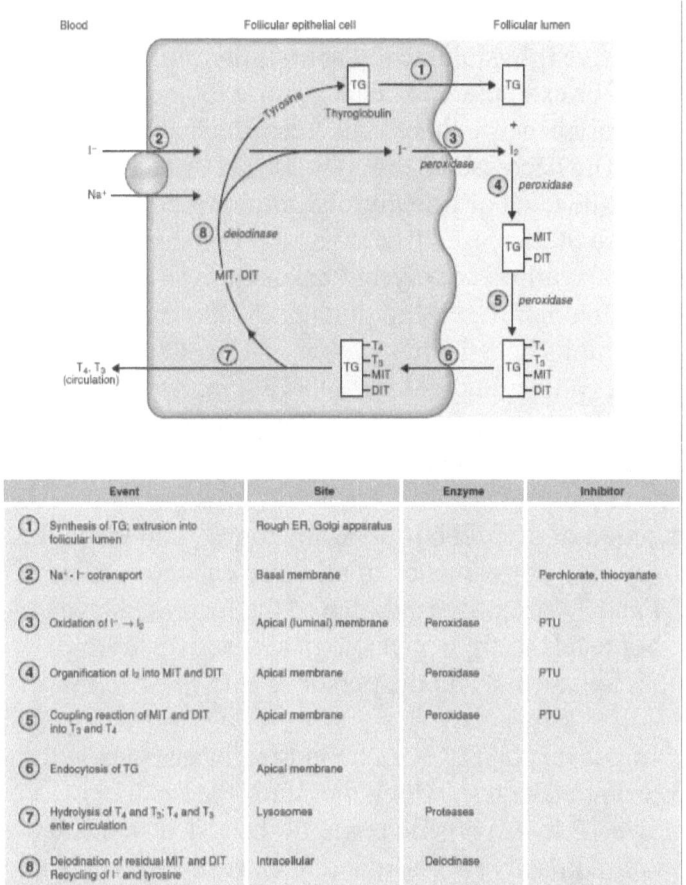

Event	Site	Enzyme	Inhibitor
① Synthesis of TG; extrusion into follicular lumen	Rough ER, Golgi apparatus		
② Na⁺ - I⁻ cotransport	Basal membrane		Perchlorate, thiocyanate
③ Oxidation of I⁻ → I₂	Apical (luminal) membrane	Peroxidase	PTU
④ Organification of I₂ into MIT and DIT	Apical membrane	Peroxidase	PTU
⑤ Coupling reaction of MIT and DIT into T₃ and T₄	Apical membrane	Peroxidase	PTU
⑥ Endocytosis of TG	Apical membrane		
⑦ Hydrolysis of T₄ and T₃; T₄ and T₃ enter circulation	Lysosomes	Proteases	
⑧ Deiodination of residual MIT and DIT Recycling of I⁻ and tyrosine	Intracellular	Deiodinase	

Binding of Thyroid Hormones in the Circulation

Thyroid hormones (T4 and T3) circulate in the bloodstream either bound to plasma proteins or free (unbound). Most T4 and T3 circulates bound to thyroxine-binding globulin (TBG). Smaller amounts circulate bound to T4-binding prealbumin and albumin. Still smaller amounts circulate in the free, unbound form. Because only free thyroid hormones are physiologically active, the role of TBG is to provide a large reservoir of circulating thyroid hormones, which can be released and added to the pool of free hormone. Changes in the blood levels of TBG alter the fraction of free (physiologically active) thyroid hormones. For example, in hepatic failure, blood levels of TBG decrease because there is decreased hepatic protein synthesis. The decrease in TBG levels results in a transient increase in the level of free thyroid hormones; a consequence of increased free thyroid hormone is inhibition of synthesis of thyroid hormones (by negative feedback). In contrast, during pregnancy, the high level of estrogen inhibits hepatic breakdown of TBG and increases TBG levels. With a higher level of TBG, more thyroid hormone is bound to TBG and less thyroid hormone is free and unbound. The transiently decreased level of free hormone causes, by negative feedback, increased synthesis and secretion of thyroid hormones by the thyroid gland. In pregnancy, as a consequence of all these changes, levels of total T4 and T3 are increased (due to the increased level of TBG), but levels of free, physiologically active, thyroid hormones are normal and the person is said to be "clinically euthyroid."

Circulating levels of TBG can be indirectly assessed with the T3 resin uptake test, which measures the binding of radioactive T3 to a synthetic resin. In the test, a standard amount of radioactive T3 is added to an assay system that contains a sample of the patient's serum and the T3-binding resin. The rationale is that radioactive T3 will first bind to unoccupied sites on the patient's TBG and any "leftover" radioactive T3 will bind to the resin. Thus, T3 resin uptake is increased when circulating levels of TBG are decreased (e.g., hepatic failure) or when endogenous T3 levels are increased (i.e., endogenous hormone occupies more sites than usual on TBG). Conversely, T3 resin uptake is decreased when circulating levels of TBG are increased (e.g., during pregnancy) or when endogenous T3 levels are decreased (i.e., endogenous hormone occupies fewer sites than usual on TBG).

Activation of T4 in Target Tissues:
As noted, the major secretory product of the thyroid gland is T4, which is not the most active form of thyroid hormone. This "problem" is solved in the target tissues by the enzyme **5′ iodinase,** which converts T4 to T3 by removing one atom of I2. The target tissues also convert a portion of the T4 to **reverse T3** (rT3), which is inactive. Essentially, T4 serves as a precursor for T3, and the relative amounts of T4 converted to T3 and rT3 determine how much active hormone is produced in the target tissue.

In **starvation** (fasting), target tissue 5′ iodinase plays an interesting role. Starvation inhibits 5′ iodinase in tissues such as skeletal muscle, thus lowering O2 consumption and basal metabolic rate during periods of caloric deprivation. However, brain 5′ iodinase differs from the 5′ iodinase in other tissues and is, therefore, not inhibited in starvation; in this way, brain levels of T3 are protected even during caloric deprivation.

Regulation of Thyroid Hormone Secretion

The factors that increase or decrease the secretion of thyroid hormones are summarized in Table:

Major control of the synthesis and secretion of thyroid hormones is via the hypothalamic-pituitary axis (Fig. 9-19). Thyrotropin-releasing hormone (TRH) is secreted by the hypothalamus and acts on the thyrotrophs of the anterior pituitary to cause secretion of thyroid-stimulating hormone (TSH). TSH then acts on the thyroid gland to stimulate the synthesis and secretion of thyroid hormones.

TRH, a tripeptide, is secreted by the paraventricular nuclei of the hypothalamus. TRH then acts on the thyrotrophs of the anterior pituitary to stimulate both transcription of the TSH gene and secretion of TSH. (Recall that the other action of TRH is to stimulate the secretion of prolactin by the anterior pituitary.)

TSH, a glycoprotein, is secreted by the anterior lobe of the pituitary in response to stimulation by TRH. The role of TSH is to regulate the growth of the thyroid gland (i.e., a trophic effect) and the secretion of thyroid hormones by influencing several steps in the biosynthetic pathway. The thyrotrophs of the anterior pituitary develop and begin secreting TSH at approximately gestational week 13, the same time that the fetal thyroid gland begins secreting thyroid hormones.

TSH secretion is regulated by two reciprocal factors: (1) TRH from the hypothalamus stimulates the secretion of TSH, and (2) Thyroid hormones inhibit the secretion of TSH by down-regulating the TRH receptor on the thyrotrophs, thus decreasing their sensitivity to stimulation by TRH. This negative feedback effect of thyroid hormones is mediated by **free T3,** which is possible because the anterior lobe contains thyroid deiodinase (converting T4 to T3). The reciprocal regulation of TSH secretion by TRH and negative feedback by free T3 results in a relatively steady rate of TSH secretion, which, in turn, produces a steady rate of secretion of thyroid hormones (in contrast to growth hormone secretion, whose secretion is pulsatile).

The **actions of TSH on the thyroid gland** are initiated when TSH binds to a membrane receptor, which is coupled to adenylyl cyclase via a Gs protein. Activation of adenylyl cyclase generates **cAMP,** which serves as the second messenger for TSH. TSH has two types of actions on the thyroid gland.

(1) It increases the synthesis and secretion of thyroid hormones by stimulating *each* step in the biosynthetic pathway: I− uptake and oxidation, organification of I_2 into MIT and DIT, coupling of MIT and DIT to form T4 and T3, endocytosis, and proteolysis of thyroglobulin to release T4 and T3 for secretion.

(2) TSH has a trophic effect on the thyroid gland. This trophic effect is exhibited when TSH levels are elevated for a sustained period of time and leads to hypertrophy and hyperplasia of thyroid follicular cells and increased thyroidal blood flow.

The TSH receptor on the thyroid cells also is activated by **thyroid-stimulating immunoglobulins**, which are antibodies to the TSH receptor. Thyroid stimulating immunoglobulins are components of the immunoglobulin G (IgG) fraction of plasma proteins.

When these immunoglobulins bind to the TSH receptor, they produce the same response in thyroid cells as TSH: stimulation of thyroid hormone synthesis and secretion and hypertrophy and hyperplasia of the gland (i.e., hyperthyroidism). **Graves disease,** a common form of hyperthyroidism, is caused by increased circulating levels of thyroidstimulating immunoglobulins. In this disorder, the thyroid gland is intensely stimulated by the antibodies, causing circulating levels of thyroid hormones to be increased. In Graves disease, TSH levels are actually lower than normal because the high circulating levels of thyroid hormones inhibit TSH secretion by negative feedback.

FACTORS AFFECTING THYROID HORMONE SECRETION:

STIMULATORY FACTORS	INHIBITORY FACTORS
TSH	IODINE DEFICEINCY
THYROID STIMULATING IMMUNOGLOBULINS	DEIODINASE DEFICIENCY
INCREASED TBG LEVELS (E.G PREGNANCY)	EXCESSIVE IODINE INTAKE (WOLFF CHAIKOFF EFFECT)
	PERCHLORATE: THIOCYANATE(INHIBIT Na I COTRANSPORT)
	PROPYLTHIOURACIL INHIBITS PEROXIDASE ENZYME
	DECREASED TBG LEVELS (E.G LIVER

REGULATION OF THYROID HORMONES:

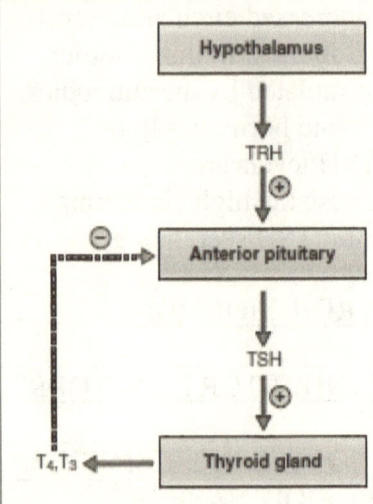

Actions of Thyroid Hormones:
Thyroid hormones act on virtually every organ system in the human body. Thyroid hormones act synergistically with growth hormone and somatomedins to promote bone formation; they increase basal metabolic rate (BMR), heat production, and oxygen consumption; and they alter the cardiovascular and respiratory systems to increase blood flow and oxygen delivery to the tissues.

The first step in the action of thyroid hormones in target tissues is **conversion of T4 to T3 by 5′-iodinase.** (Recall that T4 is secreted in far greater amounts than T3, but it also is much less active.) In an alternate pathway, T4 can be converted to rT3, which is physiologically inactive. Normally, the tissues produce T3 and rT3 in approximately equal amounts (T3, 45% and rT3, 55%). However, under certain conditions, the relative amounts may change. For example, pregnancy, fasting, stress, hepatic and renal failure, and β-adrenergic blocking agents all decrease the conversion of T4 to T3 (and increase conversion to rT3), thus decreasing the amount of the active hormone. Obesity increases the conversion of T4 to T3, increasing the amount of the active hormone. Once T3 is produced inside the target cells, it enters the nucleus and binds to a **nuclear receptor.** The T3- receptor complex then binds to a thyroid-regulatory element on DNA, where it stimulates **DNA transcription.** The newly transcribed mRNAs are translated, and new proteins are synthesized. These new proteins are responsible for the multiple actions of thyroid hormones. Other T3 receptors located in ribosomes and mitochondria mediate posttranscriptional and posttranslational events. A vast array of **new proteins** are synthesized under the direction of thyroid hormones, including Na^+-K^+ ATPase, transport proteins, β1-adrenergic receptors, lysosomal enzymes, proteolytic proteins, and structural proteins. The nature of the protein induced is specific to the target tissue. In most tissues, Na^+-K^+ ATPase synthesis is induced, which leads to increased oxygen consumption, BMR, and heat production. In myocardial cells, myosin, β1-adrenergic receptors, and Ca^{2+} ATPase are induced, accounting for thyroid hormone–induced increases in heart rate and contractility. In liver and adipose tissue, key metabolic enzymes are induced, leading to alterations in carbohydrate, fat, and protein metabolism.

The effects of thyroid hormone (T3) on various organ systems are as follows:

  Basal metabolic rate (BMR). One of the most significant and pronounced effects of thyroid hormone is **increased oxygen consumption** and a resulting increase in **BMR** and

body temperature. Thyroid hormones increase oxygen consumption in all tissues *except brain, gonads, and spleen* by inducing the synthesis and increasing the activity of the **Na+-K+ ATPase.** The Na+-K+ ATPase is responsible for primary active transport of Na+ and K+ in all cells; this activity is highly correlated with and accounts for a large percentage of the total oxygen consumption and heat production in the body. Thus, when thyroid hormones increase Na+-K+ ATPase activity, they also increase oxygen consumption, BMR, and heat production.

♦ **Metabolism.** Ultimately, increased oxygen consumption depends on increased availability of substrates for oxidative metabolism. Thyroid hormones increase glucose absorption from the gastrointestinal tract and potentiate the effects of other hormones (e.g., catecholamines, glucagon, and growth hormone) on gluconeogenesis, lipolysis, and proteolysis. Thyroid hormones increase both protein synthesis and degradation, but, overall, their effect is *catabolic* (i.e., net degradation), which results in decreased muscle mass. These metabolic effects occur because thyroid hormones induce the synthesis of key metabolic enzymes including cytochrome oxidase, NADPH cytochrome C reductase, α-glycerophosphate dehydrogenase, malic enzyme, and several proteolytic enzymes.

Cardiovascular and respiratory. Because thyroid hormones increase O2 consumption, they create a higher demand for O2 in the tissues. Increased O2 delivery to the tissues is possible because thyroid hormones produce an increase in cardiac output and ventilation. The **increase in cardiac output** is the result of a combination of increased heart rate and increased stroke volume (increased contractility). These cardiac effects are explained by the fact that thyroid hormones induce the synthesis of (i.e., up-regulate) cardiac β1-adrenergic receptors. Recall that these β1 receptors mediate the effects of the sympathetic nervous system to increase heart rate and contractility. Thus, when thyroid hormone levels are high, the myocardium has an increased number of β1 receptors and is more sensitive to stimulation by the sympathetic nervous system. (In complementary actions, thyroid hormones also induce the synthesis of cardiac myosin and sarcoplasmic reticulum Ca2+ ATPase.)

Growth. Thyroid hormone is required for growth to adult stature. Thyroid hormones act synergistically with growth hormone and somatomedins to promote bone formation. Thyroid hormones promote ossification and fusion of bone plates and bone maturation.
In hypothyroidism, bone age is less than chronologic age.

Central nervous system (CNS). Thyroid hormones have multiple effects on the CNS, and the impact of these effects is age dependent. In the **perinatal period,** thyroid hormone is *essential for normal maturation of the CNS.* Hypothyroidism in the perinatal period causes irreversible mental retardation. For this reason, screening of newborns for hypothyroidism is mandated; if it is detected in the newborn, thyroid hormone replacement can reverse the CNS effects. In **adults,** hypothyroidism causes listlessness, slowed movement, somnolence, impaired memory, and decreased mental capacity. Hyperthyroidism causes hyperexcitability, hyperreflexia, and irritability.

Autonomic nervous system. Thyroid hormones interact with the **sympathetic nervous system** in ways that are not fully understood. Many of the effects of thyroid hormones on BMR, heat production, heart rate, and stroke volume are similar to those produced by catecholamines via **β-adrenergic receptors.** The effects of thyroid hormones and catecholamines on heat production, cardiac output, lipolysis, and gluconeogenesis appear to be synergistic. The significance of this synergism is illustrated by the effectiveness of **β-adrenergic blocking agents** (e.g., propranolol) in treating many of the Symptoms of hyperthyroidism.

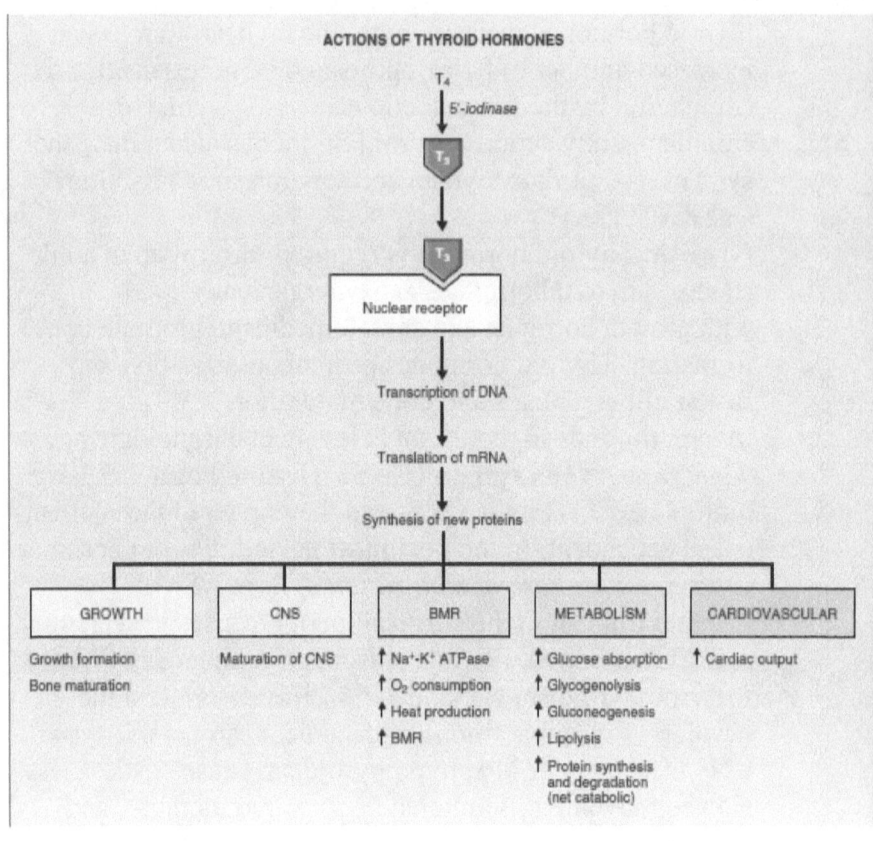

Pathophysiology of Thyroid Hormone

The most common endocrine abnormalities are disturbances of thyroid hormones. The constellation of signs and symptoms produced by an excess or a deficiency of thyroid hormones are predictable on the basis of the hormones' physiologic actions. Thus, disturbances of thyroid hormones will affect growth, CNS function, BMR and heat production, nutrient metabolism, and the cardiovascular system. The symptoms of hyperthyroidism and hypothyroidism, common etiologies, TSH levels, and treatments.

Hyperthyroidism

The most common form of hyperthyroidism is **Graves disease**, an autoimmune disorder characterized by increased circulating levels of **thyroid-stimulating immunoglobulins.** These immunoglobulins are antibodies to TSH receptors on thyroid follicular cells. When present, the antibodies intensely stimulate the thyroid gland, resulting in increased secretion of thyroid hormones and hypertrophy of the gland. Other causes of hyperthyroidism are thyroid neoplasm, excessive secretion of TRH or TSH, and administration of excessive amounts of exogenous thyroid hormones. The **diagnosis of hyperthyroidism** is based on symptoms and measurement of increased levels of T3 and T4. TSH levels may be decreased or increased, depending on the cause of the hyperthyroidism. If the *cause* of hyperthyroidism is Graves disease, thyroid neoplasm (i.e., the disorder is in the thyroid gland), or exogenous administration of thyroid hormones (factitious hyperthyroidism), then TSH levels will be decreased by negative feedback of the high levels of T3 on the anterior pituitary. However, if the *cause* of hyperthyroidism is increased secretion of TRH or TSH (i.e., the disorder is in the hypothalamus or anterior pituitary), then TSH levels will be increased.

The **symptoms of hyperthyroidism** are dramatic and include weight loss accompanied by increased food intake due to the increased metabolic rate; excessive heat production and sweating secondary to increased oxygen consumption; rapid heart rate due to up-regulation of $\beta 1$ receptors in the heart; breathlessness on exertion; and tremor, nervousness, and weakness due to the CNS effects of thyroid hormones. The increased activity of the thyroid gland causes it to enlarge, called **goiter.** The goiter may compress the esophagus and cause difficulty in swallowing.

Treatment of hyperthyroidism includes administration of drugs such as **propylthiouracil,** which inhibit the synthesis of thyroid hormones; surgical removal of the gland; or radioactive ablation of the thyroid gland with 131I–.

Hypothyroidism

The most common cause of hypothyroidism is **autoimmune destruction of the thyroid gland** (thyroiditis) in which antibodies may either frankly destroy the gland or block thyroid hormone synthesis. Other causes of hypothyroidism are surgical removal of the thyroid as treatment for hyperthyroidism, hypothalamic or pituitary failure, and I– deficiency. Rarely, hypothyroidism is the result of target tissue resistance caused by down-regulation of thyroid-hormone receptors.

The **diagnosis of hypothyroidism** is based on symptoms and a finding of decreased levels of T3 and T4. Depending on the cause of the hypothyroidism, TSH levels may be increased or decreased. If the defect is in the thyroid gland (e.g., thyroiditis), TSH levels will be increased by negative feedback; the low circulating levels of T3 stimulate TSH secretion. If the defect is in the hypothalamus or pituitary, then TSH levels will be decreased.

The **symptoms of hypothyroidism** are opposite those seen in hyperthyroidism and include decreased metabolic rate and weight gain without increased food intake; decreased heat production and cold intolerance; decreased heart rate; slowing of movement, slurred speech, slowed mental activity, lethargy, and somnolence; periorbital puffiness; constipation; hair loss; and menstrual dysfunction. In some cases, **myxedema** develops, in which there is increased filtration of fluid out of the capillaries and edema due to accumulation of osmotically active mucopolysaccharides in interstitial fluid. When the cause of hypothyroidism is a defect in the thyroid, a **goiter** develops from the unrelenting stimulation of the thyroid gland by the high circulating levels of TSH. Finally, and of critical importance, if hypothyroidism occurs in the **perinatal period** and is untreated, it results in an irreversible form of growth and mental retardation called **cretinism.**

Treatment of hypothyroidism involves thyroid hormone replacement therapy, usually T4. Like endogenous hormone, exogenous T4 is converted to its active form, T3, in the target tissues.

Goiter

Goiter (i.e., enlarged thyroid) can be associated with certain causes of hyperthyroidism and also, perhaps surprisingly, with certain causes of hypothyroidism and euthyroidism. The terms hyperthyroid, hypothyroid, and euthyroid describe, respectively, the *clinical states* of excess thyroid hormone, deficiency of thyroid hormone, and normal levels of thyroid hormone. Thus, they describe blood levels of thyroid hormone, *not* the size of the thyroid gland. The presence or absence of goiter can be understood only by analyzing the etiology of the various thyroid disorders. The central principle
in understanding goiter is that high levels of TSH and substances that act like TSH (e.g., thyroid-stimulating immunoglobulins) have a trophic (growth) effect on the thyroid and cause it to enlarge.

Graves disease. In Graves disease, the most common cause of hyperthyroidism, the high levels of thyroid stimulating immunoglobulins drive excess secretion of T4 and T3 and also have a trophic effect on the thyroid gland to produce **goiter.** Although TSH levels are decreased (by negative feedback) in Graves disease, the trophic effect is due to the TSH-*like* effect of the immunoglobulins.

TSH-secreting tumor. TSH-secreting tumors are an uncommon cause of hyperthyroidism. Increased levels of TSH drive the thyroid to secrete excess T4 and T3 and have a trophic effect on the thyroid gland to produce **goiter.**

Ingestion of T4. Ingestion of exogenous thyroid hormones, or factitious hyperthyroidism, is associated with increased levels of thyroid hormone (from the ingestion),

which causes decreased levels of TSH (by negative feedback). Because TSH levels are low there is *no* **goiter**; in fact, with time, the thyroid gland shrinks, or involutes.
Autoimmune thyroiditis. Autoimmune thyroiditis is a common cause of hypothyroidism, in which thyroid hormone synthesis is impaired by antibodies to peroxidase, leading to decreased T4 and T3 secretion. TSH levels are increased (by negative feedback), and the resulting high levels of TSH have a trophic effect on the thyroid gland to produce **goiter.**
That's right! The gland enlarges even though it is not effectively synthesizing thyroid hormones.
TSH deficiency (anterior pituitary failure). TSH deficiency is an uncommon cause of hypothyroidism, where the decreased levels of TSH cause decreased thyroid hormone secretion and *no* **goiter**.
I− deficiency. Deficiency of I− leads to transiently decreased synthesis of T4 and T3, which increases TSH secretion by negative feedback. Increased TSH levels then have a trophic effect on the gland, causing **goiter.** The enlarged gland (which is otherwise normal) can often maintain normal blood levels of thyroid hormone (due to the high TSH levels); in that case, the person will be clinically euthyroid and asymptomatic. If the gland cannot maintain normal blood levels of thyroid hormone, then the person will be clinically hypothyroid

	Hyperthyroidism	Hypothyroidism
Symptoms	Increased basal metabolic rate Weight loss Negative nitrogen balance Increased heat production Sweating Increased cardiac output Dyspnea (shortness of breath) Tremor, muscle weakness Exophthalmos Goiter	Decreased basal metabolic rate Weight gain Positive nitrogen balance Decreased heat production Cold sensitivity Decreased cardiac output Hypoventilation Lethargy, mental slowness Drooping eyelids Myxedema Growth retardation Mental retardation (perinatal) Goiter
Causes	Graves disease (increased thyroid-stimulating immunoglobulins) Thyroid neoplasm Excess TSH secretion Exogenous T_3 or T_4 (factitious)	Thyroiditis (autoimmune or Hashimoto thyroiditis) Surgery for hyperthyroidism I^- deficiency Congenital (cretinism) Decreased TRH or TSH
TSH Levels	Decreased (feedback inhibition of T_3 on the anterior lobe) Increased (if defect is in anterior pituitary)	Increased (by negative feedback if primary defect is in thyroid gland) Decreased (if defect is in hypothalamus or anterior pituitary)
Treatment	Propylthiouracil (inhibits peroxidase enzyme and thyroid hormone synthesis) Thyroidectomy $^{131}I^-$ (destroys thyroid) β-Adrenergic blocking agents (adjunct therapy)	Thyroid hormone replacement therapy

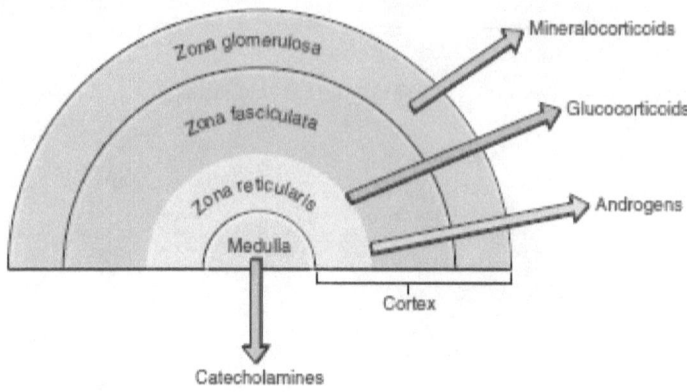

Catecholamines

THE ADRENAL CORTEX:

The zona glomerulosa produces aldosterone. The zona fasciculata and reticularis produce (cortisol) and androgens (dihydroepiandrosterone and androstenedione).

21 CARBON STEROIDS:

These include progesterone, deoxycortisone, aldosterone and cortisol. Progesterone is the precursor for others in the 21 carbon series. Hydroxylation at C -21 leads to production of deoxycorticosterone, which has mineralocorticoid (but not glucocorticoid activity). Hydroxylation at C-17 leads to the production of glucocorticoid (cortisol).

19 CARBON STEROIDS:

These have androgenic activity and are precursors to the estrogens. If the steroid have been previously hydroxylated at C-17, the C20,21 side chain can be cleaved to yield the 19 carbon steroids dehydroepiandrosterone or androstenedione in the adrenal cortex. Adrenal androgens have a ketone group at C-17 and are excreted at 17 ketosteroids in the urine. In the testes the androstenedione is converted to testosterone.

18 CARBON STEROIDS:

They have estrogenic activity. Oxidation of the A ring (aromatization) to produce estrogens occurs in the ovaries and placenta but not in the adrenal cortex or testes.

REGULATION OF SECRETION OF ADRENOCORTICAL HORMONES:

   a. **GLUCOCORTICOID SECRETION:**
      The secretion of glucocorticoids oscillates with a 24 hour periodicity or circadian rhythm. For those who sleep at night, cortisol levels are highest just before waking (8 am) and lowest in the evening (12 midnight).

      (I) **HYPOTHALAMIC CONTROL – CORTICOTROPIN RELEASING HORMONE (CRH):** CRH containing neurons are located in the para ventricular nuclei of the hypothalamus. When these neurons are stimulated, CRH is released into hypothalamic-hypophyseal portal blood and delivered to the anterior pituitary. CRH binds to the receptors on the corticotrophs of the anterior pituitary and directs them to synthesize POMC (the precursor to ACTH) and secrete ACTH. The second messenger for CRH is cAMP.

      (II) **ANTERIOR LOBE OF THE PITUITARY(ACTH):** ACTH increases steroid hormone synthesis in all zones of the adrenal cortex by stimulating cholesterol

desmolase and increasing the conversion of cholesterol to pregnenelone. ACTH also up regulates its own receptor so that sensitivity of the adrenal cortex to ACTH is increased. Chronically increased levels of ACTH cause hypertrophy of the adrenal cortex. The second messenger for ACTH is cAMP.

(III) **NEGATIVE FEEDBACK CONTROL-CORTISOL:** Cortisol inhibits the secretion of CRH from the hypothalamus and the secretion of ACTH from the anterior pituitary. When cortisol (glucocorticoid) levels are chronically elevated, the secretion of CRH and ACTH is inhibited by negative feedback.

The dexamethasone suppression test is based on the ability of dexamethasone (a synthetic glucocorticoid) to inhibit ACTH secretion. In normal persons, low dose dexamethasone inhibits or "suppresses" ACTH secretion and consequently, cortisol secretion. In persons, with ACTH secreting tumors, low dose dexamethasone does not inhibit cortisol secretion but high dose dexamethasone does. In persons with adrenal cortical tumors, neither low nor high dose dexamethasone inhibits cortisol secretion.

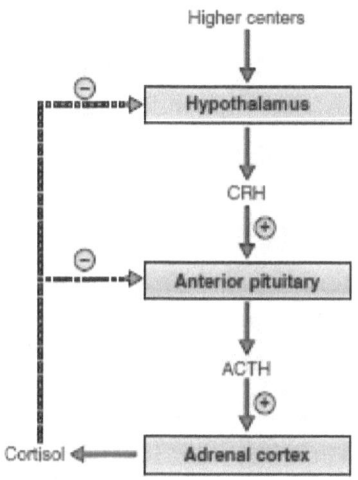

b. <u>ALDOSTERONE SECRETION:</u>

It is under control by ACTH, but is separately regulated by the renin-angiotensin system and by serum potassium.

- (i) **RENIN ANGIOTENSIN ALDOSTERONE SYSTEM:**
    - A. **DECREASE IN BLOOD VOLUME** causes a decrease in renal perfusion pressure, which in turn increases renin secretion. Renin, an enzyme, catalyzes the conversion of angiotensinogen to angiotensin I. Angiotensin I is converted to angiotensin II by angiotensin converting enzyme (ACE).
    - B. **ANGIOTENSIN ACTS ON** the zona glomerulosa of the adrenal cortex to increase the conversion of corticosterone to aldosterone.
    - C. **ALDOSTERONE** increase renal Na reabsorption, thereby restoring extracellular fluid (ECF) volume and blood volume to normal.
- (ii) **HYPERKALEMIA:** increases aldosterone secretion. Aldosterone increases renal K secretion, restoring serum K to normal.

c. **ACTIONS OF GLUCOCORTICOID (CORTISOL):**

Overall glucocorticoids are essential for the response to stress.

- (i) **STIMULATION OF GLUCONEOGENESIS:**
    Glucocorticoids increases gluconeogenesis by the following mechanisms:

a. They increase protein catabolism in muscle and decrease protein synthesis, thereby providing more amino acids to the liver for gluconeogenesis.
b. They decrease glucose utilization and insulin sensitivity of adipose tissue.
c. They increase lipolysis, which provides more glycerol to the liver for gluconeogenesis.

(ii) ANTI-INFLAMMATORY EFFECTS:
a. Glucocorticoids induce the synthesis of lipocortin, an inhibitor of phospholipase A2. (Phospholipase A2 is the enzyme that liberates arachidonate from membrane phospholipids, providing the precursor for prostaglandins and leukotriene synthesis). Because prostaglandins and leukotrienes are involved in the inflammatory response; glucocorticoids have anti-inflammatory properties by inhibiting the formation of precursor (arachidonate).
b. Glucocorticoids inhibit the production of interleukin 2 (IL-2) and inhibit the proliferation of T lymphocytes.
c. Glucocorticoids inhibit the release of histamine and serotonin from mast cells and platelets.

(iii) SUPPRESSION OF IMMUNE RESPONSE: Glucocorticoids inhibit the production of IL-2 and T lymphocytes, both of which are critical for cellular immunity.

In pharmacologic doses, glucocorticoids are used to prevent rejection of transplanted organs.

    (iv) **MAINTANENCE OF VASCULAR RESPONSIVE NESS TO CATECHOLAMINES:** Cortisol up regulates alpha 1 receptors on arterioles, increasing their sensitivity to the vasoconstrictor effect of norepinephrine. Thus with cortisol excess, arterial pressure increases: with cortisol deficiency, arterial pressure decreases.

d. **ACTIONS OF MINERALOCORTICOIDS:**
    (I) **INCREASED RENAL Na REABSORPTION:** (action on the principal cells of the late distal tubule and collecting duct).
    (II) **INCREASED RENAL K SECRETION:** (action on the principal cells of the late distal tubule and collecting duct)
    (III) **INCREASED RENAL H SECRETION:** (actions on the alpha intercalated cells of the late distal tubule and collecting duct)

e. **PATHPHYSIOLOGY OF ADRENAL CORTEX:**
    (I) **ADDISON'S DISEASE:**
    CLINICAL FEATURES ARE: Hypoglycemia, Anorexia, weight loss, nausea, vomiting, weakness, hypotension, Hyperkalemia, Metabolic acidosis, decreased axillary and pubic hair in the women, Hyperpigmentation.
    ACTH LEVELS: are increased (negative feedback effect of decreased cortisol).

TREATMENT: Replacement of glucocorticoids and mineralocorticoids

(II) **CUSHING'S SYNDROME:** It is most commonly caused by administration of pharmacologic doses of glucocorticoids and hyperplasia of the adrenal glands. It is characterized by increased androgens and cortisol levels.
CLINICAL FEATURES ARE:
Hyperglycemia, Muscle wasting, central obesity, round face, supraclavicular fat, buffalo hump, osteoporosis, striae, virilization and menstrual disorders in women and hypertension.
ACTH LEVELS: are decreased (negative feedback effect of increased cortisol).
TREATMENT: Ketoconazole and Metyrapone.

(III) **CUSHING'S DISEASE:** Due to overproduction of ACTH.
CLINICAL FEATURES ARE:
Hyperglycemia, Muscle wasting, central obesity, round face, supraclavicular fat, buffalo hump, osteoporosis, striae, virilization and menstrual disorders in women and hypertension.
ACTH LEVELS: are increased
TREATMENT: Surgical removal of ACTH secreting tumor.

(IV) **CONN SYNDROME:** It is caused by aldosterone secreting tumor

CLINICAL FEATURES ARE:
Hypertension (because aldosterone increases sodium reabsorption, which leads to increase in ECF volume and blood volume) Hypokalemia (caused by aldosterone increasing potassium secretion)Metabolic alkalosis(because aldosterone increases hydrogen secretion) and decreased renin secretion (because increased ECF volume and blood pressure inhibit renin secretion by negative feedback)
ACTH LEVELS: not affected
TREATMENT: Spironolactone (aldosterone antagonist) and surgical removal of aldosterone secreting tumor.

(V) **21 BETA HYDROLASE DEFICIENCY:**
Decreased glucocorticoids and mineralocorticoids and increased adrenal androgens. It is the most common biochemical abnormality of the steroidogenic pathway. It belongs to group of disorders characterized by adrenogenital syndrome.
CLINICAL FEATURES ARE: Virilization of women, early acceleration of linear growth, and early appearance of pubic and axillary hair, symptoms of glucocorticoid and mineralocorticoid deficiency.
ACTH LEVELS: are increased (negative feedback effect of decreased cortisol)
TREATMENT: Replacement of glucocorticoids and mineralocorticoid.

- (VI) <u>17 ALPHA HYDROLASE DEFICIENCY:</u> Decreased adrenal androgens and glucocorticoids and increased mineralocorticoids.
  <u>CLINICAL FEATURES ARE:</u> Lack of pubic and axillary hair in women, symptoms of glucocorticoids deficiency, and symptoms of mineralocorticoid excess.
  <u>ACTH LEVELS:</u> are increased (negative feedback effect of decreased cortisol)
  <u>TREATMENT:</u> Replacement of glucocorticoids and aldosterone antagonists.
- a. <u>ADRENOCORTICAL INSUFFICIENCY:</u>
  - (I) <u>PRIMARY ADRENOCORTICAL INSUFFICIENCY-ADDISON'S DISEASE:</u> It is most commonly caused by autoimmune destruction of adrenal cortex and causes adrenal crises. It is characterized by the following features:
    - A. Decreased adrenal glucocorticoids, androgens and mineralocorticoid.
    - B. Increased ACTH (Low cortisol levels stimulate ACTH secretion by negative feedback.
    - C. Hypoglycemia caused by cortisol deficiency.
    - D. Weight loss, weakness, nausea and vomiting.
    - E. Hyperpigmentation (Low cortisol levels stimulate ACTH secretion; ACTH contains the MSH fragment.
    - F. Decreased pubic and axillary hair in women (caused by deficiency of adrenal androgens)

G. ECF volume contraction, hypotension, hyperkalemia and metabolic acidosis (caused by aldosterone deficiency).

(II) SECONDARY ADRENOCORTICAL DEFICIENCY:
It is caused by deficiency of ACTH and does not exhibit hyperpigmentation (because there is deficiency of ACTH. It does not exhibit volume contraction, hyperkalemia, or metabolic acidosis (because aldosterone levels are normal).Symptoms are otherwise similar to those of Addison's disease.

ADRENAL MEDULLA:

It is a specialized ganglion in the sympathetic division of the autonomic nervous system. The cell bodies of its preganglionic neurons are located in the thoracic spinal cord. The axons of these preganglionic neurons travel in the greater splanchnic nerve to the adrenal medulla, where they synapse on the chromaffin cells and release acetylcholine, which activates nicotinic receptors. When activated, the chromaffin cells of the adrenal medulla secrete catecholamines (epinephrine and norepinephrine) into the general circulation. In contrast with sympathetic postganglionic neurons, which release only norepinephrine, the adrenal medulla secretes mainly epinephrine (80%) and a small amount of norepinephrine (20%). The reason for this difference is the presence of phenylethanolamine-N-methyltransferase (PNMT) in the adrenal medulla, but not in the sympathetic adrenergic neurons. PNMT catalyzes the conversion of norepinephrine to epinephrine, a step that interestingly requires cortisol from the nearby adrenal cortex; cortisol is supplied to the adrenal medulla in venous effluent from the adrenal medulla.

A tumor of the adrenal medulla, or pheochromocytoma, may be located on or near the adrenal medulla, or at a distant site (ectopic) location in the body. Unlike the normal adrenal medulla, which secretes mainly epinephrine, a pheochromocytoma secretes mainly norepinephrine, which is explained by the fact that the tumor is too far from the adrenal cortex to receive the cortisol that is required by PNMT.

MALE REPRODUCTIVE SYSTEM:

The male reproductive system comprises of the internal and external genital organs which can be functionally organized as:

1. ## GONADS:

Gonads or primary male sex glands are a pair of testes. The main function of the testes is to produce sperms and secrete testosterone (male sex hormones).

2. ## ACCESSORY SEX GLANDS:
    (i) ## SEMINAL VESICLE:

These are two lobulated glands situated on either side of the prostate between urinary bladder and rectum.

   a. They secrete thick alkaline fluid that mixes with the sperms as they pass into the ejaculatory ducts and urethera.
   b. The duct of each seminal vesicle joins the ductus deferens to form the ejaculatory duct.

   (ii) ## BULBOURETHERAL (COWPER'S GLANDS):

These are two pea sized glands.

   (iii) ## PROSTATE GLAND:

It is the largest accessory gland of the male reproductive system. It secretes a thin milky fluid which forms 30 % the volume of semen.

3. ## DUCTS OF MALE REPRODUCTUVE SYSTEM:
    A. **EPIDIDYMIS:** It is formed by minute convolutions of the duct of the epididymis, so tightly compacted that they appear solid. The

efferent ductus transports the sperms from the rete testis to the epididymis where they are stored. The sperms can remain viable for a month in the epididymis. Secretions of the epididymis provide nourishment to the spermatozoa and help them to mature. Non motile spermatozoa become motile after passing through epididymis.

- B. DUCTUS DEFERENS OR VAS DEFERENS: It is the continuation of the tail of epididymis. It ends by joining to the duct of seminal vesicle .It serves as a secondary storehouse for spermatozoa which will be released at the time of ejaculation.
- C. EJACULATORY DUCTS: Each ejaculatory duct is a slender tube that arises by the union of the ductus deferens with the duct of seminal vesicle. The ejaculatory ducts open as minute slit like opening into the prostatic urethra.
- D. URETHERA: The male urethra is a muscular tube that conveys urine from the internal urethral orifice of the urinary bladder to the external urethral orifice at the tip of the glans penis. It also provides exit for semen (sperms and glandular secretions).

4. SUPPORTING STRUCTURES OF THE MALE REPRODUCTIVE SYSTEM:
   a. SPERMATIC CORD: It suspends the testes in the scrotum and contains structures that pass through the inguinal canal to and from the testis viz, ductus deferens, vessels and nerves of the testis.

b. **SCROTUM:** It is considered as the outpouching of the lower part of the abdominal wall which houses testes, epididymis and lower ends of the spermatic cord. The scrotum maintains the temperature lower than the normal body temperature (about 32C) which is necessary for normal spermatogenesis.
c. **PENIS**: It is the male copulatory organ and the common outlet for urine and semen.

STRUCTURE OF TESTES:

Each testis is divided into many lobules by the fibrous septa which project from the mediastinal testes into the tunica albuginea. Each lobule consists of:

a. Seminiferous tubular compartment
b. Interstitial compartment.

SEMINIFEROUS TUBULES: The testes contain 2-3 seminiferous tubules which occupies 80-90% of volume of testes. It consists of two parts: the convoluted part and the straight part. The convoluted part form the loops and continues as two straight ends. Near the apex of the lobule the straight ends join one another to form 20-30 larger straight tubules. The straight tubules unite to form the network called rete testes. At the upper end of each testes the rete testes gives of 10-20 efferent ductules which continue into the head of epididymis.

HISTOLOGICAL STRUCTURE OF SEMINIFEROUS TUBULES:

It consists of three layers:

1. Outer capsule or tunica propria:
2. Basement membrane

3. Epithelial layer of seminiferous tubules
   a. Germ cells or spermatogonium cells: They lie in between the Sertoli cells and are arranged in an orderly fashion in 4-8 layers, which extend from the basal lamina to the lumen of seminiferous tubule. In a sexually mature individual, the spermatogenic cells of all stages of differentiation are seen arranged in an orderly manner.
   b. Supporting cells or sustentacular cells (Sertoli cells): These are irregular pyramidal cells. The base of Sertoli cells rest on the basal lamina and each cell stretches from the basal lamina to the lumen of the tubule.
      FUNCTIONS OF SERTOLI CELLS:
      (I) PHYSICAL SUPPORT AND NUTRITION: They provide physical support to maturing germ cells, nourish them and remove waste products from the germ cells.
      (II) PHAGOCYTIC FUNCTION: The residual cytoplasmic byproducts which are cast off from the spermatozoa during conversion of spermatids into sperms are phagocytized by the Sertoli cells.
      (III) MAINTENANCE OF BLOOD – TESTES BARRIER:
      The tight junction forms effective permeability barrier within the seminiferous epithelium which is defined in man as blood-testes barrier. It limits the transport of many substances from blood to seminiferous tubules.

Thus blood testes barrier protects the cells of different stages of spermatogenesis from blood borne toxic substances and from circulating antibodies.

It prevents the entry of byproducts of gametogenesis into the blood.

(iv) SECRETORY FUNCTIONS:
A. MULLERIAN INHIBITORY SUBSTANCES (MIS)
B. ANDROGENBINDING PROTEIN (ABP)
C. ESTROGEN
D. TRANSPORT PROTEINS such as transferrin and ceruloplasmin
E. PLASMINOGEN ACTIVATOR

INTERSTITIAL COMPARTMENT:

The interstitial spaces between the seminiferous tubules are filled by loose connective tissue and Leydig cells. They have endocrine function of secretion of male sex hormones (testosterone).

FUNCTIONS OF TESTES:

The two principal functions of testes are:

a. Gametogenic function (spermatogenesis) and
b. Endocrine function

SPERMATOGENESIS:

Spermatogenesis refers to the process of formation of spermatozoa from the primitive germ cells (spermatogonia).

PHASES OF SPERMATOGENESIS:

The phases of spermatogenesis are as follows:

1. Phase of mitotic division of spermatogonia: Each spermatogonium divides 5 times to form 32 spermatogonia. The division occurs in the basal compartment of the seminiferous tubules.
2. Phase of formation of primary spermatocyte by mitotic division: The 32 spermatogonia undergo mitosis to form 64 primary spermatocytes. Primary spermatocytes are large cells with large nucleus having diploid number of chromosomes (2n).
3. Phase of formation of secondary spermatocyte by meiotic division: Each primary spermatocyte undergoes meiotic division.
   a. After first reduction division (meiosis) the 64 tetraploid primary spermatocytes (4n) are converted into 128 primary spermatocytes with diploid number of chromosomes (2n)
   b. The 128 primary spermatocytes (meiosis) to form 256 secondary spermatocytes having haploid number of chromosomes (n). Therefore 50%of sperms will have X chromosomes and other 50% will have Y chromosomes.
4. Phase of formation of spermatid: Each secondary spermatocyte divides mitotically to give rise to two spermatids. Thus, a total of 512 spermatids are formed from a single spermatogonium.
5. Phase of formation of spermatozoa (spermiogenesis): The spermatids do not divide further but undergo morphological changes to form sperms or spermatozoa. The spermatid undergoes

changes in the shape and orientation of its organelles. The spermatids mature into spermatozoa in the deep folds of the cytoplasm of the Sertoli cells.

STRUCTURE OF SPERMATOZOA:

A fully formed spermatozoon comprises of following parts:

a. <u>Head:</u> It is surrounded by acrosome. Acrosome is a thick cap like structure which covers the anterior two third parts of the head. It contains a number of enzymes (hyaluroinidase, proteolytic enzymes and acid phosphatase) which helps the sperm in penetrating ovum during fertilization.

b. <u>Neck:</u> It is a narrow constricted part. It consists of a funnel shaped basal body and a spherical centriole.

c. <u>Tail:</u> It is the motile portion and is also called flagellum. It can be divided into three parts:
   (i) <u>Middle piece:</u>
   (ii) <u>Principal piece:</u>
   (iii) <u>End piece:</u>

STORAGE OF SPERMATOZOA:

About 120 million sperms are formed each day. A small quantity of them is stored in the epididymis but most of them are stored in the vas deferens and ampulla of vas deferens. They can remain stored maintaining their fertility for about a month.

MATURATION AND CAPACITATION OF SPERMATOZOA:

<u>ROLE OF EPIDIDYMIS:</u>

The fully formed spermatozoa are released into the lumen of seminiferous tubules from where they reach the epididymis .Epididymis is the site of extra testicular maturation of spermatozoa. When the sperms arrive in the epididymis they are non-motile and acquire some motility only after passing through the epididymis.

ROLE OF SEMINAL VESICLES AND PROSTATE GLAND:

The secretions of seminal vesicles and the prostate have a stimulating effect on sperm motility but the spermatozoa become fully motile only after ejaculation.

ROLE OF FEMALE GENITAL TRACT: Spermatozoa acquire ability to fertilize the ovum only after they have been in the female genital tract for some time (1-10 hours).This final step in their maturation is called capacitation.

SEMEN:

Semen or the seminal fluid refers to the fluid ejaculated during the orgasm at the time of male sexual act.

CHARACTERISTIC FEATURES:

VOLUME: The average volume of semen per ejaculation is 2.5-3.5 ml after an abstinence of two days. Volume of semen decreases with repeated ejaculations.

APPEARANCE: Its appearance is milky due to prostatic secretions.

SPECIFIC GRAVITY: It is about 1.028

REACTION: is alkaline with a pH of 7.5.The alkalinity is due to prostatic secretions. The alkaline semen brings the vaginal pH from 3.5-4 to 6-6.5, the pH at which sperms show optimal motility.

NATURE OF SEMEN: when ejaculated is liquid but soon it coagulates in vitro or in the vagina,, and finally undergoes secondary liquefaction after about 15-30 minutes. The clotting of semen soon after ejaculation helps to retain it in the vagina for sometimes. Lysis later on would release the sperms for their free movement into the uterine cavity for fertilization.

COMPONENTS OF SEMEN AND THEIR CHARACTERISTICS:

The semen comprises of following components:

1. SPERMATOZOA: The normal sperm count varies from 35 million to 200 million per ml of semen with an average of 100 million per ml.
2. SECRETIONS OF SEMINAL VESICLES: Secretions of seminal vesicles contribute 60% of the semen volume. The secretion from the seminal vesicles is mucoid and viscous fluid. It is neutral and slightly alkaline in nature. It contains fructose, phosphorylcholine, ergothionine,ascorbic acid,flavins and prostaglandins.
FUNCTIONS SUBSERVED BY SEMINAL VESICLE SECRETIONS ARE:
NUTRITION: This is for sperms after being ejaculated into female genital tract, is provided by the fructose and other nutritive substances from seminal vesicle secretions.
CLOTTING OF SEMEN: soon after ejaculation into the female genital tract occurs due fibrinogen present in the seminal vesicle

FERTILIZATION OF OVUM: may be enhanced by the prostaglandins present in seminal vesicle secretion.

3. SECRETIONS OF PROSTATE GLAND: Secretion of prostate gland forms about 10%of the total semen bulk. It contributes milky and alkaline fluid part of the semen.
FUNCTIONS SUBSERVED BY THE PROSTATIC FLUID COMPONENT OF SEMEN ARE:
MAINTANENCE OF OPTIMUM PH FOR FERTILIZATION (6-6.5):It is the function of the alkaline prostate fluid which neutralizes the acidity of vaginal secretion. At this pH, the sperms become motile and chances of fertilization are enhanced.
CLOTTING OF SEMEN: by converting fibrinogen (from seminal vesicles) into a coagulum is caused by the clotting enzymes present in the prostatic fluid.

4. SECRETION OF BULBOURETHERALGLAND: Secretion of bulbouretheral gland and other mucous glands provide consistency to the semen after puberty.
ENDOCRINE FUNCTIONS OF TESTES:

A. TESTOSTERONE: The most important testicular hormone is testosterone. Leydig cells are numerous in newborn male infants and in adult males. So, the androgens are secreted in infancy and after puberty. The androgens secretion starts decreasing after 40 years and becomes almost zero by the age of 80 years. A normal man secretes 4-9 mg of testosterone daily. More than 98% of secreted testosterone is bound to plasma proteins; 68% is bound to albumin, and 30% is bound to testosterone binding globulin also called sex steroid binding globulin. A very small percentage of the plasma testosterone is unbound. The free fraction alone is physiologically active in the target tissues.

B. <u>ANDROSTENEDIONE:</u> is an important steroid precursor for blood estrogens in men. It is secreted by the testis at a rate of 2.5 mg/day.

C. <u>DIHYDROTESTEOSTERONE:</u> is an important androgen present in the blood.

<u>ADRENAL CORTEX:</u> also secretes androgens normally testosterone, androstenedione and dehydroepiandrosterone. The action of adrenal androgens are unimportant under physiological conditions, because their quantity is insignificant.

<u>FUNCTIONS OF ANDROGENS:</u>

A. FUNCTIONS OF ANDROGENS IN FETAL PERIOD (IN UTERO): The testosterone is secreted by the fetal testes at about 2nd to 4th month of embryonic life. The functions of androgens in fetal period are:
1. EFFECT ON SEX DIFFERENTIATION IN FETUS: Gonadal differentiation is dependent on the genotype of the embryo.
2. EFFECT ON DESCENT OF TESTIS: The testes developed in the abdominal cavity are pushed into the scrotum through inguinal canal just before birth. Testosterone is necessary for this descent of testes.

B. FUNCTIONS OF ANDROGENS AT PUBERTY:
1. EFFECTS ON EXTERNAL GENITALIA: Testosterone causes pubertal enlargement of penis. Scrotum increases in size and becomes pigmented. Rugal folds appear in scrotal skin.
2. EFFECTS ON ACCESSORY SEX ORGANS: Testosterone (with or without DHT) causes enlargement of seminal vesicles. DHT promotes growth of prostate and stimulates prostatic secretions.

C. EFFECT ON PSYCHE:
1. PSYCHOLOGICAL DIFFERENTIATION: A brief exposure of fetal hypothalamus to androgens (from its own testes) during early embryonic period causes male pattern of sexual behavior during puberty. It occurs due to constant secretion of pituitary gonadotropins.
2. LIBIDO: During puberty testosterone initiates sexual drive (libido) and erectile function (potency)
3. AGGRESSIVE BEHAVIOR: Testosterone produces aggressive behavior and interest in the opposite sex.

D. ANABOLIC AND GENERAL GROWTH PROMOTING EFFECTS:

Testosterone causes nitrogen retention in the body and causes accelerated growth of the body and skeletal muscles in particular. Androgens increase the rate of linear growth of the bones causing a rapid increase in stature at puberty.

E. FUNCTIONS OF ANDROGENS IN ADULTS:
  1. HAIR GROWTH: Androgenic patterns of hair growth are maintained. With increasing age, male baldness may be initiated.
  2. PSYCHE: Behavioral attitudes and sexual potency are maintained in post pubertal adults.
  3. BONE: Bone loss and osteoporosis are prevented by androgens in adult males.
  4. SPERMATOGENESIS: It is maintained in adulthood by testosterone along with FSH. The testosterone acts on both Sertoli cells and germ cells and thus maintains spermatogenesis.
  5. HEMATOPOIESIS: Testosterone stimulates erythropoiesis. Therefore accounts for the greater hemoglobin concentration and RBC count in males.
  6. EFFECTS ON CIRCULATING AND STORED BODY FATS: Testosterone increases circulating levels of low density lipoproteins (LDL) cholesterol and decreases plasma high density lipoproteins (HDL) cholesterol.

7. REGULATION OF GONADOTROPIN SECRETION: Androgen suppression of LHRH and LH by negative feedback effect.

CONTROL OF TESTICULAR FUNCTIONS:

The two main functions of testes viz spermatogenesis and secretion of testosterone are controlled by the hypothalamus hypophyseal testicular axis.

CONTROL OF SPERMATOGENESIS:

The hypothalamic hypophyseal testicular axis controlling the spermatogenesis is as follows:

1. STIMULATORY CONTROL:
    a. ROLE OF HYPOTHALAMUS: At puberty hypothalamic cells become more mature and their sensitivity for circulating sex hormones (negative feedback) decreases so much that there is a pulsatile release (8-14 pulses per day) of gonadotropin releasing hormone (GnRH) from the hypothalamus. The GnRH stimulates anterior pituitary to secrete LH and FSH.
    b. ROLE OF ANTERIOR PITUITARY: The anterior pituitary control spermatogenesis through the

gonadotropic hormones (FSH and LH) and growth hormones.

(i) FSH stimulates cells of Sertoli cells which play following roles during spermatogenesis:

Sertoli cells help in conversion of spermatids to sperms.

They secrete androgen binding protein ABP which stabilizes the high supply of testosterone to the developing germ cells in the seminiferous tubular lumen. FSH also promotes the synthesis of inhibin by Sertoli cells.

ROLE OF LH: The LH stimulates Leydig cells to cause testosterone secretion. The testosterone is required for normal spermatogenesis.

ROLE OF GROWTH HORMONE: Growth hormone specifically promotes early division of the spermatogonia themselves. In its absence, as in primary dwarfs, spermatogenesis is severely deficient or absent.

c. **ROLE OF TESTICULAR HORMONES:** Testosterone secreted by Leydig cells by paracrine effect acts on both Sertoli cells and germ cells and thus maintains spermatogenesis. It is important to note that:

Estrogen formed from testosterone by Sertoli cells (when stimulated by FSH) is probably also essential for spermatogenesis.

2. <u>FEEDBACK INHIBITORY CONTROL:</u>

The spermatogenesis is controlled by following negative feedback mechanisms

   a. Inhibin secreted by Sertoli cells are directly on the anterior pituitary and inhibits the secretion of FSH.
   b. Testosterone and estradiol inhibit LH secretion by negative feedback mechanism.

   Estradiol exerts the negative feedback effect at both the hypothalamic (GnRH) and pituitary (LH) levels.

   Testosterone has its feedback effect mainly at the hypothalamic (GnRH) level.

CONTROL OF TESTOSTERONE SECRETION:

IN FETUS:

During fetal life, human chorionic gonadotropin (HCG) secreted by placenta stimulates the development of Leydig cells in the testis of fetus and causes testosterone secretion.

IN ADULTS:

STIMULATORY CONTROL:

The hypothalamic hypophyseal testicular (Leydig cells) axis controls the secretion of testosterone in adults as;

Hypothalamus produces gonadotropin releasing hormone (GnRH) which stimulates anterior pituitary to FSH and LH.

Anterior pituitary controls the secretion of testosterone (steriodogenesis) primarily through LH.

FEEDBACK INHIBITORY CONTROL:

Plasma testosterone level is maintained at a constant level by a feedback control exerted by testosterone and estradiol independently to control LH. Testosterone negative feedback is exerted mainly on the opioidergic neurons that project to GnRH neurons.

OVERVIEW OF FEMALE REPRODUCTIVE SYSTEM:

The female reproductive system comprises internal and external genitalia which can be organized as:

PRIMARY SEX ORGANS OR OVARIES:

The primary sex organs are a pair of ovaries which corresponds with testes in males. The main functions of ovaries are:

1. To produce ova.
2. To secrete sex hormones.

ACCESSORY SEX ORGANS:

The accessory sex organs of females include internal genital organs and external genitalia.

FEMALE INTERNAL GENITALIA:

The internal genital organs include uterus, fallopian tubes and vagina.

- a. **UTERUS:** It is hollow, thick walled muscular organ, situated between the urinary bladder and rectum. It can be divided into two parts:
  (1) **BODY OF UTERUS:** It forms the upper $2/3^{rd}$ part of the uterus. Its lower limit is marked by a constriction which corresponds to narrowing of uterine cavity at internal os. Body of the uterus can be divided into two parts: Fundus is the rounded part of the body that lies superior to the opening of the fallopian tubes. Isthmus is the

relatively constricted region of the body (approx. 1 cm long) just above the cervix.

(2) <u>CERVIX OF THE UTERUS:</u> It is the cylindrical lower part which protrudes into the upper most vagina. It is approximately 2.5 cm long in an adult non-pregnant woman. Its cavity extends from the internal os to external os which opens into the vagina.

STRUCTURE OF UTERUS:

The wall of the body of uterus is consisting of three layers:

a. <u>PERIMETRIUM:</u> It is the external serosal layer.
b. <u>MYOMETRIUM:</u> It is the middle muscular layer comprising bundles of smooth muscles amongst which there is connective tissue.
c. <u>ENDOMETRIUM:</u> It is inner most layer of uterus which consists of epithelial lining and stroma.

FUNCTIONAL DIVISIONS OF ENDOMETRIUM:

Functionally the endometrium of the body of the uterus can be divided into two strata:

1. <u>STRATUM FUNCTIONALE:</u> It consists of superficial 2/3rd thickness of endometrium which undergoes monthly cyclic changes in preparation for the implantation of fertilized ovum and is shed during menstruation. This portion of endometrium is supplied by long and spiral (coiled) arteries.

2. **STRATUM BASALE:** It is the deepest 1/3rd layer of endometrium. It does not participate in cyclic changes but functions as regenerative layer. This part of endometrium is supplied by short and straight basal arteries.

b. **FALLOPIAN TUBES:** Each fallopian tube (also known as uterine tube) is approximately 10 cm long in length and 8 mm in diameter. It has a medial or uterine end which is attached to and opens into the uterus and a lateral end opens into peritoneal cavity near the ovary.

PARTS:
(1) **UTERINE OR INTERSTITIAL PART:** It is the most medial part which passes through the thick uterine wall.
(2) **ISTHMUS:** It is relatively narrow and thick walled part which is just next to the uterine part. It is about 2.5 cm in length.
(3) **AMPULLA:** It is the next thin walled and dilated part of the tube.
(4) **INFUNDIBULUM:** It refers to funnel shaped lateral end of the tube. It is prolonged into a number of finger like processes known as fimbria. One fimbria is longer than the rest of the fimbriae and is attached to the outer pole of the ovary.

STRUCTURE:

Fallopian tubes consist of same three coats as of the uterus viz endometrium, myometrium and perimetrium.

FUNCTIONS:

The uterine tubes convey ova, shed by the ovaries to the uterus. Ova enter the tube as its fimbriated end. The sperms enter the uterine tube at its medial end after traversing the vagina and uterine cavity. Secretions present in the tubes provide nutrition, oxygen and other requirements for ova and spermatozoa passing through the tube. Fertilization takes place in the ampulla and the fertilized ovum travels towards the uterus through the tube. The ciliated epithelial cells lining the tube help to move ova towards uterus.

c. <u>VAGINA:</u> The vagina is a musculocutaneous tube (about 8-10 cm long) located anterior to the rectum and posterior to urethra and urinary bladder. Its upper end surrounds the lower part of cervix and its lower end i-e vaginal orifice opens into the vestibule of vagina (the cleft between the labia minora).

<u>STRUCTURE:</u> The wall of vagina consists of a mucous membrane, a muscle coat and an outer fibrous coat or adventitia.
   (1) <u>MUCOUS MEMBRANE</u> shows numerous longitudinal folds. In adult female the vaginal mucosa lined by stratified squamous epithelium. The epithelial cells are rich in glycogen and this property is estrogen dependent.
   (2) <u>MUSCLE COAT</u> is made up of an outer layer of longitudinal fibers, and a much thinner layer of circular fibers. Many elastic fibers are present among the muscle fibers. The lower end of the

vagina is surrounded by striated fibers of the bulbospongiosus muscle that form a sphincter for it.

(3) <u>ADVENTITIAL COAT</u> surrounds the muscle coat and is made up of fibrous tissue containing many elastic fibers.

<u>FUNCTIONS:</u> The vagina serves following functions:

<u>a.</u> It serves as the excretory duct for menstrual fluid.
<u>b.</u> It forms the inferior part of pelvic (birth) canal.
<u>c.</u> It receives the penis and ejaculate during sexual intercourse.

FEMALE EXTERNAL GENITALIA:

The external genitalia include mons pubis, labia majora, labia minora, clitoris, vestibule of vagina, bulbus of vestibule and greater vestibular glands. The vulva serves as:

a. A sensory and erectile tissue for sexual arousal and intercourse.
b. To direct the flow of urine.
c. To prevent entry of foreign material into the urogenital tract.

OVARIES:

<u>FUNCTIONAL ANATOMY:</u> There are two pairs of ovaries located one on each side behind and below the fallopian tubes. The ovaries are ovoid glands with a combined weight of 10-20 gm. during reproductive years, which decreases with increasing age. Each ovary

is about 3-5 cm in length and is attached to the uterus by the broad ligament and round ligament of the ovary.

STRUCTURE:

HISTOLOGICALLY, each ovary consists of the following parts

1. GERMINAL EPITHELIUM: Germinal epithelium refers to the epithelium lining the outer surface of the ovary and consists of a single layer of cuboidal cells. The germinal epithelium is a misnomer and it does not produce germ cells.
2. CORTEX: The cortex is the outer thick part of the substance of the ovary. It consists of the following tissues:
   A. TUNICAL ALBUGINEA is the outer condensation of the connective tissue present immediately below the germinal epithelium.
   B. STROMA OF THE CORTEX present deep to the tunica albuginea is made up of reticular fibers and numerous fusiform cells that resemble mesenchymal cells.
   C. OVARIAN FOLLICLES at various stages of development are scattered in the stroma. Each follicle contains a developing ovum.
3. MEDULLA:

The medulla is the inner small part of the substance of ovary. It consists of connective tissue in which numerous blood vessels (mostly veins), smooth vessels and elastic fibers are present.

HILUM:

The hilum refers to the area where ovary attaches to mesentry. It is the site of entry of blood vessels and lymphatics.

FUNCTIONS OF OVARIES:
The two principal functions of ovaries are:
1. Gametogenic function i-e oogenesis
2. Endocrine function i-e secretion of female hormones called ovarian hormones.

OOGENESIS:

Oogenesis refers to the process of formation of ova from the primitive germ cells.

PRIMITIVE GERM CELLS: When the bipotential gonads differentiate into ovaries in genetic female (44+ XX) embryo by the tenth week of gestation, the primitive germ cells increases in number by mitosis to form oogonia. OOGONIA

are the stem cells from which ova are derived. The oogonia proliferate by mitosis to form primary oocytes.

PRIMORDIAL FOLLICLES: The diploid primary oocytes become enveloped by single layer of flat granulosa cells and in this form are called PRIMORDIAL FOLLICLES.

a. After puberty the oogenesis or formation of ovum occurs in a highly cyclic fashion, once every 28 days till menopause.
b. Every month, in each ovary more than one primordial follicle start undergoing maturation process but only one reaches maturity and the rest undergoes atresia at different stages of development. Thus throughout the whole normal reproductive life of about 30 years(from

13-42 years) about 450 ova are expelled and the remainder degenerate.

c. The different stage of maturation of primordial follicles into graffian follicles is called (folliculogenesis).

PHASES OF FOLLICULOGENESIS:
1. PRIMORDIAL FOLLICLES are the fundamental reproductive units of ovary. At the time of puberty both ovaries contain 3, 00,000 primordial follicles.
   a. Primordial follicles are formed in fetal life. Each primordial follicle consists of the primary oocyte in prophase of the first meiotic division surrounded by a single layer of spindle shaped cells called the granulosa cells.
   b. Both the granulosa cells and the primary oocyte are enveloped in a thin membrane called basal lamina.
   c. The granulosa cells believed to provide nutrition to the ovum and also secrete oocyte maturation inhibiting factor (OMF) which keeps the ovum in immature stage till puberty.
2. PRIMARY FOLLICLE: The primary follicle is formed when the primordial follicle undergoes following developmental changes:
   a. Granulosa cells, which are flat in primordial follicle become columnar and undergo mitotic division to from a multilayered stratum granulosum.

b. Oocyte enlarges and becomes about 20 micron in size.
   c. Zona pellucida, a homogenous membrane appears consisting of glycoprotein between the granulosa (follicular) cells and the oocyte. With the appearance of zona pellucida the follicle is now referred to as a multilaminar primary follicle.
3. SECONDARY FOLLICLE form from the primary follicle when:
   a. Granulosa cells undergo further proliferation.
   b. Oocyte further increases in size up to 100 microns.
   c. Theca folliculi is formed outside the basal lamina from the spindle shaped cells from the stroma of cortex in ovary. The theca folliculi consists of an inner rim of secretory cells called theca interna and an outer rim of thickly packed fibers and spindle shaped cells called theca externa (that merges with the surrounding stroma)
4. TERTIARY FOLLICLE: After proliferation the granulosa cells start secreting follicular fluid, this causes cavity to be formed in the stratum granulosum which is called antrum or follicular cavity. The fluid filled in the antrum is called liquor folliculi which also contains estrogen. The granulosa cells

continue to proliferate and the size of follicle is increased.

5. GRAFFIAN (ANTRAL) FOLLICLE: After about 7th day of sexual cycle one of the tertiary follicle increases in size in response to gonadotropins (FSH and LH) and forms the mature follicle called graffian follicle. A fully mature graffian follicle is characterized by:
   a. Size of the follicle increases markedly to about 2-5 mm. The growth of the graffian follicle is accomplished by granulosa and theca proliferation.
   b. Antrum becomes larger
   c. Theca internal becomes more prominent
   d. Formation of secondary oocyte. Just prior to ovulation, the primary oocyte of the fully matured graffian follicle completes first meiotic division (which began in the fetal life at about 28 weeks of gestation i-e before birth) and forms the secondary oocyte with a haploid nucleus and the first polar body.

ENDOCRINE FUNCTIONS OF THE OVARY:

The endocrine functions of the ovaries are to produce female sex hormones which include:

1. Estrogens
2. Progesterone

ESTROGENS:

Estrogens are C-18 steroids. The naturally occurring estrogens include:

a. Estradiol: It is the principal and physiologically most potent estrogen. Ovarian estradiol accounts for more than 90% of the circulating estrogen.
b. Estrone: It is a weak ovarian estrogen
c. Estriol: It is the degradation product of estradiol and estrone. It is the weakest of all naturally occurring estrogens.

FUNCTIONS OF ESTROGENS:

REPRODUCTIVE ACTIONS:

AT PUBERTY:

a. Growth and development of genital organs:
   (i) Ovaries increase in size and complete ovarian cycles start which are characterized by folliculosis, ovulation and corpus luteum formation.
   (ii) Fallopian tubes become functional and show certain changes such as epithelium becomes more ciliated, motility of fallopian tubes also increases at ovulation to transport shedded gametes.
   (iii) Uterus enlarges in size; endometrium gets thickened due to increase in stroma and blood flow. The rhythmic cyclic changes (proliferative and secretory) occur with onset of menstrual cycle.

- (iv) Cervix: also enlarges and with onset of menstrual cycle, endocervix undergoes cyclic changes.
- (v) Vagina: increases in size, Its epithelial increases in height
- (vi) External genitalia: Increase in size of clitoris, labia majora and labia minora increase in size and get widened.

APPEARANCE OF SECONDARY SEX CHARACTERISTICS:

Estrogen is responsible for appearance of secondary sexual characteristics.

<u>IN AN ADULT WOMAN</u>: Estrogens along with progesterone regulate the ovarian cycle, menstrual cycle and cyclic changes in the cervix, vagina and fallopian tubes in non pregnant state.

- a. It play an important role in maintenance of pregnancy and then during parturition
- b. It is important for breast development.

OTHER ACTIONS:

- a. <u>EFFECTS ON BONES:</u>
  - (i) Estradiol accelerates the linear growth of bones at puberty by its osteoblastic activity.
  - (ii) Estradiol enlarges the hip and widens the inlet of the pelvic bone to facilitate child birth.
- b. <u>EFFECTS ON METABOLISM:</u>
  - (i) <u>PROTEIN METABOLISM</u>: Estrogens cause positive nitrogen balance due to growth promoting effect.

- (ii) **FAT METABOLISM:** Estrogens causes fat deposition in subcutaneous tissues, in the breasts and the thighs.
- c. **WATER AND ELECTROLYTE BALANCE:** It causes salt and water retention and result premenstrual tension in some women.
- d. **EFFECT ON VASCULATURE:** In general, estrogens have vasodilator and antivasoconstrictor effect.
- e. **EFFECT ON BEHAVIOR:** It increases libido in human females.
- f. **EFFECT ON SKIN:** Estrogens make the skin soft and more vascular. It makes the sebaceous glands secretion thin. Therefore synthetic estrogens are used for the treatment of acne.

PROGESTERONE:

Progesterone is a C-21 steroid meant for maintenance of pregnancy.

FUNCTIONS OF PROGESTERONE:

The physiological changes of progesterone can be grouped as reproductive actions and other actions.

REPRODUCTIVE ACTIONS:
- a. **ACTIONS ON UTERUS:** The progesterone is responsible for the secretory phase of the endometrial cycle and prepares the endometrium to receive the zygote. It decreases the uterine motility.
- b. **ENDOCERVIX:** The cervical secretions become thick and viscid and ferning pattern disappears.
- c. **VAGINA:** Vaginal epithelium becomes thickened, cornified and infiltrated with leucocytes.

d. **FALLOPIAN TUBES:** Progesterone increases the epithelial cell secretions rich in nutritive materials to provide nutrition to shedded ovum, incoming sperms or to zygote if fertilization occurs.
e. **BREAST:** Progesterone causes lobular and alveolar growth of the breasts.
f. **DURING PREGNANCY:** the main function of the progesterone is to maintain pregnancy.

OTHER ACTIONS:

a. **THERMOGENIC EFFECT:** Progesterone is known as a thermogenic steroid, increases the basal body temperature by 0.5* C in post ovulatory phase.
b. **EFFECT ON CNS:** Progesterone alters the secretion of various neurotransmitters in the hypothalamus and other areas of the brain and thereby decreases the appetite and produces somnolence.
c. **EFFECT ON RESPIRATION:** Progesterone increases the sensitivity of the respiratory center to carbon diaoxide stimulation. Due to this fact the pACO2 is slightly less in woman during luteal phase of the sexual cycle.
d. **EFFECT ON FAT METABOLISM:** Progesterone decreases the serum HDL. Thus it acts as a proathrogenic agent.

OTHER OVARIAN HORMONES:

a. **INHIBIN:** It is a polypeptide that inhibits the FSH release.
b. **ACTIVIN:** It is also a polypeptide and its action is to activate FSH secretion from the anterior pituitary.

c. <u>RELAXIN</u>: Relaxin is a polypeptide produced by the corpus luteum and other sites include: uterus, placenta and mammary glands and in males from the prostate gland. Its main role is during pregnancy as it relaxes pubic symphysis and pelvic joints, softens and dilates the uterine cervix and facilitates delivery.

   <u>In non pregnant state:</u> It is released from the corpus luteum and endometrium during secretory phase and its function is not known.

   <u>In males:</u> relaxin is present in the semen and helps in the sperm motility.

d. <u>OVARIAN ANDROGENS</u>: A small amount of testosterone is also secreted by the ovaries during biosynthesis of estrogen and progesterone but the main source of androgens in females is the adrenal cortex. The androgens are responsible for acne vulgaris, libido and pubic hair.

<u>FEMALE SEXUAL CYCLE:</u>

The sexual life span of a female can be divided into three phases:

1. <u>BEFORE PUBERTY:</u> During this period primary and accessory female sex organs remain quiescent.
2. <u>PUBERTY TO MENOPAUSE:</u> With the onset of puberty the female sexual cycle starts, which repeats every 28 days. The occurrence of first menstrual cycle is called menarche. The permanent stoppage of menstrual cycle is called menopause, which occurs at the age of about 45-50 years. The period between menarche and menopause is called

reproductive period. During this period females have rhythmic sexual cycles.
3. <u>POSTMENOPAUSAL PERIOD:</u> It extends after menopause (45-50 years) to rest of the life. During this period the female sexual cycle ceases.

Female sexual cycle refers to monthly rhythmic sexual cycle during the normal reproductive period.

4. <u>COMPONENTS OF HUMAN FEMALE SEXUAL CYCLE:</u> During each female sexual cycle, rhythmic changes occur in the ovaries and accessory organs – uterus, cervix and vagina.
5. <u>DURATION OF FEMALE SEXUAL CYCLE:</u> it is usually 28 days. But under physiological conditions it may vary between 20 and 40 days. Traditionally the first day of the menstrual bleeding is considered as the first day of female sexual cycle.

OVARIAN CYCLE:

Ovarian cycle refers to rhythmic changes occurring in the ovaries during each female sexual cycle of about 28 days. During each cycle a single mature ovum is released from the ovary. Ovarian changes occurring during the female sexual life completely depend on the gonadotropic hormones (FSH and LH) which are secreted by the anterior pituitary. The ovarian cycle can be divided into three phases:

a. Preovulatory phase or follicular phase
b. Ovulation
c. Post ovulatory phase or luteal phase.

PREOVULATORY PHASE: This phase extends from the fifth day of the cycle till the time of the ovulation (which takes place at about 14th day of the cycle). Thus this phase generally lasts for 8-9 days but may vary from 10-25 days.

Changes in the ovary during this phase are mostly under the influence of FSH from the anterior pituitary. LH also helps in maturation of the follicle in the later part of follicular phase.

During this phase of each cycle some 10-15 primordial follicles start maturing, but only one follicle matures fully and the rest undergo atresia at different stages of development.

OVULATION: Ovulation refers to release of secondary oocyte from the ovary (following rupture of graffian follicle) into the peritoneal cavity. It usually occurs 14 days after the onset of menstruation.

DETERMINATION OF OVULATION TIME:

The ovulation time can be measured by the following indirect methods:

1. FROM BASAL BODY TEMPERATURE: The basal body temperature falls slightly just before ovulation and increases slightly after ovulation. Therefore the time of ovulation can be determined by measuring the morning temperature from rectum and vagina.
2. FROM HORMONAL EXCRETION IN URINE: The urinary excretion of end products of estrone, estradiol increases to a peak at the time of ovulation and that of end products of progesterone like pregnenediol increases after ovulation. Therefore,

time of ovulation can be determined by estimating their urinary levels for few days during mid period of menstrual cycle.

3. FROM HORMONAL LEVELS IN PLASMA: The plasma content of FSH, LH, estrogen and progesterone is measured during mid period of menstrual cycle and time of ovulation is determined from following observations:
   a. LH and estrogen levels are increased and FSH level is decreased at the time of ovulation.
   b. Progesterone level is increased after ovulation
4. BY ULTRASOUND SCANNING: The process of ovulation can be recorded.

POST OVULATORY PHASE:

This phase is also called the luteal phase of ovarian cycle and is remarkably constant period of 14 days. This phase is characterized by following events:

FORMATION OF CORPUS HEMORRHAGICUM: Following ovulation the outer wall of the graffian follicle collapses and promptly fills with blood forming the so called corpus hemorrhagicum.

FORMATION OF CORPUS LUTEUM: Soon the granulosa cells and theca cells of the follicle lining begin to proliferate, and the clotted blood is rapidly replaced with yellowish lipid rich luteal cells. This process is called lutenization and the total mass of the cells is now called corpus luteum. LH is responsible for lutenization.

FORMATION OF CORPUS ALBICANS: If there is no fertilization and pregnancy does not occur, the corpus luteum begins to regress after 24th day of the sexual cycle and is eventually replaced by whitish scar tissue called the corpus albicans. This involution occurs due to falling levels of FSH and LH and also the hormone inhibin secreted by the luteal cells. With the involution of the corpus luteum on 26th day of the normal female sexual cycle, the levels of estrogen, progesterone and inhibin fall. This removes feedback inhibition of anterior pituitary consequently the secretion of FSH and within few days the LH secretion begins and the next ovarian cycle is initiated.

CORPUS LUTEUM OF PREGANANCY: However if the ovum released is fertilized and pregnancy occurs, then the corpus luteum formed during postovulatory phase persists and serves as the major source of estrogen and progesterone till the 3rd month of pregnancy when the placenta takes over its endocrine functions.

ENDOMETRIAL CYCLE: Endometrial cycle refers to the cyclic changes occurring in the endometrium during active reproductive period (menarche to menopause) in females leading to recurrent monthly bleeding per vaginum (menstruation). These cyclic changes in the endometrium are brought about by the cyclic production of estrogens and progesterone by the ovaries.

PHASES OF ENDOMETRIAL CYCLE:

The endometrial cycle of 28 days can be divided into three phases:

a. Menstrual phase (1st-5th)
b. Proliferative phase(6th-14th day)
c. Secretory phase(15th -28th day)

PROLIFERATIVE PHASE: It follows the phase of menstruation after which only a thin basal layer of original endometrium is left. Hormone responsible for changes in the endometrium during this phase is estrogen secreted by the developing graffian follicle in the ovary. Thus, proliferative phase of endometrial cycle co-incides with the follicular phase of ovarian cycle. Changes in endometrium which occurs during proliferative phase:

a. Thickness of endometrium which is less than 1 mm at the end of menstrual phase increases to 3-4 mm at the end of proliferative phase.
b. Angiogenesis in the stratum functionale leads to proliferation of the blood vessels which becomes the spiral arterioles of blood vessels that profuse the stratum functionale.
c. Endometrial glands are stimulated to grow. The glands contain glycogen but they are non-secretory.

SECRETORY PHASE:

Hormone responsible for changes in the endometrium during this phase is both estrogen and progesterone secreted by the corpus luteum formed after ovulation. Thus the secretory phase of the endometrial cycle coincides with the luteal phase of the ovarian cycle.

Changes in the endometrium which occur during this phase are:

a. There is elongation and coiling of endometrial mucous glands. These glands become secretory and secrete viscous fluid containing glycogen.
b. Blood supply of endometrium further increases as progesterone promotes spiraling of blood vessels.

c. Two characteristic features of endometrium in secretory phase thus are prominent corkscrew shaped glands and increased vascularity.
d. Thickness of endometrium increases to 5-6mm at the end of secretory phase. Thus the thickened endometrium with large amounts of nutrients is ready to provide appropriate conditions for implantation of ovum during this phase.
e. If fertilization does not occur and there is no pregnancy, the corpus luteum in the ovary involutes to form corpus albicans and on the day 26th of the menstrual cycle, the levels of estrogen and progesterone fall suddenly and mark the end of secretory phase of endometrial cycle.

MENSTRUAL CYCLE:

The menstrual cycle of the endometrial cycle is also called bleeding phase. The average duration of this phase is 3-5 days. About 24 hours before the end of the menstrual cycle there is a sharp decline in the plasma levels of estrogen and progesterone, which is responsible for the menstrual bleeding.

a. Endometrial debris contains sloughed necrosed off tissue, blood, serous fluid and large amounts of prostaglandins and fibrolysins.
b. Average amount of blood loss during each menstrual cycle is 30 ml.
c. Menstrual blood immediately gets clotted inside the uterine cavity but soon gets liquefied by fibrolysins present in the endometrial debris.

d. During menstrual phase about 2/3rd of the superficial endometrium is sloughed off and only a thin basal layer (2mm thick is left).

CYCLIC CHANGES IN THE CERVIX:

The mucosal lining of the cervix also shows certain cyclical changes during sexual cycle.

DURING MENSTRUAL PHASE:

The mucosa of cervix does not undergo desquamation (shedding off) like that of endometrium.

DURING PROLIFERATIVE PHASE:

The secretions of the mucosal cells of endocervix become thin, watery and alkaline. At the time of ovulation the cervical mucus is thinnest and its elasticity is maximum. It can be stretched like a long thin elastic thread up to a 8-12cm. The mucus also produces a characteristic fern like pattern when a drop of mucus is spread on the glass slide and allowed to dry (Fern test).

This characteristic nature of cervical mucus favors the transport of sperms in the female genital tract and makes the conditions favorable for fertilization.

DURING SECRETORY PHASE:

Under the influence of progesterone, cervical secretions decrease in quantity and become thick, tenacious and cellular and fern pattern is not seen. These changes make a plug and prevent the entry of sperm through cervical canal.

FERN TEST:

The fern pattern of cervical mucus in proliferative phase and its disappearance in secretory phase is indicative of ovulatory cycle, whereas the persistence of fern pattern throughout the cycle indicates anovulatory cycle.

CYCLIC CHANGES IN VAGINA:

Vaginal canal is lined by stratified squamous epithelium which is highly sensitive to estrogen. Vaginal epithelium undergoes following cyclic changes in endometrial cycle.

In proliferative phase: vaginal epithelium becomes thickened and cornified.

In secretory phase: Under the influence of progesterone vaginal epithelium proliferates and gets infiltrated with leucocytes and the vaginal secretions become thick and viscid.

OTHER CHANGES DURING SEXUAL CYCLE:

Hormonal oscillations during sexual cycle through mainly effect ovaries, uterus, cervix and vagina but some change have also been observed in the fallopian tubes, breast and in the body weight.

Changes in the fallopian tubes are as follows:

1. During follicular phase, there occurs increase in the number of cilia of epithelial cells and their rate of beating.
2. At the time of ovulation the motility of fallopian tubes increases.
3. During luteal phase, under the influence of progesterone, there occurs an increase in the secretions of epithelial cells. This provides nutrition to the ovum, incoming sperm and the zygote if fertilization occurs.

Changes in the breast:

Some women complain of feeling of fullness and tenderness in the breasts. These symptoms have been related to the proliferation of lobules and duct system under the influence of estrogen and progesterone. All these symptoms regress during menstrual cycle.

Premenstrual weight gain:

Many women experience feeling of heaviness near the end of the cycle. This effect is due to salt and water retention caused by the estrogen. The feeling of heaviness disappears during menstruation phase.

HORMONAL CONTROL OF THE FEMALE SEXUAL CYCLE:

The hypothalamo –hypophyseal –gonadal axis regulates the cyclic changes occurring during female sexual cycle.

ROLE OF HYPOTHALAMUS:

Hypothalamus regulates the secretion of gonadotropins (both FSH and LH) through the gonadotropin releasing hormone (GnRH). The GnRH reaches the anterior pituitary through the hypothalamo-hypophyseal portal system where it is stored as small granules. It stimulates the anterior pituitary cells to release gonadotropins.

ROLE OF ANTERIOR PITUITARY:

The anterior pituitary plays a role in female sexual cycle regulation by releasing gonadotropins (FSH and LH). Gonadotropin in turn regulates the ovarian cycle i-e formation of graffian follicle, ovulation and formation of corpus luteum.

REGULATION OF GONADOTROPINS:

The secretion of both FSH and LH is regulated by:

a. <u>GONADAL HORMONES</u>: The gonadal hormones (estrogen and progesterone) regulate gonadotropin secretion by their feedback effect. Depending on relative plasma level of these hormones the effect may be positive or negative or both positive and negative.
   - (I) ESTROGENS: in moderately high plasma concentration (just before ovulation) inhibits the release of FSH by negative feedback effect) and promotes LH secretion (by positive feedback effect).
   - (II) HIGH LEVELS OF ESTROGEN AND PROGESTERONE: in mid luteal level phase inhibit the secretion of FSH and LH (by negative feedback effect).
   - (III) LOW LEVELS OF GONADAL HORMONES: (during menstruation phase) increase the secretion of both FSH and LH by positive feedback effect.
   - (IV) The feedback effect (positive or negative) of ovarian hormones is brought about by its action either directly on anterior pituitary or through hypothalamus.
   - (V) Oral contraceptives are preparations containing high concentration of estrogen and progesterone. These drugs inhibit gonadotropin release by negative feedback effect and prevent ovulation.

b. <u>HUMAN CHORIONIC GONADOTROPIN:</u> It is a glycoprotein secreted by syncytiotrophoblasts during early pregnancy (12-16 weeks of gestation).Like LH, HCG also maintains the functional state of corpus luteum and thus elevate gonadal hormones resulting in inhibition of gonadotropin release.
c. <u>PROLACTIN:</u> It is a mammotropic hormone secreted from anterior pituitary during lactation. It inhibits GnRH release and thus lowers the basal secretion of FSH and LH (cause for lactation amenorrhea).
d. <u>ACTIVIN:</u> It is structurally quite similar to inhibin (secreted from the ovary).It is synthesized in the cells of anterior pituitary. It stimulates the synthesis and release of FSH by autocrine and paracrine actions.

<u>ROLE OF OVARIES:</u> Ovaries play a role in regulation of ovarian cycle and endometrial cycle by secreting gonadal hormones (estrogen and progesterone).

a. <u>ESTROGENS:</u> In each sexual cycle the plasma concentration of estrogen starts rising from first day of the cycle and reaches to its peak just before ovulation (at 12-13th day) called estrogen surge. Estrogen through positive feedback effect is responsible for ovulation due to LH surge. Estrogen is responsible for the proliferative phase of the endometrial cycle.
b. <u>PROGESTERONE:</u> After ovulation there occurs formation of corpus luteum and the progesterone concentration starts rising. Therefore, in the luteal

phase of ovarian cycle level of both estrogen and progesterone are high, but progesterone rises markedly. Progesterone prepares the estrogen primed endometrium for implantation. Thus, it is responsible for secretory phase of endometrial cycle.

PHYSIOLOGY OF PREGNANCY:

Physiology of pregnancy is mainly concerned with maternal adaptations to provide ideal atmosphere for fertilization, nutrition to the growing fetus, and safe child birth. The physiology of pregnancy can be discussed under following headings:

1. Fertilization and implantation
2. Formation of placenta and its functions
3. Physiologic changes during pregnancy
4. Applied aspects

FERTILIZATION AND IMPLANTATION:

FERTILIZATION:

Fertilization refers to fusion of male and female gametes (i-e spermatozoon and ovum). It takes place in the middle segment (ampulla) of the fallopian tube. It involves following events:

1. **TRANSPORT OF GAMETES:**

Before fertilization, the ovum and sperms reach the ampulla for fertilization.

TRANSPORT OF OVUM:

At the time of ovulation the ovum is directly expelled into the peritoneal cavity and then enters the fallopian tube. The contractions of smooth muscle fibers present in the wall of fallopian tube also help in transport of the ovum.

TRANSPORT OF SPERMS IN THE FEMALE GENITAL TRACT:

After ejaculation, several million sperms (average-200 million sperms per ejaculation) get deposited in the vagina. After ejaculation normal sperm shows flagellar movements in the fluid medium at a rate of 1-4 mm/min. Therefore, in 30-6- minutes, they are able to reach the fallopian tube.

2. SPERM CAPACITATION:

Sperm capacitation refers to the process that makes a sperm to fertilize an ovum. Immediately after ejaculation in female genital tract the sperm undergoes certain changes, which enable it to fertilize an ovum. It takes about 1-10 hours(capacitation period).Sperm capacitation occurs due to removal of certain factors, which normally remain quiescent in male genital tract.

These are:

CHOLOESTEROL CONTENTS OF THE ACROSOMAL MEMBRANE:

In the female genital tract the cholesterol contents of acrosomal membrane decreases and it becomes weak leading to easy release of enzymes from the head.

CALCIUM IONS:

The membrane of sperm becomes permeable to calcium ions. The influx of Ca acts by two ways:

It makes the flagellar movements of the sperms more strong and whipish (hyper activation of sperms) and secondly it triggers the release of enzymes from the acrosome.

3. FUSION OF GAMETES:

The fusion of ovum and sperm involves the following steps:

a. <u>CHEMOATTRACTION:</u> Chemoattraction of the sperms to ovum occurs by substances produced by the ovum.
b. <u>PENETRATION OF SPERM THROUGH OVUM COVERINGS</u>: It is made possible by release of enzymes hyaluroinadase and other proteolytic enzymes present on the acrosome of the sperm. The binding of sperm to zona pellucida glycoprotein (ZP3) triggers acrosomal reaction.
   (i) Acrosomal reaction: It involves release of acrosin (protease enzyme) from anterior membrane of acrosome of the sperm.
   (ii) Only one sperm can enter into the oocyte, and further entry of sperms is prevented by the activation of ovum.

<u>IMPLANTATION:</u>

(i) Implantation of a fertilized ovum involves following steps:
(ii) Formation of Blastocyst:
   a. The fertilized ovum starts dividing immediately and is called morula (16 cell stage) and blastocyst (100 cell stage). Blastocyst on cut section shows inner cell mass surrounded by a layer of cells called trophoblast, which is covered by zona pellucida.
   b. The trophoblast layer consists of an inner layer (cytotrophoblast) and an outer (syncytiotrophoblast). The

syncytiotrophoblasts secrete proteolytic enzyme that digest and liquefy the endometrial cell.

(iii) Transportation of blastocyst in uterine cavity:

In next 3-4 days blastocyst then erodes and burrows into the endometrium. Then blastocyst goes deeper and deeper into the uterus mucosa till whole of it lies within the endometrium.

(iv) Decidual reaction:

After implantation the endometrium is called decidua. The stroma cells of endometrium get enlarged become vacuolated and filled with glycogen and lipids. These cells are called decidual cells. The stored glycogen and lipids are the source of nutrition for the embryo till placenta takes up the function. Therefore this change in stroma cell is called decidual reaction.

PLACENTA AND PREGNANCY TESTS:
PLACENTA:

Placenta is a temporary organ found during pregnancy. It is an important link betweenthe mother and the fetus. When fully formed the placenta is a disc shaped structure has a diameter of 15-20 cm and weighs about 500 gm.

After birth of the baby, the placenta is shed off along with decidua.

THE PLACENTAL MEMBRANE:

The maternal and fetal bloods do not mix with each other. They are separated by a placental membrane, made up of the layers of the wall of the villus. From the fetal side:

a. Endothelium of fetal blood vessels and its basement membrane.
b. Surrounding mesenchymal tissue (connective tissue)

c. Cytotrophoblast and its basement membrane.
d. Syncytiotrophoblast.
e. The total area of the membrane varies from 4m2 -14 m2. Its thickness is 0.025 mm in the beginning and in the later part of pregnancy it is reduced to 0.02 mm.

FUNCTIONS OF PLACENTA:

The fully functional placenta develops by the end of third month (12 weeks) of pregnancy. Placenta serves mainly three functions:
a. Hormonal secretion (endocranial functions of placenta)
b. Transport of substances between mother and fetus, and
c. Protection of the fetus.

HORMONE SECRETION:

The syncytiotrophoblast of the placenta serves as an endocrine gland. The hormones secreted by placenta are:
a. Human chorionic gonadotrophins(HCG)
b. Human chorionic sommatotrophins(HCS)
c. Human chorionic thritropin(HCT)
d. Placental progesterone
e. Placental estrogens
f. Relaxin

1. <u>Human chorionic gonadotrophin.</u> Human chorionic gonadotrophin (HCG) is a polypeptide. It is secreted by syncytiotrophoblast, soon after fertilization it is detected in the maternal blood as early as 6-8 days after conception, and reaches its peak between 60-90 days of gestation. After this the concentration falls to al very low level and just before labor its level falls to zero. Its approximate peak value in human maternal blood normal pregnancy is 5mg/ml.

PHYSIOLOGIC EFFECTS OF HCG ARE:
a. HCG is a luteotropic hormone. Its action is similar to LH of anterior pituitary hence called second luteotropic hormone. It maintains the functions of the corpus luteum up to 7 weeks after conception until fetoplacental unit is able to synthesize its own estrogen and progesterone.
b. HCG stimulates fetal testes in male fetus to secrete testosterone prior, to fetal pituitary LH secretion. This testosterone and MRF secreted by fetal testes is responsible for development of male genital organs and descent of testes during intrauterine life.

CLINICAL IMPORTANCE (APPLICATION) OF HCG: Is the presence of HCG in the urine forms the basis of all the pregnancy tests. HCG appears in the urine as early as 10 days after gestation with 99% accuracy. If fetus dies early then HCG disappears from the blood as well as from the urine.

2. **HUMAN CHORIONIC SOMMATOTROPHIN:** The syncytiotrophoblast cells of placenta also secrete large amount of human chorionic sommatotropin (HCS). HCS is protein in nature and structurally resembles to growth hormone.

PLASMA CONCENTRATION:
The secretion of HCS begins at 5th week of pregnancy. It increases gradually throughout pregnancy and its plasma concentration is directly proportional to the weight of the placenta. Its peak reaches at term and peak value is 15 µg/ml.

It functions as maternal growth hormone of pregnancy and causes deposition of protein in the tissues, and brings about nitrogen, calcium and potassium retention.

3. <u>HUMAN CHORIONIC THROTROPIN:</u>
Human chorionic thyrotropin (HCT) secreted by the placenta has quite similar properties to that of thyroid stimulating hormones (TSH). The physiological role is not fully understood.

4. <u>PLACENTAL PROGESTERONE:</u>
<u>SYNTHESIS:</u>
During early pregnancy it is synthesized by corpus luteum of pregnancy and then by syncytiotrophoblasts of placenta (85% of total contribution). The various facts regarding synthesis of progesterone in placenta are:
Placental syncyiotrophoblasts do not synthesize cholesterol. Therefore cholesterol is mainly derived from maternal circulation and very little is contributed by the fetus.
The fetus, placenta and mother, though they are independent, but constitute a functional unit called (fetoplacental maternal unit).
Plasma concentration:
During pregnancy plasma concentration of progesterone rises steadily throughout gestation reaching a maximum plateau at 30- 40 weeks and its level does not fall to zero like other placental hormones. Just before the onset of labor its level decreases.
PHYSIOLOGICAL EFFECTS OF PLACENTAL PROGESTERONE ARE:
   a. It helps to preserve pregnancy by promoting the growth of endometrium. It converts secretory endometrium of the luteal phase of menstrual cycle to decidual during pregnancy.
   b. It has a marked inhibitory effect on the contractions of uterus.

    c. It causes the development of alveolar system of mother's breast. It synergic action with estrogen prepares the breast for lactation after the birth of the baby.
    d. Progesterone has an immunosuppressive role in protecting the fetus.
    e. By acting as a precursor for corticosteroid synthesis by the fetal adrenal cortex it helps in growth and development of fetus.

5. **PLACENTAL ESTROGENS:**
Placental estrogens are C21 steroid hormones quantitatively oestriol is the major estrogen of pregnancy with smaller amount of estradiol and estrone.
It mediates the following effects:
    a. It causes growth and development of maternal reproductive organs(uterus increases in size, weight, length and volume both by hypertrophy and stretching of myometrium)
    b. Estrogen stimulates the development of lactiferous ductal system in the mammary glands,
    c. It stimulates hepatic synthesis of thyroxine binding globulin, steroid binding globulin and angiotensinogens. It also stimulates renin secretion.
    d. Just before term, estrogen to progesterone ratio increases and uterus is dominated by estrogen.

PHYSIOLOGIC CHANGES DURING PREGNANCY:

The normal average duration of pregnancy in human beings is 280 days (40 weeks) and is calculated from the first day of the last menstrual period or 256 -270 days from the time of ovulation. As the pregnancy progresses various types of extra demands are imposed on the mother's body by the growing fetus, which are met with by certain adaptations in almost all the organ systems of the body. These physiological changes include:

CHANGES IN THE GENITAL ORGANS:

a. **UTERUS:** To accommodate the growing fetus marked increase in the size of the uterus takes place. The enlargement is mainly due to hypertrophy and to some extent hyperplasia of the myometrial smooth muscle fibers.

b. **OVARIES:** The follicular changes and ovulation donot occur because the FSH and LH of anterior pituitary are inhibited.

c. **CERVIX:** Endocervix gets hypertrophied, the cervical glands increase in number and their secretion form a plug that closes the cervical canal, and the tough cervix gets soft.

d. **MAMMARY GLANDS:** Under the influence of various hormones the breast enlarges in early pregnancy. Hyperplasia of ductal and alveolar tissue occurs, the areola becomes pigmented and many sebaceous glands become prominent in the areola. Nipples also become larger and pigmented.

WEIGHT GAIN: A woman may gain total of 10-12 kg of weight during normal pregnancy which is contributed by:

a. Fetus 3 kg
b. Placenta and amniotic fluid 1.5 kg
c. Uterus and breast enlargement 1 kg
d. Increase in blood volume and interstitial fluid 1.5 kg
e. Fat deposition 3.5-4 kg

HEMATOGOLOGICAL CHANGES:

a. Blood volume: The total blood volume increases by 30%. The plasma volume increases relatively more than that of red blood cell volume which causes hemodilution thus there is physiological anemia of pregannacy.
b. The hematological indices show following changes:
   (I)   RBC count decreases.
   (II) Hb concentration decreases.
   (III) PCV decreases
   (IV) ESR increases
   (V)   Reticulocyte count increases
c. Plasma proteins: The total concentration of plasma proteins decreases from 7.5 to 6 gm % due to hemodilution. The fibrinogen level increases, but serum albumin markedly decreases.
d. Leucocytes: Total leucocyte count increases and may reach up to 20,000/mm3
e. Platelets: There occurs slight decrease in platelet count.
f. Coagulation factors: Pregnancy seems to be a hypercoaguable state due to increase in following :fibrinogen and factors VII, VIII, IX and X. The hypercoagulability of the blood plays significant

role of hemostasis at the time of placenta during delivery.

CARDIOVASCULAR SYSTEM CHANGES:

a. Position of the heart: The gravid uterus pushes the diaphragm upwards resulting change in the position of heart as:
  (i) Heart rate: Heart rate also increases by 10-12 beats/min
  (ii) Cardiac output increases from 5liters/min to 7 liters/min at 20 weeks of gestation.
  (iii) Blood pressure may show following changes:
    a. Systolic blood pressure: in normal pregnancy there is either no change in systolic pressure or some fall may occur.
    b. Diastolic blood pressure: decreases and by 16-20 weeks of pregnancy its value is lowest. Then it starts rising and comes back to normal.
  (iv) Blood flow: Blood flow to the skin, uterus and kidneys increases to meet the demands.
  (v) Venous pressure: The gravid uterus exerts pressure on the pelvic veins, abdominal veins and femoral veins, thus increasing the venous pressure. The rise in femoral venous pressure results in edema in feet (common occurrence).

RESPIRATORY SYSTEM CHANGES:

a. Hyperventilation: High levels of plasma progesterone during pregnancy increase the

sensitivity of respiratory neurons to CO_2 resulting in hyperventilation.
b. Gas exchange: Gas exchange across the alveoli is greatly enhanced due to marked increase in the pulmonary blood flow.
c. Oxygen consumption: Oxygen consumption of body increases by 15% to meet the demands of growing fetus and for the extra work of heart, uterus and other tissue.

URINARY SYSTEM CHANGES:

Kidney functions show following changes:

a. Renal blood flow: There is marked increase in renal blood flow due to increase in cardiac output and vasodilation.
b. Glomerular filtration rate (GFR) increases by 50% due to increase in renal blood flow and solute load.
c. Renal tubular absorptive capacity for sodium and chloride ions also increases by 50% due to high level of steroid hormones secreted by the placenta and the adrenal cortex.
d. Glycosuria is a common physiological phenomenon during pregnancy.
e. Proteinuria occurs due to increase in excretion of proteins.
f. Water balance: During later months of pregnancy excess of water is retained due to :
   (i) Decreased protein concentration
   (ii) Retention of sodium
g. Acid base balance: Hyperventilation during pregnancy results in respiratory alkalosis. Kidneys

therefore compensate for it by excreting more HCO3 ions in the urine.

GASTROINTESTINAL SYSTEM CHANGES:

a. GIT secretions: Hypochlorhydria is very common due to decreased gastric secretion
b. GIT motility: decreases under the influence of hormones resulting in delayed gastric emptying.
c. Gall bladder functions: Gall bladder increases in size and empties its content at a very slow rate.
d. Liver functions are also altered during pregnancy. The fibrinogen synthesis increases and albumin decreases thus plasma A: G ratio is also altered.
e. Morning sickness: anorexia, nausea and vomiting are very common in early pregnancy (first trimester) especially in the morning hours hence known as morning sickness. The cause for the morning sickness is not known.
f. Glucose tolerance curve: also shows disturbances. It becomes diabetic type due to glucose being rapidly absorbed from the intestine.

METABOLIC CHANGES:

a. The basal metabolic rate (BMR) of the pregnant woman increases by about 15% during later half of the pregnancy.
b. Protein metabolism: When the diet is balanced and adequate then there is nitrogen retention and positive nitrogen balance. The proteins are deposited in the uterus, breast, in the fetus, and in the placenta.
c. Carbohydrate metabolism shows following changes:

- (i) Blood glucose levels increases due to rapid absorption from the gut.
- (ii) Glucosuria is of common occurrence due to increase in GFR and decrease in renal threshold for glucose.
- (iii) Ketosis may occur due to anorexia and excessive vomiting.

d. Fat metabolism: About 3-4 kg of fat is deposited in the body during pregnancy. These occurs an increase in plasma concentration of cholesterol, phospholipids and triglycerides.

e. Mineral metabolism: depicts following changes
  - (i) Calcium and phosphorus: in normal pregnancy mother retains about 50 gm. of extra calcium and 30-40 gm. of phosphorus. These are deposited in the fetus and also retained in the mother stores (skeleton).
  - (ii) Iron metabolism: Iron requirements tremendously increase during pregnancy and lactation.

ENDOCRINE SYSTEM CHANGES:

Almost all the endocrine glands of the mother react substantially during pregnancy. Firstly due to increased metabolic load on the mother and secondly in response to the hormones produced by the placenta and fetus.

CHANGES IN THE SKIN:

a. Hyperpigmentation: occurs on the face (butterfly pattern called as chloasma), areola, nipple and midline of abdomen (linea Alba) extending from pubic symphysis to xiphisternum. The

hyperpigmentation is related to increased secretion of ACTH and MSH during pregnancy.
b. Stria gravidarum: These are linear scars present on the lower abdomen due to stretching of the skin.

PSYCHOLOGICAL CHANGES:

The nervous system shows the mild changes in the form of craving for particular types of food item, alterations in the behavior, emotions and mood. In few cases true psychosis may also develop but cause is not known.

PHYSIOLOGY OF VISION:

The wall of the eye consists of three concentric layers; an outer layer which is fibrous includes the cornea, corneal epithelium, conjunctiva and sclera. The middle layer, which is vascular, includes the iris and choroid. The inner layer is neural and contains the retina. The functional portions of retina cover the entire posterior eye, with the exceptions of blind spot, which is the OPTIC DISC. Visual acuity is highest at a central part of retina, called the macula; light is focused at a depression in the macula called the FOVEA. The eye also contains a lens, which focuses light; pigments absorb light and reduce; and two fluids, aqueous and vitreous. Aqueous humor fills the anterior chamber of the eye, and vitreous humor fills the posterior chamber of the eye. The sensory receptors for vision are PHOTORECEPTORS, which are located on the retina. They are of two types' rods and cones.

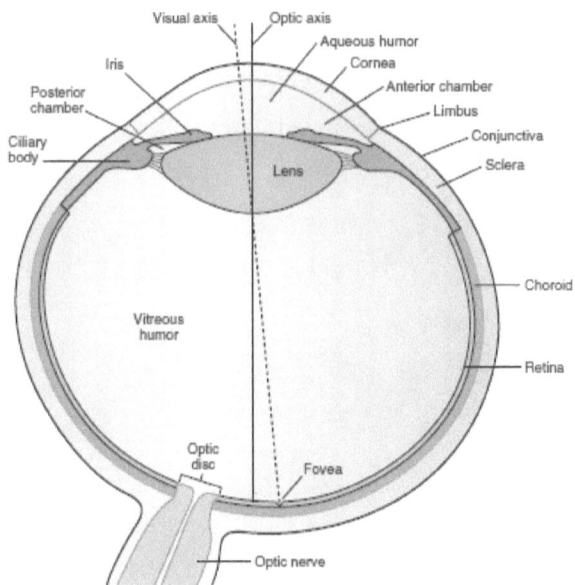

RODS: It has low acuity and does not participate in color vision, have low thresholds, are sensitive to low intensity light and function well in darkness.

CONES: they have a high threshold for light than rods, operate best in day light, provide higher visual acuity and participate in color vision. The cones are not sensitive to low intensity light.

Information is received and transduced by photoreceptors on retina and then is carried to CNS via axons of retinal ganglion cells .Some optic nerves cross at the optic chiasma, and others continue ipsilaterally. The main visual pathway is through the dorsal lateral geniculate nucleus of thalamus, which project to visual cortex.

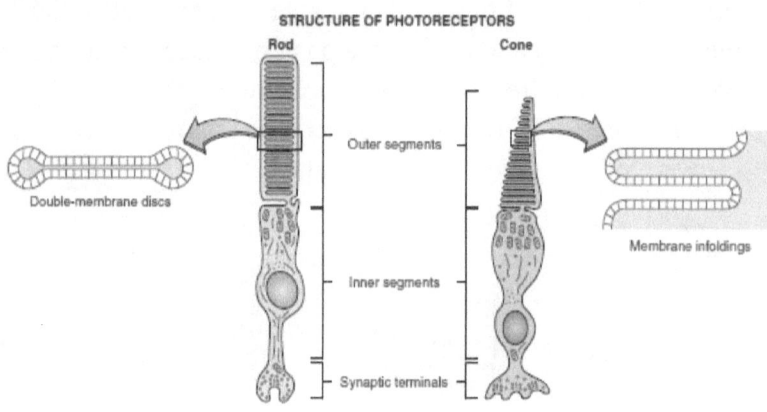

LAYERS OF RETINA:

The retina is a specialized sensory epithelium that contains photoreceptors and other cell types arranged in layers. Retinal cells include photoreceptors, interneurons (bipolar cells, horizontal cells and amacrine cells). Synapses are between cells in two plexiform layers, an outer plexiform layer and inner plexiform layer. The layers of retina are:

1. LAYER OF PIGMENT EPITHELIUM: Single layer of hexagonal cells containing melanin pigment serves as;
   a. Absorbs stray light ;reduces light scatter
   b. Phagocytose the ends of outer segments of rods which are continuously shed.
   c. Reconvert the metabolized photo pigment into a form that can be reused after it is transported back to photoreceptor.
2. LAYERS OF RODS AND CONES:
   It consists of outer segments of photoreceptors (rods and cones)
3. EXTERNAL LIMITING MEMBRANE:
   It contains numerous connections between muller cells and inner segments of photoreceptors.
4. OUTER NUCLEAR LAYER:
   It contains nuclei of rods and cones.
5. OUTER PLEXIFORM LAYER:
   It contains synapses between photoreceptors, bipolar cells and horizontal cells.
6. INNER NUCLEAR LAYER:
   It consists of cell bodies and nuclei of bipolar cells, amacrine cells and horizontal cells.
7. INNER PLEXIFORM LAYER:

It consists of synapse between bipolar cells, ganglion cells and amacrine cells.
8. <u>GANGLION CELL LAYER:</u>
It transmits visual information to brain.
9. <u>NERVE FIBER LAYER:</u>
Axons of ganglion cell layer are present here.
10. <u>INNER LIMITING MEMBRANE:</u>
Projections of Muller cells separates the retina from vitreous.

LAYERS OF THE RETINA

1. Pigment cell layer
2. Photoreceptor layer
3. Outer nuclear layer
4. Outer plexiform layer
5. Inner nuclear layer
6. Inner plexiform layer
7. Ganglion cell layer
8. Optic nerve layer

PHOTORECEPTION:

It is the transduction process in rods and cones that converts light energy into electrical energy. Rhodopsin, the photosensitive pigment is composed of OPSIN (a protein belonging to superfamily of G protein- coupled receptors) and retinal (an aldehyde of vitamin A). When light strikes the photoreceptors, retinal is chemically transformed in a process called photo isomerization, which begins the transduction.

1. Light strikes retina, which initiates photo-isomerization of retinal-11 cis retinal is converted to all Trans retinal. Now opsin is converted to METRHODOPSIN II (Regeneration of 11 cis retinal requires vit A and deficiency of vitamin A causes night blindness.
2. Metrhodopsin activates a G protein that is called TRANSDUCIN. Now transducin activates PHOSPHODIESTERASE that catalyzes conversion of cGMP to 5GMP, decreasing levels of cGMP.
3. In the photoreceptor membrane, Na channels that carry inward current are regulated by cyclic GMP.
4. In the dark, there is an increase in cGMP which produces inward Na current (or dark current) and depolarization of photoreceptor membrane. In the light, there is a decrease in cyclic GMP levels, which closes Na channels in the photoreceptor membrane, reduces inward Na current and produces hyperpolarization.
5. Hyperpolarization of photoreceptor membrane decreases the release of glutamate from the synaptic terminals of photoreceptor.

6. There are two types of glutamate receptors on bipolar and horizontal cells;
   a. Ionotropic (depolarizing and excitatory)
   b. Metatropic (hyperpolarizing and inhibitory)

   The type of receptor on the bipolar or horizontal cells determines whether the response will be depolarization (excitation) or hyperpolarization (inhibition). Decreased release of glutamate that interacts with IONOTROPIC RECEPTORS will result in hyperpolarization and inhibition of bipolar or horizontal cells (i-e decreased excitation). And decreased release of glutamate that interacts with metabotropic receptors will result in depolarization and excitation of bipolar or horizontal cells (i-e decreased inhibition causes excitation) This process will produce on-off patterns for visual fields.

STEPS IN PHOTORECEPTION

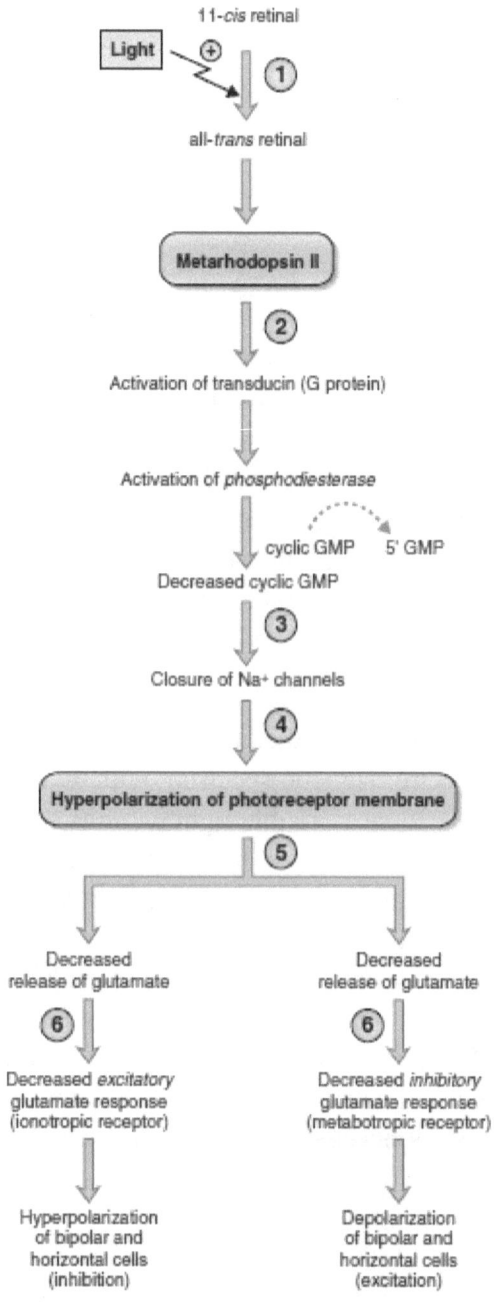

Vision, the act of seeing is extremely important to human survival. More than half of the sensory receptors are in the eye and a large part of cerebral cortex is devoted to processing visual information.

ELECTROMAGNETIC RADIATION:

Electromagnetic radiation is energy in the form of waves that radiates from the sun. There are many types of electromagnetic radiation, including gamma rays, UV light, visible light, infrared radiation, microwaves and radio waves. This range of electromagnetic radiation is known as ELECTROMAGNETIC SPECTRUM. The distance between two consecutive peaks of an electromagnetic wave is the wavelength. Wavelengths vary from short to long; for example gamma rays have wavelength smaller than a nanometer and most radio waves have wavelengths greater than a meter.

The eyes are responsible for the detection of visible light, the part of the electromagnetic spectrum with wavelength ranging from 400-700nm. Visible light exhibits colors. The color of visible light depends on its wavelength. An object can absorb certain wavelengths of visible light and reflect others; the object will appear the color of the wavelength that is reflected. For example green apple green because it reflects mostly green light and absorbs most other wavelengths of visible light. An object appears white because it reflects all wavelengths of visible light. An object appears black because it absorbs all wavelengths of visible light.

SUMMARY OF STRUCTURES OF EYEBALL:

1. **FIBROUS TUNIC:**
   a. **CORNEA:** Admits and refracts and bends the light.
   b. **SCLERA:** Provides shape and protects the inner parts.
2. **VASCULAR TUNIC:**
   a. **IRIS:** regulates the amount of light that enters the eyeball.
   b. **CILIARY BODY:** secretes aqueous humor and alters the shape of lens for near or far vision (accommodation).
   c. **CHOROID:** Provides blood supply and absorbs scattered light.
3. **NEURAL TUNIC:**
   a. **RETINA:** Receives light and converts it into receptor potentials and nerve impulses, output to brain via axons of ganglion cells which form the optic nerve.
4. **LENS:** Refracts light.
5. **ANTERIOR CHAMBER:** It contains aqueous humor that helps maintain shape of the eyeball and supplies oxygen and nutrients to lens and cornea.
6. **VITEROUS CHAMBER:** It contains vitreous body that helps maintain shape of the eyeball and keeps retina attached to the choroid.

PHYSIOLOGY OF VISION:

Light must pass through cornea, aqueous humor, pupil, lens and vitreous humor before reaching the retina. It must pass through the layers of retina to reach the photoreceptive layer of rods and cones. The outer segments of rods and cones transduce light energy from photons into membrane potentials. Photo pigments in rods and cones absorb photons and this causes a conformational change in the molecular structure of these pigments. This molecular alterations causes sodium channels to close, a hyperpolarization of membranes of rods and cones and a reduction in the amount of neurotransmitter released. Thus rods and cones release less neurotransmitter in the light and more neurotransmitter in the dark.

VISUAL PATHWAYS:

Axons from the retinal ganglion cells form the optic nerve and optic tracts, synapse in the lateral geniculate body of the thalamus and ascend to the visual cortex in the geniculcalcarine tract.

Temporal visual fields project onto nasal retina and the nasal field project onto temporal retina. Nerve fibers from each nasal hemi retina cross at the optic chiasm and ascend contralaterally. Nerve fibers from each temporal hemi retina remain uncrossed and ascend ipsilaterally. Thus fibers from left nasal hemi retina and fibers from right temporal hemi retina form the right optic tract and synapse on the right lateral geniculate body. Conversely fibers from the right nasal hemi retina form the left optic tract and synapse on the left lateral geniculate body. Fibers from the lateral geniculate body form the geniculocalcarine tract which ascends to the visual cortex (area 17 of occipital lobe). Fibers from the right lateral geniculate body form the right geniculocalcarine tract; fibers from the left lateral geniculate body form the left geniculocalcarine tract.

Lesions at various points in the optic pathway cause deficits in vision, which can be predicted by tracing the pathway. Hemianopia is loss of vision in half the visual field of one or both eyes.

If the loss occurs on the same side of the body as the lesion, it is called IPSILATERAL; if the loss occurs on the opposite side of the body as the lesion; it is called CONTRALATERAL.

OPTIC NERVE: Cutting the optic nerve cause blindness in the ipsilateral (same side) eye. Thus cutting the left optic nerve causes blindness in the left eye. All sensory information coming from that eye is lost because the cut occurs before any fibers cross at the optic chiasma.

OPTIC CHIASM: Cutting the optic chiasma causes heteronymous (both eyes) bitemporal (both temporal visual fields) hemianopia. In other words, all information is lost from fibers that cross. Thus information from the temporal field s from both eyes is lost because these fibers cross at the optic chiasma.

OPTIC TRACT: Cutting the optic tract causes homonymous contralateral hemianopia. Cutting the left optic tract results in loss of temporal visual field from the right eye (crossed) and loss of nasal visual field from the left eye (uncrossed).

GENICULOCALCARINE TRACT: Cutting the geniculocalcarine tract causes homonymous contralateral hemianopia with macular sparing (the visual field from macula is intact) Macular sparing occurs because lesions of visual cortex do not destroy all neurons that represent the macula.

Rods and cones have synaptic contacts on bipolar cells that project to ganglion cells. Axons from ganglion cells converge at optic disc to form the optic nerve, which enter the cranial cavity through optic foramen. At the optic disc, these axons acquire a myelin sheath from the oligodendrocytes of the CNS. At the optic chiasma, 60% of the optic nerve fibers from the nasal half of each retina crosses and project into contralateral optic tract. Fibers from temporal retina do not cross at the chiasm and instead pass into the ipsilateral optic tract. The optic tract contains remixed optic nerve fibers from the temporal part of the ipsilateral retina and from the nasal part of contralateral retina. Because the eye inverts image like a camera, in reality each nasal retina receives information from temporal hemi field and each temporal retina receives information from the nasal hemi field. Most fibers in the optic tract

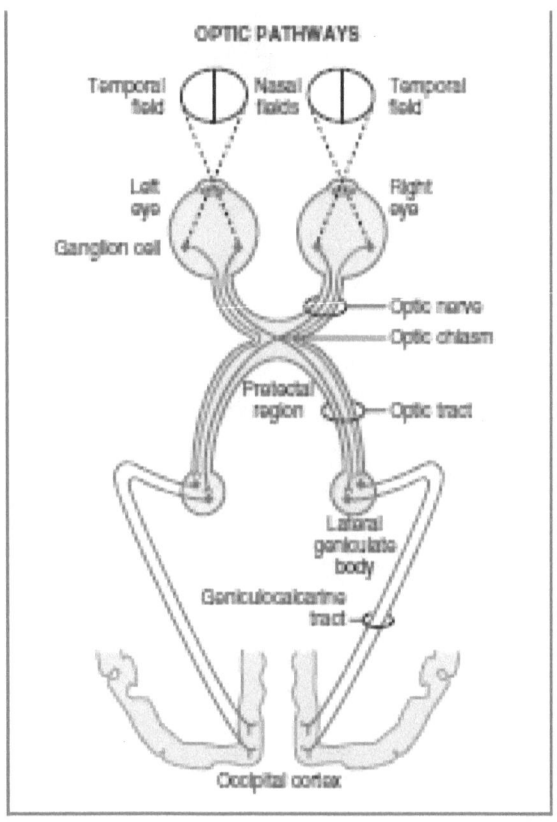

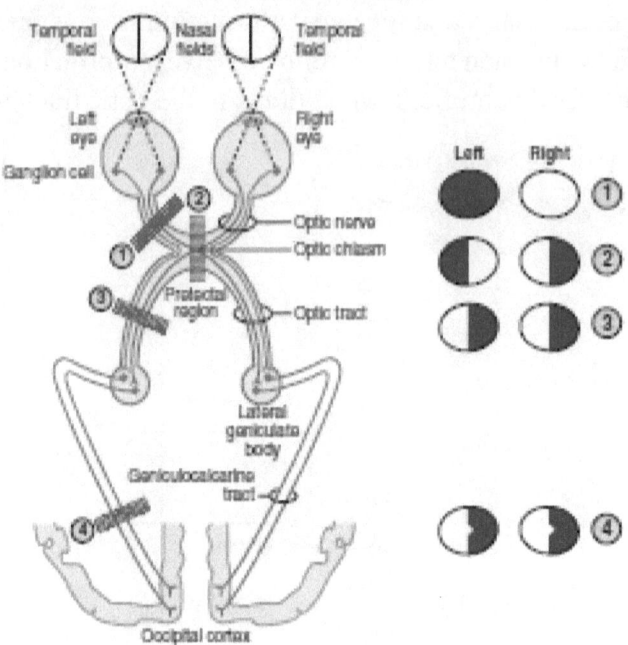

LESIONS OF OPTIC PATHWAYS

420

PHYSIOLOGY OF GUSTATION:

A chemical sense which is detected by chemoreceptors located on taste buds. Tastes are a mixture of five elementary taste qualities: salt, sweet, sour, bitter and umami (savory including monosodium glutamate).

TASTE BUDS AND RECEPTORS:

Taste receptor cells are located within taste buds on the tongue, palate, pharynx and larynx. The taste buds on the tongue are found in the taste papillae, which includes as many as several hundred taste buds. The taste buds consist of three cell types:

1. SUPPORTING CELLS: they are found among the taste receptor cells. These cells do not respond to taste stimuli, and their function is not known.
2. BASAL CELLS: these are undifferentiated cells that serve as precursors to taste receptor cells. Basal cells undergo continuous replacement. New cells, which are generated every 10 days, migrate toward the center of the taste bud and differentiate into new receptor cells. New receptor cells are needed to replace those cells that are sloughed from the tongue.

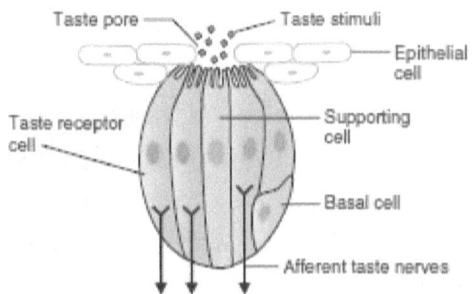

STRUCTURE OF A TASTE BUD

3. <u>TASTE RECEPTOR CELLS:</u> are the chemoreceptors of the taste system. They line the taste buds and extend microvilli in the taste pores. These microvilli provide a large surface area for detection of chemical stimuli. In contrast to the olfactory system (in which the receptor cells are the primary afferent neurons) in the gustatory system, the receptor cells are not neurons. They are specialized epithelial cells that function as chemoreceptors, transducing chemical stimuli into electrical signals. Afferent fibers innervate the taste receptor cells and transmit this information to the CNS.

    Taste buds on the tongue are organized in specialized papillae. Three types of papillae contain taste buds:

    a. <u>Circumvallate papillae:</u> are the largest in size but fewest in number. They are arranged in rows at the base of the tongue. Each circumvallate papilla is surrounded by trench, with taste buds located on the walls of the trenches. Because of their large size, approximately half the total number of taste buds is found in circumvallate papillae. The taste cells in circumvallate papillae are innervated by CN VII and IX.
    b. <u>Foliate papillae</u>: are located on the lateral borders of the tongue.
    c. <u>Fungiform papillae:</u> are scattered on the dorsum of the tongue and are most numerous near the anterior tip. The fungiform papilla is translucent with a dense blood supply, making them appear as red spots on the surface of the tongue. The

taste cells in fungiform papillae are innervated by the chorda tympani branch of CN VII.

STRUCTURE OF THE TASTE PAPILLAE

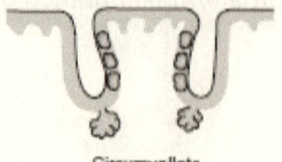
Circumvallate

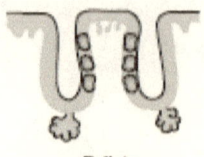
Foliate

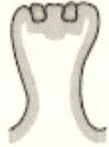
Fungiform

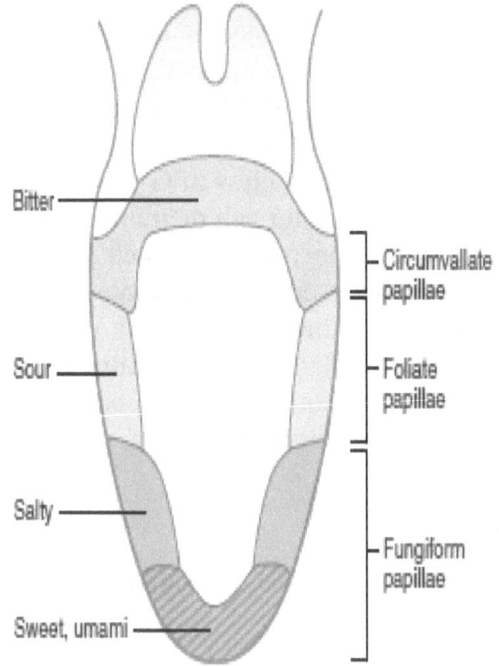

TASTE TRANSDUCTION:

Detection of the five basic taste qualities involves differential sensitivity of areas of the tongue .
Although all five taste qualities can be detected over the full surface of the tongue, different regions of the tongue do have different thresholds. The tip of the tongue is most responsive to sweet, salty, and umami, whereas the posterior tongue is most responsive to bitter, and the sides of the tongue are most responsive to sour. The chemical signals for the five taste qualities are transduced by the mechanisms shown. In most cases, transduction ultimately results in depolarization of the taste receptor membrane (i.e., a
depolarizing generator potential). This depolarization leads to action potentials in afferent nerves innervating that

portion of the tongue. For **bitter** sensation, the tastant molecules bind to G protein–coupled receptors on the taste receptor membrane and, mediated by an inositol 1,4,5-triphosphate (IP3)/Ca2+ mechanism, opens so-called transient receptor potential (TRP) channels and results in depolarization. For **sweet and umami** sensations, molecules bind to a different class of G protein–coupled receptors on the taste receptor cell membrane and, mediated by IP3/Ca2+, open TRP channels and cause depolarization. For **sour** sensation (mediated by H+), H+ enters the taste receptor through epithelial *Na+* channels (**ENaC**), leading to depolarization. For **salty** sensation (mediated by Na+), Na+ enters the taste receptor through the same epithelial Na+ channels, leading directly to depolarization.

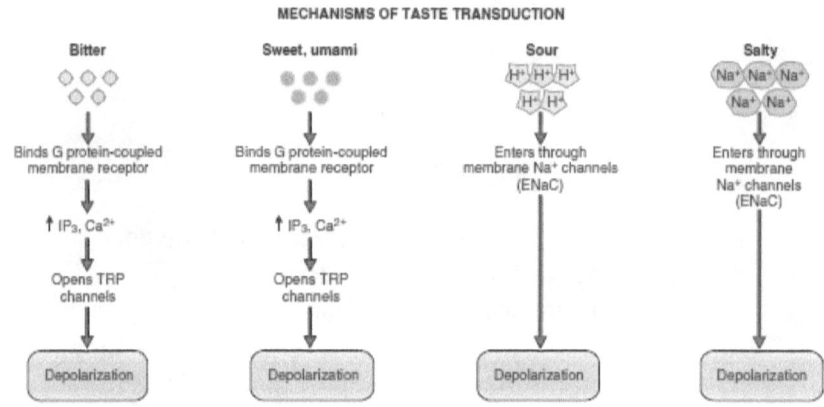

TASTE PATHWAYS:
As noted, taste begins with transduction of chemical signals in the taste receptor cells, which are located in taste buds. Transduction leads to depolarizing receptor potentials, which lead to action potentials in primary afferent neurons innervating specific regions of the tongue. Different regions of the tongue are innervated by branches of three cranial nerves. The posterior one third of the tongue (where bitter and sour sensations are most sensitive) is innervated by the

glossopharyngeal nerve (CN IX). The anterior two thirds of the tongue (where sweet, umami, and salty sensations are most sensitive) is innervated by the facial nerve (CN VII). The back of the throat and epiglottis are innervated by the vagus nerve (CN X). These three cranial nerves (CN VII, IX, and X) enter the brain stem, ascend in the **solitary tract,** and terminate on second order neurons in the **solitary nucleus** of the medulla. The second-order neurons project ipsilaterally to the ventral posteromedial nucleus of the thalamus. Third order neurons leave the thalamus and terminate in the taste cortex.

PHYSIOLOGY OF OLFACTION:

The chemical senses involve detection of chemical stimuli and transduction of those stimuli into electrical energy that can be transmitted into nervous system. Olfaction, the sense of smell is one of the chemical senses. In humans, olfaction is not necessary for life and yet it improves the quality of life and even protects against hazards.

OLFACTORY EPITHELIUM AND RECPETORS:

Odorant molecules which are present in the gaseous form reach the olfactory receptors via nasal cavity. Air enters the nostril, crosses the nasal cavity and exits into nasophyrynx. The nasal cavity contains structures called turbinates, some of which are lined by olfactory epithelium containing olfactory receptor cells. (The remainder of the epithelium is lined by respiratory epithelium. The turbinates cause the air flow to reach the upper regions of the nasal cavity.

The olfactory epithelium consists of three cell types: supporting cells, basal cells and olfactory receptor cells.

1. **SUPPORTING CELLS:** are columnar epithelial cells lined with microvilli at their mucosal border and filled with secretory granules.
2. **BASAL CELLS:** are located at the base of the olfactory epithelium and are undifferentiated stem cells that give rise to olfactory receptor cells. These stem cells undergo mitosis, producing a continuous turnover of receptor cells.
3. **OLFACPTORY RECEPTOR CELLS:** which are primary afferent neurons, are the site of odorant binding, detection and transduction. Odorant

molecules bind to receptor on the cilia, which extend into the nasal mucosa. Axons from olfactory receptor cells leave the olfactory epithelium and travel centrally to the olfactory bulb. These axons must pass through the cribriform plate at the base of the skull to reach the olfactory bulb. Thus, fractures of the cribriform plate can sever olfactory neurons, leading to olfactory disorders (e.g. anosmia).Olfactory nerve axons are unmyelinated and are the smallest and slowest fibers in the nervous system. Because the olfactory receptor cells are also primary afferent neurons, the continuous replacement of receptor cells from basal cells means that there is continuous neurogenesis.

OLFACTORY TRANSDUCTION:

Transduction in the olfactory system involves the conversion of a chemical signal into an electrical signal. that can be transmitted to the CNS. The steps in olfactory transduction are as follows:
1. Odorant molecules bind to specific **olfactory receptor proteins** located on the cilia of olfactory receptor cells. There are at least 1000 different olfactory receptor proteins (members of the superfamily of G protein–coupled receptors), each encoded by a different gene and each found on a different olfactory receptor cell.
2. The olfactory receptor proteins are coupled to adenylyl cyclase via a G protein called **Golf**. When the odorant is bound, Golf is activated, which activates **adenylyl cyclase.**
3. Adenylyl cyclase catalyzes the conversion of ATP to cAMP. Intracellular levels of cAMP increase, which **opens cation channels** in the cell membrane of the olfactory receptor that are permeable to Na^+, K^+, and Ca^{2+}.

4. The receptor cell membrane depolarizes (i.e., the membrane potential is driven toward a value in between the equilibrium potentials for the three cations, this is depolarization). This depolarizing receptor potential brings the membrane potential closer to threshold and depolarizes the initial segment of the olfactory nerve axon.
   4. Action potentials are then generated and propagated along the olfactory nerve axons toward the olfactory bulb.

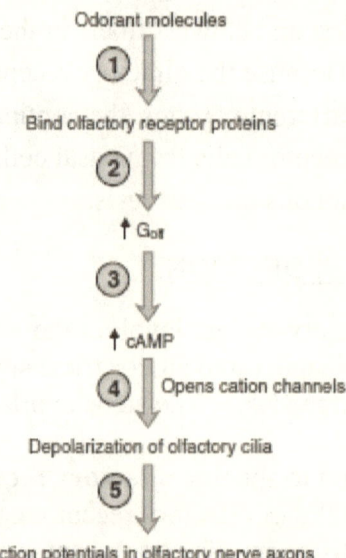

STEPS IN OLFACTORY TRANSDUCTION
Olfactory Pathways

As noted, olfactory receptor cells are the primary afferent neurons in the olfactory system. Axons from the receptor cells leave the olfactory epithelium, pass through the cribriform plate, and synapse on apical dendrites of **mitral cells** (the second-order neurons) in the **olfactory bulb.** These synapses occur in clusters called **glomeruli** . In the glomeruli, approximately 1000 olfactory receptor axons converge

onto 1 mitral cell. The mitral cells are arranged in a single layer in the olfactory bulb and have lateral dendrites in addition to the apical dendrites. The olfactory bulb also contains granule cells and periglomerular cells (not shown). The granule and periglomerular cells are inhibitory interneurons that make **dendrodendritic synapses** on neighboring mitral cells. The inhibitory inputs serve a function similar to that of the horizontal cells of the retina and may provide lateral inhibition that "sharpens" the information projected to the CNS.Mitral cells of the olfactory bulb project to higher centers in the CNS. As the olfactory tract approaches the base of the brain, it divides into two major tracts,
a lateral tract and a medial tract. The **lateral olfactory tract** synapses in the primary olfactory cortex, which includes the prepiriform cortex. The **medial olfactory tract** projects to the anterior commissure and the contralateral olfactory bulb.

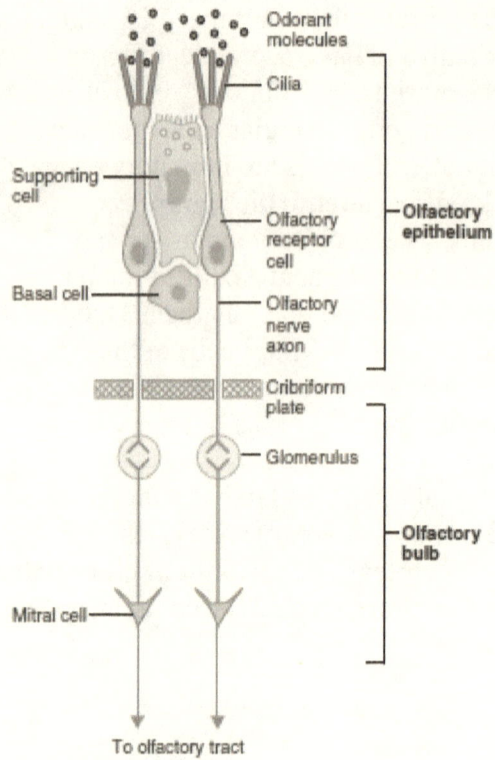

OLFACTORY PATHWAYS

AUDITION:

Sense of hearing involves transduction of sound waves into electrical energy, which then can be transmitted in the nervous system. Sound is produced by waves of compression and decompression, which are transmitted in elastic media such as air or water. These waves are associated with increases (compressions) and decreases (decompressions) in pressure. The units for expressing pressure are decibels (dB). Sound frequency is measured in cycles per second or hertz (Hz). A pure tone results from sinusoidal waves of a single frequency.

Most sounds are mixtures of pure tones. Human ear is sensitive to tones with frequencies 20 and 20,000 Hz. Most sensitive between 2000-5000 Hz. Usual ranges of frequencies in human speech is between 300 and 3500 Hz and sound intensity is about 65 dB, >100 dB (damage the auditory apparatus)> 120dB (pain).

STRUCTURES OF THE EAR:

<u>EXTERNAL EAR:</u> It consists of pinna and auditory canal. Its function is to direct sound waves into the auditory canal. External ear is filled with air.

<u>MIDDLE EAR:</u> Tympanic membrane and a chain of auditory ossicles called Malleus, incus and stapes. The tympanic membrane separates the external ear from the middle ear. An oval window and a round window lie between the middle ear and inner ear. The stapes has a footplate, which inserts into oval window and promotes interface between middle ear and inner ear. The middle ear is air filled.

INNER EAR: It consists of bony labyrinth and a membranous labyrinth. The bony labyrinth consists of three semicircular canals (lateral, posterior and superior). The membranous labyrinth consists of series of ducts called the SCALA VESTIBULI, SCALA TYMPANI AND SCALA MEDIA.

The cochlea and vestibule are formed from the bony and membranous labyrinths. The COCHLEA which is a spiral shaped structure composed of three tubular canals of ducts, contains the organ of corti. The organ of corti contains the receptor cells and is the site of the auditory transduction. The inner ear is fluid filled and fluid in each duct has a different composition. The fluid in the scala vestibule and scala tympani is called PERILYMPH which is similar to extracellular fluid. The fluid in the scala media is called ENDOLYMPH, which has a high K concentration and low sodium (Na) concentration. Thus endolymph has a composition similar to intracellular fluid.

STRUCTURE OF THE EAR:

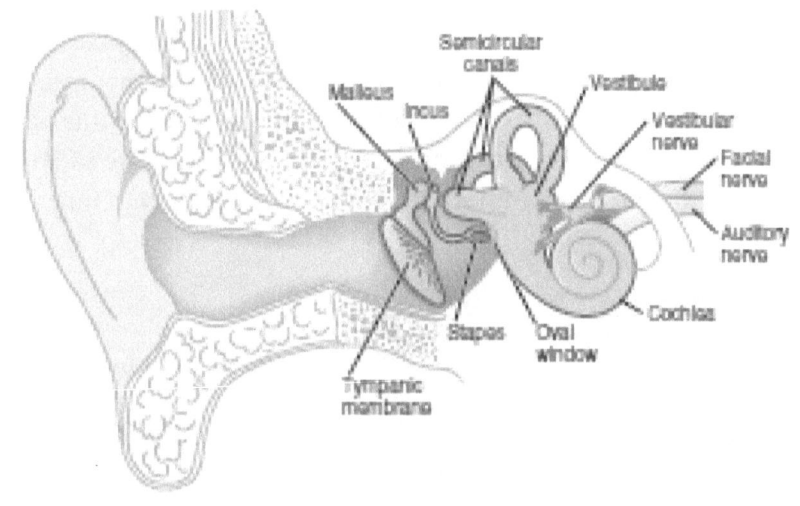

AUDITORY TRANSDUCTION:

Auditory transduction is the transformation of sound pressure into electrical energy. Many of the structures of the ear participate directly or indirectly in this transduction process. External and middle ear are air filled, and the inner ear which contains organ of corti is fluid filled. Before transduction can occur, sound waves travelling through air must be converted into pressure waves in fluid. The acoustic impedance of fluid is much greater than that of air. The combination of tympanic membrane and ossicles serves an impedance matching device that makes this conversion.

IMPEDANCE MATCHING:

It is accomplished by the ratio of large surface area of tympanic membrane to the small surface area of oval window and mechanical advantage offered by the lever system of ossicles.

The external ear directs sound waves into auditory canal, which transmits sound waves onto tympanic membrane. When sound waves move the tympanic membrane, the chain of ossicles also moves, pushing the foot plate of stapes into oval window and displacing the fluid in inner ear.

COCHLEA AND ORGAN OF CORTI:

Cochlea contains the sensory transduction apparatus, the organ of corti. The cross section of cochlea shows 3 chambers: scala vestibuli, scala media and scala tympani. Each chamber is fluid filled, the scala vestibule and scala tympani with perilymph and scala media with endolymph. The scala vestibule is separated from the scala media by Reissner's membrane. The basilar membrane separates scala media from scala tympani.

STRUCTURE OF COCHLEA AND ORGAN OF CORTI

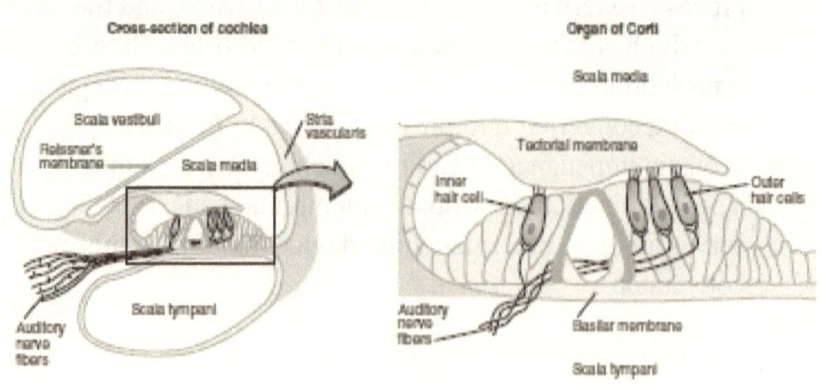

The organ of corti lies on the basilar membrane of cochlea. The organ of corti lies on the basilar membrane of the cochlea and is bathed in the endolymph contained in the scala media. Auditory hair cells in the organ of corti are sites of auditory transduction. The organ of corti contains 2 types of receptor cells, inner hair cells and outer hair cells. There are fewer hair cells arranged in single rows. Outer hair cells are arranged in parallel rows and are more numerous than inner hair cells.

Cilia protruding from hair cells are embedded in the tectorial membrane. Thus the bodies of hair cells are in contact with basilar membrane, cilia of hair cells are in contact with tectorial membrane. The nerves that serve the organ of corti are contained in the eighth nerve. The cell bodies of these nerves are located in spiral ganglia and their axons synapse at the base of hair cells. These nerves will transmit information from auditory hair cells to the CNS.

STEPS IN AUDITORY TRANSMISSION:

1. Sound waves are directed toward the tympanic membrane and as the tympanic membrane vibrates, it causes the ossicles to vibrate and the stapes to be pushed into the oval window. This movement displaces fluid in the cochlea. The sound energy is amplified by two effects: The lever action of the ossicles and the concentration of sound waves from the large tympanic membrane onto the small window. Thus, sound waves are transmitted and amplified from the air filled external and middle ears to the fluid filled inner ear, which contains the receptors.
2. Sound waves are transmitted to the inner ear and cause the vibration of the organ of corti.
3. The auditory hair cells are mechanoreceptors which are located on the organ of corti. The base of the

hair cells sits on the basilar membrane, and the cilia of the hair cells are embedded in the tectorial membrane. The basilar membrane is more elastic than the tectorial membrane. Thus, vibration of the organ of corti causes bending of cilia on the hair cells by as shearing force as the cilia push against the tectorial membrane.

4. Bending of the cilia produces a change in K conductance of the hair cell membrane. Bending in one direction produces an increase in K conductance and hyperpolarization; bending in the other direction produces decreases in K conductance and depolarization.

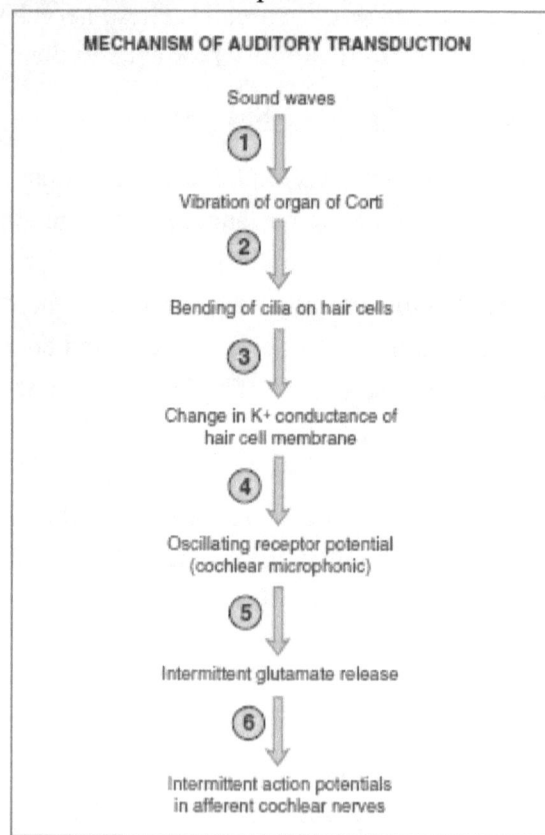

5. These changes in membrane potential are the receptor potentials of the auditory hair cells. The oscillating receptor potential is called the COCHLEAR MICROPHONIC POTENTIAL.
6. When hair cells are depolarized, the depolarization opens voltage –gated Ca channels in the presynaptic terminals of the hair cells. As a result, Ca enters the presynaptic terminals and causes release of glutamate which functions as an excitatory neurotransmitter, causing action potentials in the afferent cochlear nerves that will transmit this information to the CNS. When the hair cells are hyperpolarized, the opposite events occur, and there is decreased release of glutamate.
7. Thus, oscillating depolarizing and hyperpolarizing receptor potentials in the hair cells cause intermittent release of glutamate, which produces intermittent firing of afferent cochlear nerves.
8. The base of the basilar membrane is nearest the stapes and is narrow and stiff. Hair cells located at the base respond best to high frequencies. The apex of basilar membrane is wide and compliant .Hair cells located at the apex respond best to low frequencies.
9. Thus basilar membrane acts as a sound frequency membrane analyzer, with hair cells positioned along the basilar membrane responding to different frequencies. This spatial mapping of frequencies generates a tonotopic map which then is transmitted to higher levels of auditory system.

AUDITORY PATHWAYS:

Information is transmitted from hair cells of organ of corti to afferent cochlear nerves. The cochlear nerves synapse on neurons of dorsal and ventral cochlear nuclei of medulla, which send out axons that ascend in the CNS. Some of these axons cross to contralateral side and ascend in the lateral leminiscus (primary auditory tract) to inferior colliculus. Other axons remain ipsilateral. The two inferior colliculi are connected via the commissure of the inferior colliculus. Fibers from the nuclei of inferior colliculus ascend to the medial geniculate nucleus of thalamus. Fibers from the thalamus ascend to the auditory cortex. The tonotopic map generated at the level of organ of corti, is presented at all the levels of CNS. Complex feature discrimination (e.g. ability to recognize a patterned sequence) is the propensity of auditory cortex.

Because some auditory fibers are crossed and some are uncrossed, a mixture of ascending nerve fibers represent both ears at all levels of CNS. Thus lesions of cochlea of one ear will cause ipsilateral deafness. However, more central unilateral lesions do not cause deafness because some of the fibers transmitting information from that ear have already crossed to the undamaged side.

INTENSITY OF SOME COMMON SOUNDS:

Whisper: 30dB

Normal conversation: 60 dB

Rock music: 90 dB

Discomfort of ear: 120dB

Pain in the ear: 140dB

IMPEDANCE MATCHING MECHANISM:

The air filled middle ear conducts sound waves mechanically to the fluid filled internal ear through the ossicular system. Effective transfer of sound energy from an air to a fluid medium is difficult because most of the sound is reflected as a result of different mechanical properties of the two media, i-e impedance matching.

Nature has compensated for it by providing impedance matching mechanism to middle ear by following mechanisms:

1. Lever action of ossicles increases the force of movement by 1.3 times.
2. Hydraulic action of tympanic membrane is exerted because effective vibratory area of the tympanic membrane (above 45mm2) is much greater than the stapes-oval window. Surface area (about 3.2 mm2). This size difference, thus amplifying the pressure exerted on the oval window (14 folds).
3. Curved membrane effect: Movements of tympanic membrane are more at the periphery than at the center where malleus hand is attached. This too provides leverage.

Thus above three mechanisms together increase the sound pressure 18 folds (i-e 14x1.3). In this way the impedance mismatching between air filled middle ear and fluid filled inner ear is mostly compensated.

ATTENUATION REFLEX:

It is also called tympanic reflex or acoustic reflex which reduces sound pressure amplitude. Stimulus for this reflex is loud sound. Reflex activity: The two muscles of middle ear (tensor tympani and stapedius) contract reflexively in response to intense sound.

Contraction of tensor tympani pulls the malleus in wards whereas contraction of stapedius muscle pulls stapes outward. These two opposing forces make the ossicular system very rigid and therefore it fails to vibrate with sound waves. Thus sound is not allowed to enter inner ear (i-e is attenuated or intensity is reduced by 30-40dB). It prevents occurrence of damage to cochlea from the intense sounds like that of loud music, of jet aircraft etc.

ENCODING OF SOUND:

Encoding of sound frequencies occurs because different auditory cells are activated by different frequencies. The frequency that activates a particular hair cell depends on the position of that hair cell along the basilar membrane. The base of the basilar membrane is nearest the stapes and is narrow and stiff. Hair cells located at the base respond best to high frequencies. The apex of the basilar membrane is wide and compliant. Hair cells located at the apex respond best to low frequencies. Thus, the basilar membrane acts as a sound frequency analyzer, with hair cells positioned along the basilar membrane responding to different frequencies. This spatial mapping of frequencies generates a tonotopic map, which then is transmitted to higher levels of the auditory system.

PLACE THEORY: Incoming sounds from the environment are in a spectral representative form, extracted by the inner ear. The inner ear serves as a tuned resonator that passes the spectral representation to the brain stem and then to the auditory cortex via the auditory nerve. The basilar membrane of the ear resonates the sound with a corresponding characteristic frequency or CF. For instance, if a sound stimulus has a tone of 300 Hz, the part of the basilar membrane that has a CF of 300 Hz would be stimulated. This process is also called frequency place mapping.

Critics of place theory argue that most often, characteristic frequencies are hard to determine below 120 Hz. Perception of sound stimuli accounting for low frequencies is associated with frequency theory.

FREQUENCY THEORY: It assumes that auditory nerve can fire at rates of 20-20,000 times /sec. Because the frequency range of human hearing is 20-20,000 Hz. This became clear that an individual nerve fiber can fire at rates of between 300-500 times per second. The frequency of the nerve impulses of the auditory nerve corresponds to the frequency of a tone, which allows us to detect its pitch. The entire basilar membrane is activated by sound waves at different waves. Clearly the firing rate limitations of single neurons could not account for human perception of frequencies up to 20,000 Hz if one were to relay on frequency theory.

ENCODING OF LOUDNESS: The perception of loudness of a sound correlates with the number of active auditory neurons and their rate of firing. More intense sounds cause large vibrations that are spread across a larger area of the basilar membrane, thereby involving more hair cells and activation of more auditory neurons. Loudness is also correlated with the rate of action potential generation because large distortions of hair cells produce larger receptor potentials, which increases action potential frequency in auditory neurons.

Encoding of sound intensity (loudness) occurs at the level of cochlear nerves by the following mechanisms:

a. Increase in frequency of firing of auditory nerve fibers.
b. Increase in number of nerve fibers stimulation
c. Stimulation of inner hair cells.

APPLIED ASPECTS:

MASKING: It is a phenomenon in which pressure of one type of sound decreases the ability of ear to hear another type of sound.

HEARING LOSS: It refers to impairment of hearing and its severity may vary from mild to profound.

DEAFNESS: It is a condition in which there is little hearing or no hearing at all.

TYPES OF HEARING LOSS:

a. **CONDUCTIVE:** Any disease process which interferes with the conduction of sound from external ear to cochlea causes conductive hearing loss. Hearing loss is partial and never complete because skull bones conduct sound waves to the cochlea (bone conduction) and basilar membrane can be set to vibration.
b. **SENSORINEURAL:** It results from lesions of cochlea (sensory type) or 8th cranial nerve and its

central connections (neural type). Usually the hearing loss is complete.

TINITUS: It is a ringing sensation in the ear. It is caused by Irritative stimulation of either of inner ear or the vestibulocochlear nerve.

AUDIOMETRIC TESTS:

Audiometry refers to measurement of auditory acuity (sharpness of hearing) using the audiometer.
Pure tone audiometry is performed in a sound proof room. Each ear is tested separately. (AC) thresholds are measured for tones of 125, 250, 500, 1000,2000,4000,8000 Hz and bone conduction thresholds for 250, 500, 1000, 2000 and 4000 Hz. In a normal person, both for air and bone conduction is at zero dB and there is no A-B gap. The amount of intensity that has to be raised above the normal level is a measure of degree of hearing loss at that frequency. It is charted in the form of a graph called audiogram. Threshold of bone conduction (BC) is a measure of cochlear function. Difference in thresholds of air and bone conduction (A-B gap) is a measure of degree of conductive deafness.

HEARING TESTS: These two tests are performed with tuning forks of different frequencies (250-512 Hz). They are useful in distinguishing conductive deafness from sensorineural deafness.
RINNE TEST: Air conduction (AC) of the ear is compared with bone conduction (BC).
In normal individuals the Rinne's test is positive.
In conductive deafness, the Rinne's test is negative.
In complete nerve deafness, both bone conducted and air conducted sounds are not perceived.

WEBER'S TEST: Bone conduction is compared on both sides.
Normally the sound is heard equally in both ears.
In conductive hearing loss, the sound is lateralized (better heard) towards the affected ear. This is because the masking effects of environmental noise is absent in the affected ear.
In sensorineural hearing loss, the sound is lateralized towards the better ear, because the sound is reaching the normal cochlea through bone.